How To Report Statistics in Medicine

Publications from the BMJ Publishing Group are available to members through the American College of Physicians.

Our *Resources for Internists* catalog and ordering information for the American College of Physicians and BMJ Publishing Group are available from:

Customer Service Center
American College of Physicians
Independence Mall West
Sixth Street at Race
Philadelphia, PA 19106-1572
215-351-2600
800-523-1546, ext. 2600

HOW TO REPORT STATISTICS IN MEDICINE

ANNOTATED GUIDELINES FOR AUTHORS, EDITORS, AND REVIEWERS

Thomas A. Lang, MA

Manager, Medical Editing Services
Department of Scientific Publications
The Cleveland Clinic Foundation
Cleveland, Ohio

Michelle Secic, MS

Senior Biostatistician
Department of Biostatistics and Epidemiology
The Cleveland Clinic Foundation
Cleveland, Ohio

With a Foreword by
Edward J. Huth, MD, MACP
Editor Emeritus, Annals of Internal Medicine

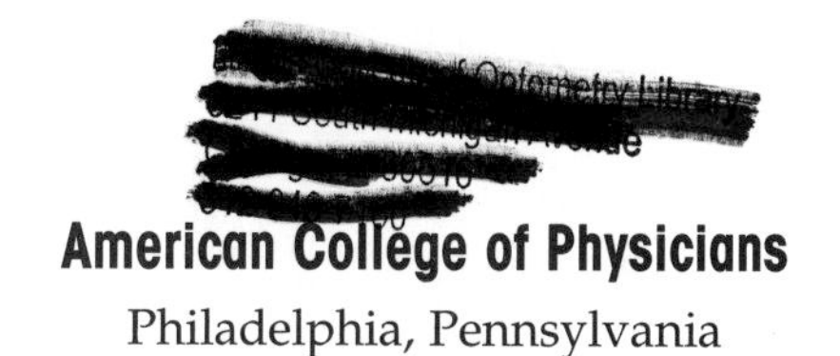

American College of Physicians
Philadelphia, Pennsylvania

Acquisitions Editor: Mary K. Ruff
Manager, Book Publishing: David Myers
Administrator, Book Publishing: Diane M. McCabe
Production Supervisor: Allan S. Kleinberg
Production Editor: Victoria Hoenigke
Interior and Cover Design: DiDona Design

Printed in the United States of America.
Composition by Techsetters, Inc.
Printing/binding by Port City Press

American College of Physicians
Independence Mall West
Sixth Street at Race
Philadelphia, PA 19106-1572

Library of Congress Cataloging-in-Publication Data

Lang, Thomas A. (Thomas Allen)
How to report statistics in medicine: annotated guidelines for authors, editors, and reviewers / by Thomas A. Lang and Michelle Secic.
p. cm. – (Medical writing and communication)
Includes bibliographical references.
ISBN 0-943126-44-4
1. Medical statistics. 2. Medical writing. I. Secic, Michelle. 1967- . II. Series.
RA409.L357 1997
610′.72–dc20 96-30333
CIP

97 98 99 00 01 02 / 9 8 7 6 5 4 3 2 1

To Toni and Colin, for the real meaning of significance; and to Kathy F. Grupe, who long ago pointed a novice editor in the right direction.

TAL

To my close family and friends: John, for his constant love, support, and composure as my partner through every aspect of our lives; my father, Joseph, and my mother, Barbara, for their pride and encouragement; Joe, for his advice and leadership; Gina, for her kindness, sincerity, and concern; Dawn, for her loyalty and confidence; Rick, Jessi, and R.J., for the joy they have brought into my life; Mama and Tata, for always being there for me; Shari, for her guidance; and Dawn, Gina, Kim, and Roberta, for their unconditional friendship.

MS

CONTENTS

A Note to the Reader

My books are water; those of the great geniuses are wine—everybody drinks water.

Mark Twain (1)

Both fine wines and biostatistics are characterized by complexities and subtleties that are truly appreciated only by the relatively few people who devote the time to master them. To these readers, we extend our apologies; this book was not written for you. Rather, it was written for a much larger group of readers: those who thirst for a basic understanding of statistics, but who do not aspire to appreciate the nuances. This is a book about reporting and interpreting statistical presentations, not about understanding theories of probabilities or mathematical concepts. This is a book for water drinkers.

It is exceedingly difficult to explain many statistical concepts in terms that are both technically accurate and easily understood by those with only a cursory knowledge of the topic. Thus, if our explanations do not include some of the finer points of a topic or if they have bypassed some distinction of meaning, it is because we believe that such fine points and distinctions would detract from an explanation otherwise adequate for most readers.

The medical examples in this book were created to illustrate statistical concepts. As such, the vast majority are hypothetical and should be accepted as teaching devices and not as medical fact.

1. Joseph M, editor. *Man is the Only Animal that Blushes . . . or Needs to. The Wisdom of Mark Twain*. New York: Random House; 1970.

FOREWORD

The need for quantitative evidence in medical judgments has been seen for at least two millennia. In the second century AD, Galen noted that

> [the empiricists] say that a thing seen but once cannot be accepted nor regarded as true, neither what was seen a few times only. They believe something can only be accepted and considered true, if it has been seen very many times, and in the same manner every time.

But for centuries this view was almost entirely ignored. Then, a bit more than 150 years ago, Pierre Charles-Alexandre Louis raised a closely related point:

> Let us bestow upon observation the care and time which it demands; let the facts be rigorously analyzed in order to a just appreciation of them; and it is impossible to attain this without classifying and counting them; and then therapeutics will advance not less than other branches of science.

Louis cannot be considered the father of medical statistics in its present state, but less than a century passed before the pioneers in modern biological and medical statistics—Karl Pearson and Ronald Fisher—began to set standards for quantitative evidence. The power of statistical methods became clearer and clearer during the following years. Adequate study design and statistical analysis began to lead to conclusions of great import for the health of all of us, as in the studies of Wynder and Graham and Doll and Hill on tobacco smoking and carcinoma of the lung. Today even the physician who knows nothing about statistical methods expects to find in reports of clinical trials of drugs statistical evidence for what they conclude.

Unfortunately, what passes before our eyes as statistical analysis and reporting does not always represent the proper use of statistical methods or the clear and adequate reporting of statistical findings. Editors of journals and their peer reviewers may catch statistical shortcomings in the papers they consider for publication, but the review system is not always infallible in judging statistical evidence and how it is presented. Hence, authors who know their duty to try to meet high standards of scientific reporting must offer the strongest possible statistical evidence. However, this by itself is not enough; they must also strive to report this evidence clearly enough to convince even the most critical readers that the evidence is reliable and adequate. But up until now, authors have had available little published guidance in how to most effectively report their statistical data. Several biomedical style manuals have carried short sections on publication style for statistical data, but these have assumed that authors know enough about statistical reporting to do it clearly and convincingly. Now Lang and Secic, the authors of this manual, bring valuable specific and detailed help to authors who wish to make their papers as statistically convincing as possible. And authors are not the only persons who can profit from what they recommend. There are also the peer reviewers who may be uncertain of what standards for statistical reporting they should apply to papers they review. The same probably can be said of at least some editors who are ill informed on statistics and who are not fortunate enough to have statisticians on their staffs. The rest of the medical community—the readers of journals, other physicians, nurses—will eventually profit from Lang and Secic's advice when it is applied by authors and editors. And most important, there is the benefit that will trickle down in time to patients, who are the reason why our profession exists.

Edward J. Huth
Editor Emeritus, **Annals of Internal Medicine**

PREFACE

Standards governing the content and format of statistical aspects should be developed to guide authors in the preparation of manuscripts.

J.R. O'FALLON ET AL. (1)

Among the first physicians to have considered the implications of statistical probability in medical research is Donald Mainland, MD, of Dalhousie University, Halifax, Canada. He appears to have been the first to report statistics, in articles published in the *Canadian Medical Association Journal* and in the *British Medical Journal* in the 1930s (2,3). Since then, medical research has increasingly adopted the principles of experimental design and statistical analysis, with the result that biostatistics has emerged as a distinct field of study. Biostatistics has been essential in moving medical research from anecdotal case reports to experiments with control groups, and finally to the large-scale, randomized controlled trials that are now the preferred standard for scientific proof.

But there is a problem. Studies of the statistical quality of journal articles have consistently found high error rates in the application, reporting, and interpretation of statistical information, in even the most respected medical journals. Since the first such study—the earliest we found was published in 1959—error rates as high as 80% have been found, again, even in major medical journals (4–19). "These reviews [of statistical errors] reveal a remarkable and depressing consistency, with typically around fifty percent of reviewed papers being found to contain clear statistical errors" (20). Further, a large portion of these errors are so great as to cast doubts on the validity of the author's conclusions (6, 21).

At the same time, most of these errors are related to topics included in most introductory statistics books. It seems strange indeed that a problem seemingly so important, so widespread, and so long-standing should continue, despite apparently being so basic in nature.

Curiously, despite several calls to the contrary (1, 17, 20, 22–24), no comprehensive guidelines or reference books have been available to aid in statistical reporting. Several sets of general guidelines have been published in biomedical journals (20, 25–30), but we believe that they are too general in nature, too limited in scope, and too specialized in vocabulary to be useful to most authors and editors. Obviously, statistical reporting errors will likely continue without the widespread adoption of suitable reporting guidelines.

Thus, our purpose in writing this book is to provide a set of detailed, comprehensive, and understandable guidelines for reporting statistical information in medicine. Further, we tried to make the guidelines more accessible to nonstatisticians through explanations and examples and by organizing the guidelines according to how they are used in a text rather than by the mathematical principles on which they are based.

As a result, this book is not a statistics book in the usual sense. We are not concerned with teaching research design, statistical theory or methods, or the calculations of statistical tests. We consider here only the presentation of statistical information in scientific publications and discuss some related concepts that should help put these presentations into perspective. We urge authors and researchers to collaborate with biostatisticians in all phases of research, but we also believe that one need not be a statistician to present or interpret elementary statistics correctly. One does need ready access to accurate, complete, and understandable information to do so, however. This book was written to help provide this access.

More than 60 years ago, the same Dr. Mainland who started it all expressed our hopes for the future of statistical reporting (2):

> . . . progress would be made if some fundamental ideas were more clearly understood, namely, that the principles underlying statistical methods are relatively simple, that the commonest methods are easy to learn, that the methods can be used as an instrument without a deep knowledge of their mathematical structure, that the methods do not impart a fictitious accuracy or an artificial quality to the results, and that these methods tend very often to show that conclusions are not so definite as the unaided observer would think they were. If these things were understood, the methods would be much more commonly used, and, more important still, workers would come to recognize when they should appeal to the statistician. This in turn would hasten the coming of the day when a consultant statistician will be considered necessary in every medical centre.

It is a truism of medical writing that in clarifying the meaning, we coincidentally reveal it. If our book will help clarify statistical analyses, it may also improve the way medical research is conducted and interpreted.

Tom Lang
Michelle Secic

REFERENCES

1. **O'Fallon JR, Duby SD, Salsburg DS, Edmonson JH, Soffer A, Colton T.** Should there be statistical guidelines for medical research papers? Biometrics, 1978;34(4):687-95.
2. **Mainland D.** Chance and the blood count. Can Med Assoc J. 1934;(June):656-8.
3. **Mainland D.** Problems of chance in clinical work. Br Med J. 1936;2:221-4.
4. **Hall JC, Hill D, Watts, JM.** Misuse of statistical methods in the Australasian surgical literature. Aust N Z J Surg. 1982;52:541-3.
5. **Schor S, Karten I.** Statistical evaluation of medical journal manuscripts. JAMA. 1966;195(13):1123-8.
6. **Glantz SA.** Biostatistics: how to detect, correct and prevent errors in the medical literature. Circulation. 1980;61(1):1-7.
7. **Lionel ND, Herxheimer A.** Assessing reports of therapeutic trials. BMJ. 1970;3(723):637-40.
8. **Altman DG.** Statistics in medical journals: developments in the 1980s. Stat Med. 1991;10(12):1897-913.
9. **White SJ.** Statistical errors in papers in the British Journal of Psychiatry. Br J Psychiatry. 1979;135:336-42.
10. **Gore SM, Jones IG, Rytter EC.** Misuse of statistical methods: critical assessment of articles in BMJ from January to March 1976. BMJ. 1977;1(6053):85-7.
11. **Freiman JA, Chalmers TC, Smith H Jr, Kuebler RR.** The importance of beta, the type II error and sample size in the design and interpretation of the randomized control trial. Survey of 71 negative trials. N Engl J Med. 1978;299(13):690-4.
12. **Reed JF, Slaichert W.** Statistical proof in inconclusive "negative" trials. Arch Intern Med. 1981;141(10):1307-10.
13. **Gardner MJ, Altman DG, Jones DR, Machin D.** Is the statistical assessment of papers submitted to the British Medical Journal effective? BMJ. 1983;286(6376):1485-8.
14. **MacArthur RD, Jackson GG.** An evaluation of the use of statistical methodology in the Journal of Infectious Diseases. J Infect Dis. 1984;149(3):349-54.
15. **Avram MJ, Shanks CA, Dykes MH, Ronai AK, Stiers WM.** Statistical methods in anesthesia articles: an evaluation of two American journals during two six-month periods. Anesth Analg. 1985;64(6):607-11.
16. **Godfrey K.** Comparing the means of several groups. N Engl J Med. 1985;313(23):1450-6.
17. **Pocock SJ, Hughes MD, Lee RJ.** Statistical problems in the reporting of clinical trials. A survey of three medical journals. N Engl J Med. 1987;317(7):426-32.
18. **Smith DG, Clemens J, Crede W, Harvey M, Gracely EJ.** Impact of multiple comparisons in randomized clinical trials. Am J Med. 1987;83(3):545-50.
19. **Gotzsche PC.** Methodology and overt and hidden bias in reports of 196 double-blind trials of nonsteroidal antiinflammatory drugs in rheumatoid arthritis. Control Clin Trials. 1989;50(9):356.
20. **Murray GD.** Statistical aspects of research methodology. Br J Surg. 1991;78(7):777-81.
21. **Yancy JM.** Ten rules for reading clinical research reports [Editorial]. Am J Surg. 1990;159(6):553-9.
22. **Shott S.** Statistics in veterinary research. J Am Vet Med Assoc. 1985;187(2):138-41.
23. **Hayden GF.** Biostatistical trends in Pediatrics: implications for the future. Pediatrics. 1983;72(1):84-7.
24. **Altman DG, Bland JM.** Improving doctors' understanding of statistics. J R Statis Soc A. 1991;154:223-67.
25. **Altman DG, Gore SM, Gardner MJ, Pocock SJ.** Statistical guidelines for contributors to medical journals. BMJ. 1983; 286(6376):1489-93.
26. **International Committee of Medical Journal Editors.** Uniform requirements for manuscripts submitted to biomedical journals. N Engl J Med. 1991;324:424-8.
27. **Elenbaas RM, Elenbaas JK, Cuddy PG.** Evaluating the medical literature. Part II: Statistical analysis. Ann Emerg Med. 1983;

12(10):610-20.
28. **Murray GD.** Statistical guidelines for The British Journal of Surgery. Br J Surg. 1991; 78(7):782-4.
29. **Sumner D.** Lies, damned lies—or statistics? J Hypertens. 1992;10(1):3-8.
30. **Journal of Hypertension.** Statistical guidelines for the Journal of Hypertension. J Hypertens. 1992;10(1):6-8.

ACKNOWLEDGMENTS

We especially thank the following friends and colleagues for reviewing earlier drafts of our manuscript:

Daniel R. Browning, MA, MS
Computer-Assisted Reporting Specialist
Pioneer Press
Saint Paul, Minnesota

Michael Kutner, PhD
Chairman, Department of Biostatistics and Epidemiology
The Cleveland Clinic Foundation
Cleveland, Ohio

Ken Murray, MD, MS, MT (ASCP)
Medical Director, Independent Practice Association
Physician in Private Practice
Studio City, California
Clinical Assistant Professor of Family Medicine
University of Southern California
Los Angeles, California

Flauren Ricketts, MS
Instructor, Department of Mathematics
Normandale Community College
Bloomington, Minnesota

We owe a special debt of gratitude to Ed Huth, MD, MACP, who suggested that we submit our manuscript to the American College of Physicians. His encouragement of this project —which included agreeing to write the Foreword—was most welcome. We also thank Frank Davidoff, MD, FACP; R. Brian Haynes, MD, PhD, FRCP; Patricia Houston,

MD, MPH; Stephen Lock, MD; and Margaret Winker, MD, who graciously examined earlier drafts of the manuscript. Their comments, both verbal and written, were most appreciated.

Special thanks also to our colleagues in the Department of Biostatistics and Epidemiology, especially Dave P. Miller, MS; Nancy Obuchowski, PhD; Edward Mascha, MS; and Ming Tan, PhD, and in the Department of Scientific Publications, especially Cassandra Talerico, MA, and Jackie Werner. Finally, a number of people at the American College of Physicians deserve our sincere thanks for transforming our manuscript into a book: Diane M. McCabe, David Myers, Vicki Hoenigke, Allan Kleinberg, and Mary K. Ruff.

All of the people named above contributed substantially to the production of this book. Any errors that remain are, unfortunately, ours.

INTRODUCTION

The presentation of statistical guidelines should not be confused with statistical education.

S. L. GEORGE (1)

This book is not a statistics book in the usual sense. Rather, it is a guide to understanding and presenting statistical information. An earlier draft was titled *A Field Guide to the Statistical Flora and Fauna of the Biomedical Research Paper*. That is, we have written a book on wildflower identification and appreciation and not a book on plant biology, so to speak.

As indicated by its title, this book was written for authors, editors, and reviewers who prepare or evaluate biomedical research articles for publication. It should also be of value to students who are learning about biostatistics and medical research. It is divided into four parts:

Part 1, Annotated Guidelines for Reporting Statistical Information, is organized into 15 chapters that correspond to 15 general applications of biostatistics. These chapters were created to help nonstatisticians find the appropriate guidelines more easily. The guidelines themselves were derived from an extensive review of the clinical literature (see the Bibliography). The guidelines are usually accompanied by explanations, hypothetical examples, and cautions that aid in understanding, evaluating, and applying them correctly. Many guidelines are duplicated because we believe that they should be more readily available to readers than cross-referencing allows them to be. Authors and editors should refer to these guidelines when preparing manuscripts for publication.

We stress that these guidelines are just that: guidelines, not requirements.

Part 1 contains guidelines, subguidelines, cautions, methods of checking, and cross-references to related information. For example:

Subguidelines are given for special cases of the main guideline.

Potential problems identify possible reporting or interpretation problems associated with the guideline.

Methods of checking describe ways to verify or to question statistical presentations.

Related information cross-reference supplemental chapters, guidelines, tables, and figures within this text.

Part 2, Guide to Statistical Terms and Tests, is designed to help readers of scientific articles understand statistical information. Entries are descriptions of what the terms or concepts mean in the context of medical research; they are not intended to be mathematically or theoretically pure definitions. All are written to be understood by readers with only a basic knowledge of statistics. Readers who wish more detailed information should consult statistical texts.

Part 3, An Unannotated, Referenced List of Guidelines, is supplied for readers already familiar with statistical concepts, who will use the book primarily as a reference tool in writing, editing, and reviewing scientific articles.

Four appendices in Part 4 are included to assist in reporting: Appendix 1: Checklists for Reporting Clinical Trials; Appendix 2: Mathematical Symbols and Notation; Appendix 3: Rules for Presenting Numbers in Text; and Appendix 4: Spelling of Statistical Terms and Tests.

The bibliography contains the articles and books on which the guidelines are based.

The index uses a wide selection of terms and many cross-references to help readers find information.

REFERENCE

1. **George SL.** Statistics in medical journals: a survey of current policies and proposals for editors. Med Pediatr Oncol. 1985;13(2):109-12.

Differences Between Clinical and Statistical Significance

It has been said that a fellow with one leg frozen in ice and the other leg in boiling water is comfortable—on average.

J.M. Yancy (1)

One of the most common errors in reporting and interpreting medical research is the failure to distinguish between clinical and statistical significance. (Because in medical writing "significant" is reserved for its statistical meaning, we have used the phrase "clinical importance" throughout this book to refer to "clinical significance.") In general, a **clinically important finding** is a conclusion that has implications for patient care. A **statistically significant finding**, on the other hand, is a conclusion that there is evidence against the null hypothesis—that there is a low probability of getting a result as extreme or more extreme than the one observed in the data, given that the null hypothesis is true.

By itself, a statistically significant finding can have little to do with the practice of medicine. Similarly, a clinically important finding in a single case probably does not establish a biological relationship. A finding that is both clinically important and statistically significant is valuable because we are more likely to believe that the finding is the result of a biological process shared by a group of patients and that it is perhaps amenable to measurement, explanation, prediction, and control.

We call to your attention several aspects of the distinction between statistical significance and clinical importance:

1. Statistical significance essentially reflects the influence of chance on the outcome; clinical importance reflects the biological value of the outcome.

In general, *small differences between large groups* can be statistically significant but clinically meaningless. A difference of 0.02 kg in the weights of two groups of adults is not likely to have any clinical importance even if such a difference would have occurred by chance less than 1 time in 100 ($P < 0.01$) or even less than 1 time in 100 000 ($P < 0.00001$).

It is also true that *large differences between small groups* can be clinically important but not statistically significant. In a study of 20 patients in which even 1 patient dies, the death is clinically important, whether or not it is statistically significant. The important question is whether the sample is large enough to detect a clinically important difference if, in fact, such a difference existed. This question is one of statistical power.

2. Statistics are derived from groups of individuals; medicine is practiced on specific individuals.

Because statistics is based on probability, not on biology, it is concerned with populations and not individual patients. Physicians who treat individual patients on the basis of medical research are in a real sense "playing the odds": They are hoping that what has been true for a group of similar patients will be true for one particular patient.

3. Statistical conclusions require adequate amounts of data to be valid; medical decisions must often be made with insufficient data.

Statistical comparisons involving small samples often have low statistical power. That is, researchers often do not collect enough information to be reasonably confident to conclude whether, say, a new treatment is as good as or better than the standard treatment. A study reporting a negative or statistically nonsignificant result for which the statistical power is low is actually not negative at all: it is inconclusive. For the same reason, when no statistically significant differences are found between the baseline values of small treatment and control groups, it is inappropriate to conclude that the groups are equivalent: absence of proof is not proof of absence.

4. Statistical answers are probabilistic; medical treatment requires committed decisions.

Statistics incorporates the notion of probability. When a result would be expected to occur by chance less than, say, 1 time in 1000 (that is, $P < 0.001$), the result nevertheless could be the result of chance; it is simply not probable that chance is the explanation. The result obtained in a sample is also an estimate of what might be expected to occur in the larger population. Although a 95% confidence interval provides a measure of precision for this estimated result, it, too, is a probabilistic statement and not a sure thing.

5. Statistical analysis always requires measurement; medicine sometimes requires intuition.

Science is measurement. Unfortunately, not everything in medical science is easily measured: depression, pain, quality of life; even the more physical aspects of life, such as liver function or cardiac health, are not easily quantified. Measurements and probability statements can be of great help in medicine, but they are not yet able to replace experience, perceptiveness, and intuition in many cases.

6. The statistical and clinical applications of the term *normal* are often confused and vague.

In statistics, the term *normal* generally refers to a distribution of values that forms a symmetric bell-shaped curve. Data are said to be *normally distributed* if they form such a distribution when graphed. In medicine, the term *normal* is often used casually to mean common, acceptable, or healthy.

These two definitions unfortunately are often combined to define clinically normal as a characteristic with a commonplace value in a normal distribution of values for the characteristic. That is, values that occur in the middle 95% of the values collected from a healthy population are usually considered to be normal by definition, and those that occur in the lowest 2.5% and the highest 2.5% are considered to be abnormal.

Such definitions are statistical, however, not clinical. In its best clinical use, the term *normal* is a value that is associated with only a small likelihood of disease or disability, no matter where the value lies on the distribution of values. Likewise, the term *abnormal* is a value associated with a high likelihood of disease, no matter where the value lies on the distribution.

REFERENCE

1. **Yancy JM.** Ten rules for reading clinical research reports [Editorial]. Am J Surg. 1990; 159(6):553-9.

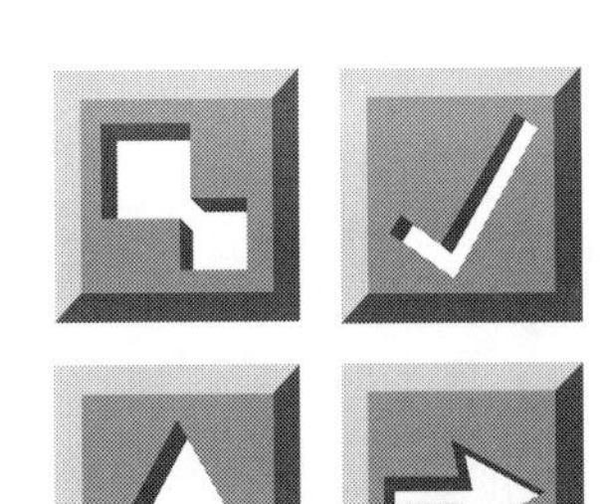

Part 1

Annotated Guidelines for Reporting Statistical Information

Chapter 1

ASKING QUESTIONS AND FINDING ANSWERS

Reporting Research Designs and Activities

...the most important issues in biostatistics are not expressed with statistical procedures. The issues are inherently scientific, rather than purely statistical, and relate to the architectural design of the research, not to the numbers with which the data are cited and interpreted.

A.R. FEINSTEIN (1)

Statistical analyses must be understood in the context of the larger research effort. The research question, study design, sampling techniques, and data collection methods determine which statistical procedures are appropriate and how and when these procedures are applied to the data. Thus, for statistical guidelines to be useful, they must be accompanied by guidelines for reporting research designs and activities.

The guidelines below can be applied to several types of research designs, especially randomized controlled clinical trials. Not all guidelines apply to every study. They are listed approximately in the order in which they should be addressed in the scientific article. The subheadings used in this chapter are also appropriate for inclusion in scientific articles.

The guidelines that follow address a broad range of issues that may arise in reporting original research. They are also described in detail to make them understandable to as wide an audience as possible. In these respects, they differ from other published lists of guidelines. They are also different from, but compatible with, guidelines recently proposed to implement the concept of "structured reporting." ***(See Appendix 1: Checklists for Reporting Clinical Trials.)***

GUIDELINES ADDRESSED IN THE INTRODUCTION

1.1 State the purpose of the study. Identify the relationships that were studied and the reasons for studying them.

The importance of stating the purpose of a research project is obvious, but such a statement is sometimes missing from research reports. Often, the author is working in a specialized field and assumes that anyone reading the article will know why the work was undertaken. Sometimes the purpose is simply left unstated, and sometimes research evolves until the original purpose has been forgotten.

In two excellent articles, Schwartz and Lellouch (2) and Simon and colleagues (3) make a compelling argument that the purpose of therapeutic studies should be either explanatory or pragmatic—but not both. **Explanatory studies** or **efficacy studies** are driven by *the need to understand* a disease or therapeutic process. Such studies are best conducted under "optimal" or "laboratory" conditions that allow tight control over patient selection, treatment, and follow-up. **Pragmatic studies** or **effectiveness studies,** on the other hand, are driven by *the need to make clinical decisions.* These studies are usually conducted under "normal" conditions that reflect the circumstances under which medical care is usually provided. Thus, it is useful to identify whether the study was designed to be explanatory or pragmatic (4). Many medical research studies do, however, have elements of both of these purposes. When this is the case, the purpose of each hypothesis should be kept in mind when interpreting the results.

Other authors distinguish among **pathophysiologic studies,** whose results are not directly applicable to patient care, **epidemiologic studies,** whose results are applicable to large populations, and **therapeutic studies,** whose results can be generalized to patients with characteristics similar to those in the sample studied (5).

Heterogeneous samples are more typical of pragmatic studies, whereas more homogeneous samples usually indicate explanatory studies (6). The heterogeneity of the sample should be appropriate for the primary comparison and for the type of study.

It may also be appropriate to identify the funding source of the research and any restrictions placed on the study (7,8). The source of research funds is customarily disclosed to the journal editor on the title page of the submitted manuscript. The journal, in turn, usually prints the name of the funding source in a footnote on the first or last page of the published article. Although the funding source is not typically given in the introduction of a scientific article, a case can be made that it should be.

1.2 If the study was designed to test one or more a priori hypotheses, state the hypotheses.

Good science is characterized by a "clear statement of a testable question" (9). When the testable question is asked before the study is designed and conducted, it is called an **a priori hypothesis.** In this case, the results can be interpreted in light of the question. When questions are asked after the data have been collected, either because the initial purpose of the study was not clear or because the questions were suggested by the data, the analysis is termed **post hoc,** or after-the-fact. The results of post hoc analyses should usually be considered as exploratory or speculative because data collected to answer one question may not be appropriate to answer another.

Identify any planned subgroup or secondary analyses and distinguish between the primary and secondary hypotheses.

1.3 State how the original data may be obtained for reanalysis and the format in which the data are stored.

Research data are usually difficult and expensive to collect. If they can be used for additional studies or reanalyzed, much time, effort, and money can be saved. The argument has also been made that data collected by studies funded by public agencies, such as the National Institutes of Health or the National Science Foundation, should be available to the public. Many researchers are reluctant to release their data, however, presumably from the fear that others will find fault with the study or reach different conclusions.

In its Instructions for Authors, the *Journal of the American Medical Association* (JAMA) requires that authors agree to the following as a condition of publication: "If requested, I shall produce the data upon which the manuscript is based for examination by the editors or their assignees" (10). Such an approach fosters scientific exchange and provides a means of investigating claims of scientific misconduct.

Data are often stored in large computer databases. Reporting the name of the database or spreadsheet software program (such as ORACLE, Datalex, Paradox, FoxPro, Excel, and so on) and the operating system of the associated computer system (such as Unix or Windows) aids other researchers in assessing the availability and usefulness of the data to meet their needs.

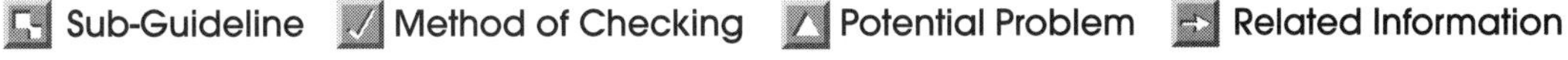

GUIDELINES ADDRESSED IN THE MATERIALS AND METHODS

The Study Focus

1.4 Specify the observational or experimental unit(s) of interest.

An observational or experimental unit of interest is the subject of the study. It is important to identify these observational units and to avoid mixing units. For example, observations may be made of several patients, who might have two or more tumors; each tumor may undergo multiple biopsies; each biopsy may produce several specimens; and each specimen may be stained to detect any of several cell types. Results could be reported as the number of cells, the number of slides, the number of biopsies, the number of tumors, or the number of patients, and it is important to keep these units separate.

Some areas of medicine that are prone to mixing observational units are:

- Ophthalmology (number of eyes versus number of patients)
- Orthopedics (number of arms or legs versus number of patients)
- Dentistry (number of teeth versus number of patients)

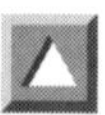

In studies where observational units may be mixed, be aware that some of the observations may be paired because these studies often involve multiple observations on individual patients. For example, in a study of 11 ears from 7 patients, 4 patients will have observations on both ears; these observations are paired by definition ***(see also Guideline 1.11).***

1.5 Describe the population studied and to which the results are to be generalized.

A description of the population of interest is necessary so that readers can confirm the appropriateness of the sample and know to which groups the results may pertain. The description should include relevant demographic, diagnostic (including the stage of disease), prognostic, and comorbid factors (11–14). In addition, major subgroups of interest in the population should be identified (15).

EXAMPLES:

- The population of interest consists of all patients with end-stage liver disease and a history of alcoholism who are being considered for liver transplantation.

- All pregnant women with abnormal ultrasound results during the third trimester of pregnancy were eligible for the study.
- We were interested in the use of bicycle helmets by children under the age of 18 from urban and suburban families of lower, middle, and upper socioeconomic status.

1.6 Provide operational definitions for all explanatory variables (independent variables, contributory variables, risk factors, predictive variables, or prognostic factors) and all response variables (dependent variables, endpoints, or outcomes).

An **operational definition** is one that describes a variable in observable or measurable terms. For example, "hypotensive, normotensive, and hypertensive" could be defined operationally by the range of systolic blood pressure, in millimeters of mercury, that establishes each group. It may be helpful to list the variables studied in the text or in a table.

Specify the unit of measurement for each variable (for example, mm, kg, mg/dL).

Use established definitions and measures if possible to make comparing studies easier (16–18).

Quantify study participants' exposure to presumed causal agents (12,19,20). For example, in cancer studies, the exposure to cigarette smoke may be quantified by the estimated number of "pack years" reported by study participants.

Operational definitions may not always adequately measure the variable in question. Some concepts, such as visual acuity, lend themselves to operational definitions. Other variables, such as depression, may be more difficult to define. "Participants were considered to be depressed when their score on the Depression Inventory was less than 50" is an operational definition of depression, but how well this definition actually represents depression may be open to discussion.

1.7 Specify the minimum change or difference in the response variable(s) that is considered to be clinically important.

Specifying the nature of a clinically important outcome before the study begins helps to avoid bias in interpreting the results and keeps the research focused on clinical importance, as opposed to statistical significance.

The size of a clinically important difference is also one of the factors in a power calculation, which helps determine sample size.

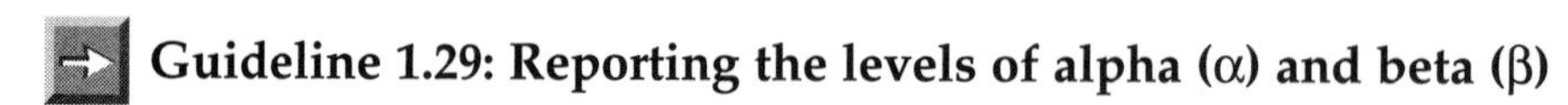

Guideline 1.29: Reporting the levels of alpha (α) and beta (β)

1.8 Indicate whether the study was approved by the appropriate Institutional Review Board(s) and whether animal subjects were treated according to approved guidelines.

One of the most important ethical considerations in biomedical research is the treatment of human and animal subjects. Human subjects must generally be treated in accordance with the principles set forth in the *World Medical Association Declaration of Helsinki* as revised in 1989. Animal subjects must generally be treated in accordance with guidelines issued by the US National Institutes of Health (NIH) contained in *The Care and Use of Laboratory Animals,* National Institutes of Health, Washington, D.C., Publication No. 80-23, as revised in 1989, or in accordance with the *Principles of Laboratory Animal Care* formulated by the National Society for Medical Research.

The Study as Planned

1.9 Describe the study design.

At a minimum, indicate whether the study was

- **Observational** or **experimental.** An observational study does not involve an intervention or a manipulation, whereas an experimental study does.
- **Retrospective** or **prospective.** In a retrospective study, data are collected before the research question is posed; in a prospective study, the research question is posed before the data are collected.
- A **randomized (or controlled) clinical trial,** which is a special type of prospective study (either observational or experimental) in which participants have been randomly assigned to treatment or control groups to help prevent bias.

When describing a study design, use as many of the terms in Table 1.1 as apply.

TABLE 1.1 A Classification of Study Designs (Adapted from Saunders 1990).

Observational Studies

Descriptive studies (includes case reports of single patients and patient series)
Retrospective case-control studies (includes studies of causation, incidence, and risk factor identification)
Cross-sectional (survey or prevalence) studies (includes studies of disease characterization, diagnosis, and staging)
Prospective cohort studies (includes studies of the causes and incidence of disease, natural history or prognosis studies, and risk factor identification)
Retrospective cohort studies
Longitudinal studies

Experimental Studies

Controlled trials
Parallel or concurrent control groups (with or without random assignment)
Sequential controls (includes self-controls and cross-over trials)
External (historical) controls
Studies without control groups

1.10 Describe fully the treatment under study and the protocol under which it was administered.

In addition to a complete description of the treatment, the indications for initiating, modifying, and discontinuing treatment should be described (21) as well as the details of diagnosis and management (22). State also the planned duration of treatment.

For studies involving medications, identify the following (23):

- Generic and brand name of the drug
- Manufacturer's name and location
- Dosage form (for example, tablet, capsule, ointment)
- Route of administration (for example, oral, intravenous injection, transdermal)
- Dose administered (use SI or metric units)
- Frequency of administration
- Results of bioavailability studies (3,11,24) (**Bioavailability** is the degree to which a substance is available to the target tissue after administration. Stomach acids can reduce the bioavailability of drugs taken orally, for example.)
- Results of any safety studies (indicate whether the drug is safe)
- Results of any efficacy studies (indicate whether the drug is effective when taken as prescribed)

If applicable, also report the following:

- Strength of the medication
- Concentration in the "vehicle" or delivery medium, if the drug is in a solution
- Rate of administration (for intravenous administration)
- Duration of administration
- Conditions under which the drug is begun or withdrawn

For studies involving surgical technique, report the following:

- Details of the surgery (18)
- Training, skill, and experience of the surgeons (24)

For equipment used in treatment, identify the following:

- Name and model number
- Manufacturer's name and location
- Function and technical specifications

Was the duration of treatment long enough to be meaningful (11)?

1.11 If the groups are to be paired, report the criteria and rationale for the pairing.

To help reduce variation between experimental and control groups, participants can be paired or matched on one or more variables. For example, to study the effects of diet on heart disease, participants might be paired by age and sex to reduce the variation in heart disease associated with these characteristics. Each group would then contain equal numbers of men of the same ages and women of the same ages. **Self-controls,** in which each participant serves as his or her own control (for example, in a preoperative-to-postoperative comparison), also produce paired data.

The paired design is often ignored in subsequent analyses (25,26). Because paired participants are analyzed together, the loss of one member of the pair results in the loss of data from both members. To reduce such losses of data, the paired design may be abandoned, and data from all participants are simply pooled in their respective groups. The aggregate values for each group are then compared, the matching between pairs is inappropriately ignored, and the advantage of pairing is lost ***(see also Guideline 4.8).***

Research designs using paired samples should be analyzed with statistical tests for paired data ***(see also Table 4.2).***

1.12 Describe any potential confounding variables and the methods used to control for them.

Confounding variables are those that alter or obscure the relationship between the explanatory and response variables. Confounding variables can be controlled for by appropriate research designs or examined for their effect on the outcome with statistical analyses, but in either case they must be identified.

EXAMPLES:

- Pairing subjects by age and sex attempts to ensure that these variables will be equally distributed in the experimental and control groups and so will not confound the results.
- Random assignment seeks to avoid the confounding bias of physician assignment or patient preference.
- Statistical techniques, including multiple linear regression and multiple logistic regression, can be used to assess confounding variables.

Chapter 7: Reporting Regression Analyses, and Chapter 8: Reporting Analyses of Variance (ANOVA)

1.13 Identify the study setting and the source of study participants.

Reporting the setting in which a study is conducted helps to put the research into perspective. For example, county hospitals may provide different services than private rehabilitation hospitals and may treat patients with different socioeconomic characteristics. "Of particular importance is whether the setting is the general community, a primary care or referral center, private or institutional practice, ambulatory or hospitalized care" (4,18,27–29).

It may also be appropriate to describe the referral pattern of patients (30,31). Patients who are referred to, and who are admitted to, a tertiary care center may differ from those who present to a physician in private practice or to a community hospital. This **referral filter bias** is especially important in studies in which the incidence or prevalence of disease and disability are factors, such as studies of diagnostic tests. Tertiary care centers are more likely to see more patients and sicker patients and are more likely to have the human and technical resources to detect rarer conditions more often.

For retrospective studies of registries or special databases, include a brief description of the following:

- The original purpose of the registry and the dates of any major revisions to its structure or purpose
- The scope of the registry, including the number of records, the extent of information in each record, and the inclusive dates of the data contained in the registry
- How the registry is managed: the personnel and procedures for collecting, screening, entering, and extracting the data contained in the registry
- The methods for ensuring the accuracy and completeness of the data
- If possible, the results of the most recent verification of the data including the error rate

Administrative databases rarely contain data on clinical severity or functional outcomes (3,32). For example, administrative databases may record only the presence or absence of coronary artery disease, not the severity of the disease, which may be required for clinical studies.

Data compiled for billing or claims purposes often contain errors and omissions in clinically important areas (3,32).

1.14 Specify how the sample size was determined. If the sample size was determined in combination with a power calculation, give the details of the calculation.

In some studies, especially retrospective ones, sample size is determined by how many patients with a certain diagnosis were encountered in a given time or how many records were available. In other studies, the number of participants can be set by the researcher. In this case, a good sample will be large enough to provide reliable conclusions (11) but not so large that participants will be needlessly put at risk (33,34) or that resources are wasted by collecting more data than necessary.

Ideally, sample size should be chosen with the aid of a statistical power calculation. In general, statistical power indicates the ability of a statistical test to detect a difference of a given size. Statistical power depends on several factors, including sample size. The relationships among the factors included in a power calculation are illustrated in **Table 4.1** (p. 69).

Is the sample size adequate for the question under study? The ability to detect clinically important findings assumes, among other things, that the sample size was adequate (35).

1.15 Specify the sampling technique.

If all subjects of interest can be studied, there is no need to sample. Instead, the entire population of interest can be evaluated, in a process called a **census.** For example, the victims of the 1976 outbreak of what was eventually called legionnaires' disease constituted a census. Most populations are too large and too widely dispersed for a census to be performed, so they must be **sampled.** Because most statistical techniques depend on randomly selected samples, how a population is sampled is critical to the quality of the study.

Some common sampling techniques are:

- **Random selection** from the population (that is, each participant has an equal probability of being included in the study)
- All participants presenting for treatment who meet the inclusion criteria during a given time interval
- **Convenience,** at the experimenter's discretion
- **Self-selection,** by participants who volunteer
- **Blocking,** where each treatment is represented the same number of times within each block to reduce the total sample size. For example, each of three skin tests could be performed in a "block" on each of 15 patients. Thus, 45 observations can be obtained from only 15 patients.
- **Matching or pairing,** in which participants are chosen to "match" other participants on the basis of similar characteristics (usually demographic variables) in the attempt to reduce variability between groups.
- **Stratification,** in which a population is first divided into subgroups on the basis of one or more characteristics thought to affect the outcome and then the subgroups are sampled (36). (This process is sometimes referred to as **oversampling** because some subgroups are sampled more heavily than others to obtain the desired number of participants.)

  Stratified sampling allows researchers to balance important characteristics evenly between experimental and control groups to reduce bias and to permit the analysis of important subgroups. For example, in studying the effect of handedness on cognitive functioning, researchers may have to oversample left-handed people, who comprise only about 20% of the population. Stratification, if not dealt with in the design, can also be dealt with in the statistical analysis by adding the stratification factor as one of the explanatory variables.

1.16 Give the inclusion and exclusion criteria for the study.

Inclusion criteria are the explanatory variables of interest to the researcher (such as diagnosis, age, and so on); exclusion criteria are poten-

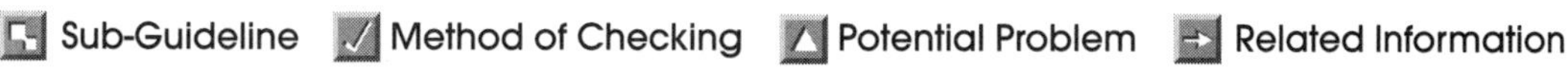
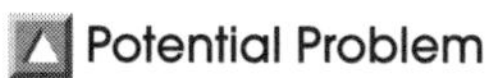
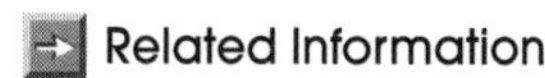

tial confounding variables that the researcher wishes to avoid (such as pregnancy or comorbidities). Both sets of criteria must be specified to ensure the integrity of the sampling process and the generalizability of the results to the population of interest. It may be useful to list these criteria.

Specify how patients were diagnosed or assessed with the criteria (37).

For retrospective (archival) studies, specify the procedure used to identify the records of the population studied (28).

Extensive protocol eligibility criteria have a substantial impact on the numbers and types of patients enrolled in clinical trials (38). The number of exclusion criteria can be large: one study of nine multicenter cancer trials found that the average number of exclusion criteria was 23 (38).

A study with a large number of inclusion or exclusion criteria is more likely to be an explanatory study than a pragmatic study ***(see also Guideline 1.1).***

1.17 Describe the circumstances under which informed consent was obtained.

Because much research involving human subjects must be conducted with their informed consent, how they are approached for their consent, by whom, and under what conditions may determine whether they participate in the study. A description of the approach will help determine whether any undue pressure or circumstance may have affected the decision to participate. (The most common reason eligible patients do not participate in a trial is that their physicians prefer a particular therapy and recommend that they not participate (38).)

1.18 Specify how study participants were assigned to experimental groups (treatment or control groups).

Control groups generally are one of two types:

- **Historical controls** are study participants who have been studied at another time and usually in a different place. For example, the characteristics of infants born in one hospital may be compared with published data for those born in another. Data from the study in question may be compared with data from these historic controls, but it may be difficult to determine whether any resulting differences are the result of the treatment or of the inherent differences between the two groups.

- **Concurrent controls** are study participants who were treated as controls during the same period in which the experimental group was treated. Sometimes, these controls are **hospital controls** who are patients hospitalized for reasons unrelated to the study in question. Their proximity to the study population makes them attractive as controls, but only if their medical conditions are unrelated to the study in question.

Give the rationale for the use of hospital or historic controls (36).

For randomized controlled trials, specify the method of random assignment.

Participants who have been **randomly assigned** (the term "randomized" as a verb is not preferred) to a treatment or to a control group have an equal probability of being assigned to a given group. The purpose of random assignment is to prevent **selection bias,** or systematic variation in the assignment of patients, by introducing chance, or random variation, into the selection process.

Unbiased methods of random assignment include assignment with a table of random numbers or with a computer program that generates random numbers. Methods of random assignment prone to bias include alternating assignment or assignment by birth date or hospital admission number.

A concept related to random assignment is **allocation concealment,** which is the attempt to prevent selection bias by concealing the assignment sequence until allocation. If assignment can be predicted, patients may be maneuvered, intentionally or unintentionally, into a particular assignment. For example, if the randomization sequence indicates that patient No. 23 will receive the experimental intervention, allocation concealment will remove the ability to position a specific patient to be No. 23.

One common way to implement allocation concealment is to separate those who have the assignment sequence from those who make the assignments. In such a case, the researcher would call the data coordinating center of the study to receive the assignment each time a participant was enrolled in the study. Another common way to conceal assignment is to seal each individual assignment in an opaque envelope. The envelopes, one for each study participant, are then given to the researcher, to be opened when the assignment is made.

In fact, studies without random assignment and studies in which the allocation was inadequately concealed tend to find larger differences in treatment than studies with random assignment and successful concealment, indicating that selection bias probably does affect study results (39,40).

"Masking" (blinding) in a randomized controlled trial, a related concept for keeping group assignment secret, is also important in reducing bias (*see Guideline 1.19).*

State whether patients were enrolled in the trial before random assignment (41).

State the typical time between assignment and the beginning of treatment (shorter is better) (25,42).

"Haphazard" assignment is not random assignment (13,22,41,43).

1.19 Specify the technique of masking (blinding), if applicable.

Masking (the term is preferred to *blinding*) reduces bias by preventing patients, caregivers, and even statisticians from knowing who is in the experimental group and who is in the control group. Because the experimenters' and participants' expectations and the placebo effect can bias a study, it is important to describe the method of masking and to report whether the masking was effective. Patients really do try to guess to which group they have been assigned, as do their caregivers.

In a single-masked study, generally only the patients are masked. In a double-masked study, the patients and data collectors (the caregivers, investigators, or both) are masked, although the data evaluators (the investigators, biostatisticians, or both) are not. Although such studies are rare, in a triple-masked study, the patients, data collectors, and data evaluators are masked.

1.20 Describe fully any placebo medications, sham procedures or surgeries (in animal studies), or alternative or concomitant treatments received by control groups.

For studies involving control groups receiving alternative treatments, report the following:

- Nature and intensity of the alternative or concomitant treatments
- Source of the placebo or the details of its preparation
- Degree to which the placebo matches the experimental medication in appearance, taste, and texture
- Details of sham operations performed on animals

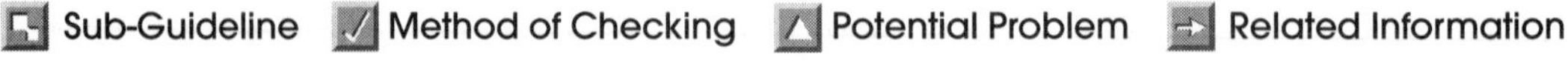

1.21 Describe the methods of data collection or measurement.

The quality of the data can be affected by how they are collected. For example, blood pressure readings taken by a nurse may differ from those taken by an electronic monitor; the interpretation of an echocardiogram evaluated visually by a cardiologist may not be the same as the interpretation based on a computerized assessment.

When data consist of observations or judgments, identify the following:

- Training and experience of the evaluator(s)
- Conditions under which the observations were made (for example, was the evaluator masked?)
- Whether the observations were structured with a checklist

For equipment used in data collection, identify the following:

- Name and model number
- Manufacturer's name and location
- Reagents
- Analytic method
- How and whether the device was calibrated
- Limits of the device's sensitivity or resolution (26,44–46)
- Accuracy of the measurements provided

1.22 Describe the planned nature and duration of follow-up efforts.

Many biological effects take time to appear. Studies often have a **follow-up period** during which participants are monitored periodically after a medical or surgical treatment. The length of the follow-up period and the thoroughness of the follow-up examinations are thus important to report if all the implications of the treatment are to be identified. It may also be important to report who performed the follow-up examinations.

Is the follow-up period long enough to allow clinically meaningful observations? (47,48)

1.23 Describe any quality-control methods used to ensure completeness and accuracy of data collection.

To ensure the quality of the data, many studies, especially large randomized controlled trials, use devices such as a central registration system and impartial review of data by an outside party (15,49). In particular, this second-party review should ask three questions about each study participant (15):

- Was the subject eligible for the study?
- Was the protocol followed? (Is there objective evidence of adherence to the protocol?) (17,50,51)
- Were major endpoints documented?

Data collected for one purpose may not be suitable for another.

1.24 Describe the administrative structure of multicenter trials.

Multicenter trials (especially the larger, multiyear "mega-trials") are by nature complex and subject to logistic and administrative problems that can affect the quality of the study. Procedures for handling data, verifying adherence to the protocol, and resolving differences in clinical practices should be described to establish the credibility of the study.

Statistical Methods

1.25 Describe the comparisons to be made and the statistical procedures to be used for making them.

The Uniform Requirements for Manuscripts Submitted to Biomedical Journals summarizes the overall intent of statistical reporting: "Describe statistical methods with enough detail to enable a knowledgeable reader with access to the original data to verify the reported results" (15,34,52).

Preferably, the statistical comparisons to be made in a study are specified before the data are collected. However, the choice of a specific statistical test often depends on the qualities of the data themselves (usually whether continuous data were normally distributed or not), so the specific test often cannot be stated in advance. In such cases, the general class of procedure (for example, tests of association, paired group comparisons, survival analysis) to be used can be given, generally in the last paragraph of the Materials and Methods section under the heading of Statistical Methods. The specific procedure (for example, the chi-square test, the *t* test, Cox proportional hazards analysis) actually used in the study should then be given in the Results section, along with the results of the analysis.

1.26 State whether the statistical analysis will be on the basis of intention-to-treat.

Intention-to-treat analysis is a method of adjusting for bias caused by participants leaving the study. Medical necessity sometimes precludes patients from completing the study as planned, but sometimes patients may leave the study *because* of the treatment under study. If so, the results will be based only on those participants who responded well. To reduce this potential bias, the results are first analyzed on the basis of **intention-to-treat,** in which the outcomes of all patients are analyzed with the group to which they were originally assigned, whether or not they completed the protocol. Additional analyses are often then performed on only those patients who completed the trial as planned.

1.27 Describe any planned interim analyses and any stopping rules for the study.

Many clinical studies are conducted over long periods, and interim analyses of the data are often performed to monitor progress and to detect problems. The release of interim results needs to be handled carefully because this knowledge by patient care personnel can bias the study. For this same reason, researchers should be careful if they report interim results at scientific meetings or to the media before the results are clear and the conclusions can be supported (53). Interim analyses may also invoke the multiple testing problem, which must be taken into account before sound conclusions can be drawn (***see also Guideline 1.28***).

Guidelines 5.7 to 5.9: Interim analysis of accumulating data

Also associated with interim analyses are statistical "stopping rules" for ending a study. If the interim results indicate that the treatment is either highly effective or obviously inferior or harmful, the study may need to be stopped. Clearly, if patients are unnecessarily put at risk, the study should be stopped. However, "An early significant result can occur as a result of statistical fluctuations or because of large real differences between treatments. It is only with additional follow-up that one can determine whether the initial reported conclusions are sustained and are not attributed to unusual statistical fluctuations" (15).

1.28 Specify any procedures used to control for the multiple testing problem.

The more statistical analyses performed on the same data, the more likely some *P* values will wrongly be accepted as indicating a biological relationship. If P values below 0.05 are considered to be statistically significant, meaning that 5 times in 100 the difference is attributed to, say, a treatment when in fact the treatment is not different from placebo, then 5 of every 100 P values—1 in 20—will likely be misleading. To compensate for this multiple testing problem, researchers may adjust the **alpha level** (the threshold level of statistical significance, usually 0.05), and the adjustment technique should be reported. For example, a more conservative alpha, say, 0.01, may be used.

Chapter 5. The Multiple Testing Problem

1.29 Report the levels of alpha (α) and beta (β) (or statistical power, $1 - \beta$).

Two kinds of errors are possible when making conclusions from a hypothesis test:

1. *Rejecting* the null hypothesis of no difference when in fact there is no difference, such as concluding that a treatment is effective when, in fact, it is not (**type I error**).
2. *Accepting* the null hypothesis of no difference when in fact there is a difference of the specified size, such as concluding that a treatment is *not* effective when, in fact, it is (**type II error**).

The **alpha level** is the probability, set by the researcher, of making a type I error. It is the threshold value for statistical significance. P values smaller than the alpha level are statistically significant; values greater than alpha are not. Typical alpha levels are 0.05 and 0.01.

Beta is the probability, also set by the researcher, of making a type II error. It is usually set at 0.1 or 0.2, indicating a 10% or a 20% risk of making a type II error, respectively. Beta is usually expressed as "statistical power," which is computed as $1 - \beta$. Thus, statistical powers of 0.8 or 0.9 are typical.

Guideline 4.4: Statistical power

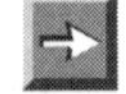

1.30 Report whether statistical tests were one- or two-tailed.

Two-tailed statistical tests are more conservative than one-tailed tests because they require a larger treatment effect to achieve the same level of statistical significance (that is, the same P value). One-tailed tests are often used when the "direction" of the difference is known in advance, as is the case when other research indicates that Group A will always have an endpoint larger than that of Group B.

Because the two types of tests produce different P values for the same data, the type of test must be specified. The rationale for using a one-tailed test should also be given.

Guideline 4.7: One- and two-tailed tests

1.31 Identify the statistical package or program used to analyze the data.

Identifying the statistical package used in the statistical analysis is important because, although commercial programs generally are validated and updated, privately developed programs may not be. In addition, not all statistical software uses the same algorithms or default options to compute the same statistics. As a consequence, the results may vary from package to package.

GUIDELINES ADDRESSED IN THE RESULTS

The Study as Conducted

1.32 Specify both the beginning and ending dates of the data collection period and give the reasons for selecting those dates.

It is important to place the study in time, especially retrospective studies based on existing data. Technological advances, changes in patient care procedures, and differences in reporting practices at different times can affect the outcomes and interpretations of a study.

For retrospective studies, identify the data accrual period; that is, give the dates during which the data were originally collected as opposed to the dates when they were abstracted for study.

1.33 When possible, provide a schematic summary of the study showing the number and disposition of participants at each stage.

A schematic summary is a diagram that depicts the research design and helps readers identify the groups by their size at each stage of the research **(Figures 1.1, 1.2, and 1.3).**

Give the number of participants who

- Were eligible but who were not approached for participation
- Were evaluated for participation but did not meet the inclusion criteria

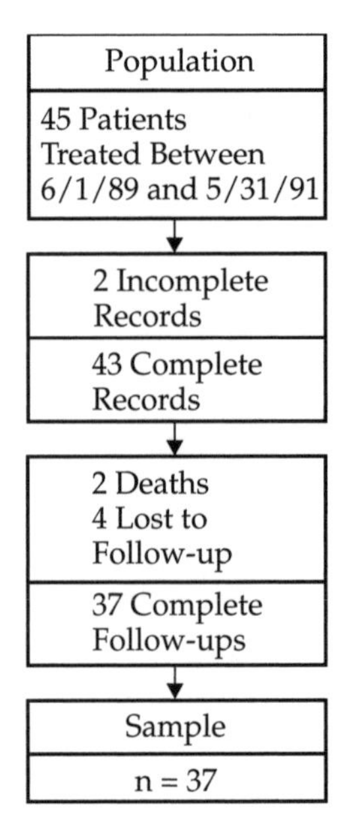

FIGURE 1.1 A schematic summary of a retrospective or chart study that included a follow-up component.

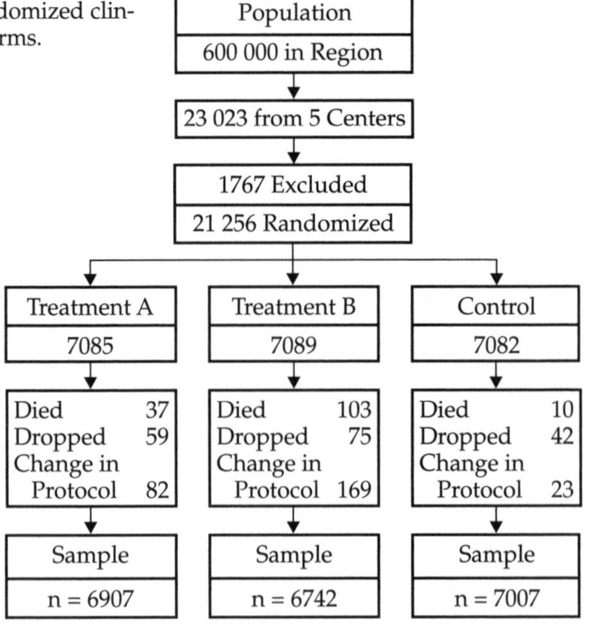

FIGURE 1.2 A schematic summary of a randomized clinical trial with three treatment arms.

FIGURE 1.3 A schematic summary of a crossover drug study.

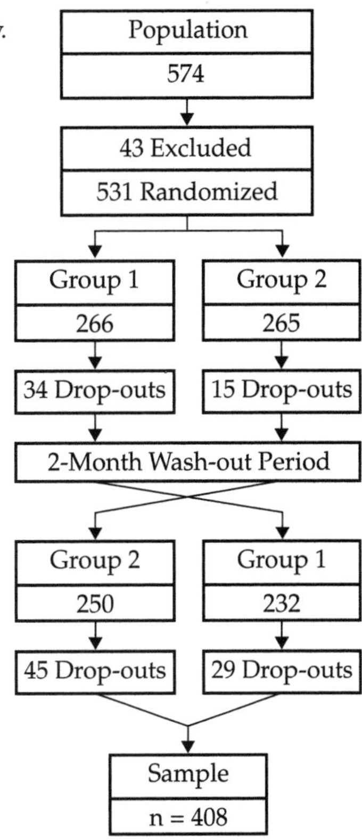

- Were evaluated for participation but declined to participate
- Did not complete the treatment (the **withdrawals** or **"drop-outs"**)
- Completed the treatment but were lost to follow-up
- Completed the treatment and the follow-up period

1.34 When appropriate, describe the subjects who were eligible and available but who were not approached to participate in the study.

Indicating the size and characteristics of the potential sample pool (the population) will help readers assess whether the sample is representative of the population.

1.35 When appropriate, describe the subjects who were evaluated for participation but who did not meet the inclusion criteria.

Patients not meeting the inclusion criteria may need to be described to determine whether one type of patient is being inappropriately excluded

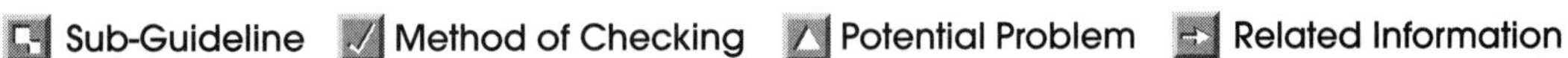

from the study. The proportion of evaluated patients not meeting the inclusion criteria can also be large. Begg (38) cites four cancer studies in which the proportion of excluded patients ranged from 44% to 76%.

1.36 Describe the subjects who were approached but who declined to participate in the study.

Subjects who agree to participate in a study may differ in important ways from those who decline to participate: they may be more likely to take risks, more desperate for a cure, or more comfortable with the health care system. For this reason, it is important to describe nonresponders so that potential differences can be identified. In some circumstances, it may also be helpful to describe the information given to prospective subjects and how they were approached for participation in the study (37,54).

Guideline 1.17: Describe the circumstances under which informed consent was obtained

1.37 Describe the participants who were enrolled in the study but who did not complete it (the withdrawals or "drop-outs").

Patients may leave or be dropped from a study for any of several reasons, some of which may bias the interpretation of the results (17):

- They experienced an unsatisfactory treatment effect.
- The protocol was violated for whatever reason.
- Data were lost or an administrative error was made.
- Reasons unrelated to the study necessitated their departure.
- They may simply have disappeared during the follow-up period.

It may be important to report the point in the study at which patients dropped out as well as their reasons for doing so.

Studies with high drop-out rates (about 15% or more) should be interpreted cautiously (24). High drop-out rates may indicate serious problems with the treatment under investigation, problems with the conduct of the study, or large losses of data.

1.38 Describe the participants who completed the treatment but who were lost to follow-up.

Participants lost to follow-up are likely to be those least satisfied with the results of the therapy. Describing their characteristics as of the last examination may help determine whether that is the case.

Rarely do follow-up efforts include 100% of the participants (55).

Studies in which more than about 15% of the participants who completed the treatment but who were lost to follow-up, for whatever reason, should be interpreted cautiously (15,31,34,50,56,57).

1.39 Describe the actual nature and duration of follow-up efforts.

Confirm whether the follow-up efforts went as planned and describe any important deviations from the plan.

1.40 Describe the participants who completed the course of treatment and the follow-up examinations.

The sample is the focus of the investigation and should be described completely. The baseline values of the sample on all the explanatory variables of the study should be summarized by treatment group.

1.41 Indicate how representative the sample is of the population of interest.

The sample must be representative of the population of interest if the results of the study are to be generalized appropriately.

1.42 Indicate the similarities and differences between the control group(s) and the experimental group(s) at baseline.

If the control and experimental groups are similar in characteristics related to the response variable at baseline, then any differences in the response variable can be more easily attributed to the treatment under study. Differences in baseline characteristics can often be adjusted for statistically, but only if they are known. Thus, baseline characteristics, such as age, weight, gender, clinical status, and so on, should be reported in the text or in a table.

However, it may not be necessary to report the *P* values for baseline comparisons in randomized trials (58). In such trials, any differences between groups on baseline variables will be the result of chance because participants were assigned to groups at random. (The purpose of random assignment is not to balance the groups on these variables—stratified sampling would do that—but to ensure that any imbalances are not the result of systematic bias.) Baseline comparisons do need to be made, however, to identify any statistical imbalances that may need to be adjusted for in the final multivariable model ***(see Chapters 7 and 8)***. If *P* values are

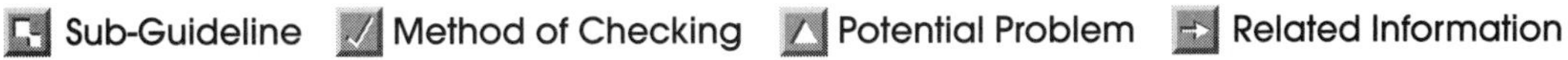

reported for baseline comparisons in a randomized trial, they should be interpreted only as measures of the strength of the imbalance between the groups and not as evidence of bias.

The experimental and control groups should, however, be examined to identify any clinically important imbalances in, say, the means of explanatory variables, whether or not these imbalances are statistically significant.

Group equivalency at baseline cannot necessarily be assumed when no statistically significant differences are found for any of the variables. Baseline measurements of groups are often compared with hypothesis tests (*P* values) to determine whether they differ significantly. However, the statistical power of these comparisons to detect clinically important differences may be so low that differences large enough to be clinically important are not identified.

Guideline 5.2: Establishing group equivalency

1.43 Indicate whether allocation concealment and masking (blinding) were successful.

Masked (blinded) studies are frequently not masked at all because participants or caregivers discover to which group the participant has been assigned (4). Patients and caregivers sometimes go to great lengths to circumvent the allocation and masking processes to manipulate or to discover the group assignment (40). When they are successful, they introduce potentially harmful biases in the form of different expectations, different degrees of adherence to the protocol, and confounding of the random assignment process. Schulz and colleagues (39) reported that studies with inadequately concealed assignment had results (odds ratios, in this case) that were 41% larger than similar studies with adequate concealment.

If masking failed, it may be appropriate to indicate the point in the study at which the failure occurred.

1.44 For observations based on judgments, provide a measure of consistency or agreement among the evaluators.

Many "measurements" in medical research are judgments or observations that cannot be measured objectively, such as the interpretation of radiographs or electrocardiograms. In such cases, two or more evaluators generally review the same image and give their opinions, which can then be combined to create a measure of agreement.

> **EXAMPLE:** Suppose two radiologists evaluate 25 radiographs for the presence or absence of a fracture. If they make the same judgment on 23 of the 25 radiographs, their judgments can be said to be "concordant" 92% (23 of 25) of the time and "discordant" 8% of the time.
>
> Measures of correlation or agreement (such as Pearson's product-moment correlation, *r*; the kappa statistic) may also be appropriate for indicating the degree of agreement among judges.

Study Outcomes

1.45 Present the results of the study.

When reporting the results of a study:

- First, present the data and the analyses of the primary comparison(s), that is, the results of the question that motivated the study (16,56,59–61). Summarize the data for the primary comparison with descriptive statistics (62,63).
- Second, report all other clinically relevant outcomes, whether expected or not.
- Third, describe any secondary or post hoc analyses that yielded interesting results.

Presenting the results of the primary comparison first not only satisfies readers' expectations but helps avoid claims of **data dredging,** a practice that may lead to presenting the most interesting (usually statistically significant) findings first in the belief that such findings are more important than the primary comparison that motivated the work.

✓ **Verify that the denominators of fractions and percentages are for the appropriate unit of observation.** A 30% response rate, for example, has different implications depending on whether it is 16 of 48 patients or 16 of 48 eyes in 24 patients.

→ **Guideline 1.4: Specify the observational or experimental units(s) of interest**

Chapter 2. Reporting Data and Descriptive Statistics

Chapter 15. Reporting Outcomes in Clinically Applicable Terms

Guideline 5.4: Differentiate between primary and secondary analyses

1.46 Report absolute (and relative, if desirable) changes or differences for all primary endpoints.

An **absolute difference** is the actual difference between measurements expressed in the units of the difference. For example, if the mean weight of a group dropped from 72 kg to 65 kg, the absolute difference is 7 kg. The **relative difference** is expressed as a percentage; here, the percent change is 9.7% (7 kg/72 kg = 9.7%). Because a change from, say, 2 kg to 1 kg is the same percent reduction as a change from 2000 kg to 1000 kg, reporting a 50% decrease for both examples, although accurate, can be misleading; hence, the absolute difference becomes important.

Guidelines 2.2 to 2.4: Reporting percentages

It may be appropriate to report the percentage of patients who improved (or not), rather than just the mean improvement score for all patients treated (16,24).

1.47 Report (95%) confidence intervals for changes or differences in the primary endpoints.

The results of a study are actually estimates of what might be expected if the treatment were to be given to the entire population of interest. **Confidence intervals** indicate the precision of such an estimate. The larger the confidence interval, the less precise the estimate.

> **EXAMPLE:** The statement that a drug reduced intraocular pressure by an average of 10 mm Hg (95% CI = 5.5 to 14.5 mm Hg) means, in essence, that if the study were to be repeated 100 times with a sample of the same size and characteristics, 95 of these trials would probably show a mean decrease of pressure between 5.5 and 14.5 mm Hg.

Chapter 3. Reporting Estimates and Confidence Intervals

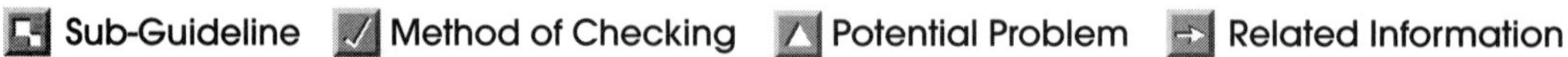
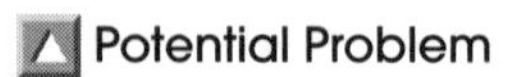

1.48 Report actual *P* values for all primary analyses.

The traditional reporting of *P* values—indicating only that $P < 0.05$—simply indicated whether the results were "statistically significant" or not. But *P* values of 0.051 and 0.049 should be interpreted similarly, despite the fact that the 0.051 is greater than 0.05 and is therefore not "significant" and that the 0.049 is less than 0.05 and thus is "significant." Reporting actual *P* values avoids this problem of interpretation.

P values should be reported to no more than two significant digits, and $P = 0.001$ is the smallest value that needs to be reported. *P* values less than 0.001 should be reported as $P < 0.001$.

Chapter 4. Reporting *P* values

1.49 Whenever possible, present the main findings of the study in figures or tables.

Not only do figures and tables save space, they can often present more information more clearly than can text. Avoid duplicating the information in the figures and tables in the text. Instead, in the text, call attention to that part of the figure or table that indicates the finding or pattern of interest.

Clinical studies may have some or all of the following tables:

- A table comparing the baseline demographic and clinical measurements (the explanatory variables) of the groups. Clinically important differences between the groups ("imbalances") should be identified and tested to determine whether the imbalance affected the outcome of interest. In trials in which assignment is not random, the imbalance should be tested statistically to determine whether a systematic bias may have occurred in group assignment.
- A table comparing the groups on any other explanatory variables, such as differences in the number of procedures performed, the time needed to complete surgery, and so on.
- A table comparing the results (the response variables) of the primary comparisons. Here, both clinically and statistically significant differences should be identified.
- Tables presenting the results of secondary or subgroup analyses.

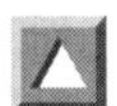

Figures and tables used to record or analyze data during a study are not necessarily the best for communicating the results of a study. Figures and tables to be published should be constructed to emphasize important trends or findings that will help readers understand the research.

Poorly constructed charts and graphs can visually misrepresent relationships among data (64). Be especially aware of where the zero point is on each axis and the increments in which the scales of each axis are drawn. Quantities are most easily compared with lines or columns drawn from a common baseline; comparisons with areas (circles of different sizes, for example) are much harder to interpret.

1.50 When feasible, report statistical findings with enough detail to allow subsequent reanalysis or meta-analysis.

It may be difficult to decide how much detail to include in reporting results. Some clinical studies are small enough that reporting raw data is possible and even desirable, but most are not. Authors should remember that an article is no longer only a report of their research, it is also a source of data for other researchers. For example, the standard errors of estimates (usually odds ratios) are crucial for meta-analyses and may need to be reported.

1.51 Report any potential confounding or interactive effects.

In addition to treatment-related effects, results can be affected by two other, often unanticipated, effects: **interactive** or **synergistic effects** caused by the interaction of the variables under study and **confounding effects** that can alter or obscure the relationship of interest. These processes should be considered and reported if they are observed.

EXAMPLES:

- Alcohol and barbiturates each depress central nervous system activity. However, sub-lethal doses of alcohol and barbiturates, when taken together, can be lethal; their *interactive or synergistic* effect is greater than the sum of their individual effects. This interaction can be described, and should be detected by, appropriate statistical techniques ***(see also Figure 7.3, p. 118)***.
- A study of two medical education instructional packets found that residents completing one packet had better scores on the evaluation test than those who completed the other. However, further investigation indicated that the clinical instructors using the supposedly stronger packet were more supportive of their residents than were the instructors using the other packet, thus *confounding* the conclusion that the stronger packet actually resulted in higher test scores.

1.52 Indicate the degree to which study participants adhered to the protocol and explain any exceptions or deviations from the protocol.

For a study to have validity, participants must adhere to the protocol. Sometimes patient-care staff administer the treatment according to the protocol, and sometimes participants themselves are responsible for following the protocol. In either case, deviations from the protocol can introduce bias, so the degree to which the protocol was followed is important. (The term *adherence* is preferred to *compliance* as less authoritarian.)

1.53 Report all potential treatment-related side effects and adverse events.

Good science, as well as scientific ethics, requires that all negative side effects or adverse consequences of a treatment be reported in full. It may be helpful to specify the timing or circumstances under which each major side effect occurred.

For studies of medications, describe or reference standard toxicity or adverse effects grading scales if possible (16).

Report the therapeutic and adverse effects of each dosage together to facilitate comparison (4).

1.54 Describe the treatment of outlying values.

Extreme values, or **outliers,** add variability and uncertainty to results and are therefore often "inconvenient." It is unethical to ignore outlying values in statistical analyses or to avoid reporting them. It may be appropriate to analyze the data twice, once with the outliers and once without, to determine their effect on the overall results, but such a practice should be acknowledged.

1.55 Account for all observations and explain any missing data.

To avoid charges of selective reporting, all observations should be accounted for.

Check for inconsistencies in the presentation of data. Data may be missing if:

- Reported totals do not equal the sum of the values given in the text and in tables (that is, check all addition).

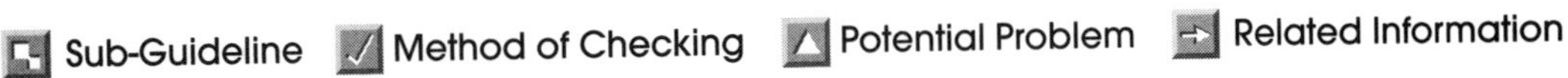
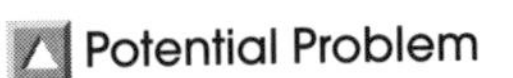
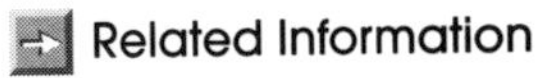

- Percentages cannot be reproduced from the numbers given.
- Tables have blank cells.
- Ratios have different denominators (indicating that the group size has changed).
- The number of data points in a graph does not equal the number of observations given in the text.

1.56 Report any anecdotal evidence or observations that might contribute to a more accurate or complete understanding of the study or its results.

"There are other methods of proof besides the mathematical; equally, we may mislead ourselves by figures alone" (65). As long as medicine is both art and science, the observations and insights of careful researchers will be important. (However, the plural of "anecdotal" is not "data"!)

GUIDELINES ADDRESSED IN THE DISCUSSION (COMMENT)

1.57 Discuss the implications of the primary analyses first.

The order of topics addressed in the Discussion should correspond to that in the Results. The primary comparison should be discussed first. Secondary analyses of interest should be discussed later and should be presented as exploratory.

1.58 Distinguish between clinical importance and statistical significance.

Someone once said that "group means do not present for treatment." Results that are statistically significant but not clinically important add nothing to patient care.

In studies with large samples, minor and even trivial differences can be statistically significant (66).

In studies with small samples, nonstatistically significant differences can be clinically important (66).

1.59 Discuss the results in the context of the published literature.

Placing the results in the context of existing knowledge helps readers to interpret the work. Describing the similarities and differences in the results of several studies—and, if possible, explaining these similarities and differences—is essential to scientific progress.

It is also helpful to address the potential implications of the results for clinical practice and future research. (It is rarely necessary to include the sentence: "More research is needed." It is often useful, however, to indicate what questions need to be investigated further.)

Scan the dates of the references to determine the timeliness or currency of the literature reviewed.

1.60 Discuss the generalizability of the results.

The purpose of any single research study is to produce results that can apply to the population of interest. The population of interest should be defined by the inclusion and exclusion criteria. However, the more specific the definition of a population and the more tightly controlled the experiment, the more difficult it may be to generalize the results to a larger, more heterogeneous population outside the controlled environment of medical research, in the day-to-day activities of health care. The ability to generalize the results of a study is affected by whether it is fundamentally an explanatory or a pragmatic study.

Guideline 1.1: State the purpose of the study

Limitations of the Study

1.61 Discuss any weaknesses in the research design or problems with data collection, analysis, or interpretation.

Disclosure of weaknesses or limitations may be difficult, but honesty is an integral part of science. Identifying difficult areas in research may help other investigators to avoid similar problems.

Conclusions

1.62 Limit conclusions to those supported by the results of the study.

Unsupported conclusions are more common in the scientific literature than one would think. Some researchers even playfully refer to this problem as "type III error" (67). Whereas type I error is essentially accepting a difference that should be rejected and type II error is essentially rejecting a difference that should be accepted, "type III error" is reaching a conclusion that is not supported by the research. (Some authors even refer to a type IV error—reaching what eventually is shown to be a correct conclusion but for the wrong reasons (68).)

"Equal emphasis must be given to positive and negative findings of equal scientific merit" (69). Although the situation is changing, the scientific literature is heavily weighted toward studies reporting statistically significant findings (or "positive" studies). Ideally, the literature would reflect competent research efforts addressing clinically important questions, regardless of the nature of the findings.

Results of secondary or post hoc analyses should be presented as exploratory (70). Post-hoc analyses may be difficult to interpret because the study was designed to answer a different question.

Conclusions should be based on fact and logic, not supposition or speculation. Document evidence to support all claims and arguments.

Studies using surrogate endpoints should be interpreted with caution: a change in a risk factor does not necessarily mean a change in the underlying condition (71,72). Surrogate endpoints are outcomes that are believed to be related to disease states but that are not the disease. For example, serum cholesterol levels are related to heart disease, but drugs that reduce serum cholesterol may not necessarily reduce the incidence of heart attack. Serum cholesterol is a surrogate endpoint in this case, and therefore the link between cholesterol-lowering drugs and heart attacks is indirect and needs to be interpreted cautiously.

1.63 List the conclusions of the study and describe their implications.

Listing the conclusions helps authors identify them specifically and allows readers to find them more easily. Discussing the implications of the conclusions helps to put the results of the study in perspective.

List conclusions; do not restate results. Conclusions should describe the clinical implications of the results.

REFERENCES

1. **Feinstein AR.** Clinical biostatistics XXV. A survey of the statistical procedures in general medical journals. Clin Pharmacol Ther. 1974;15(1):97-107.
2. **Schwartz D, Lellouch J.** Explanatory and pragmatic attitudes in therapeutical trials. J Chronic Dis. 1967;20(8):637-48.
3. **Simon G, Wagner E, Vonkorff M.** Cost-effectiveness comparisons using real world randomized trials: the case of new antidepressant drugs. J Clin Epidemiol. 1995;48(3): 363-73.
4. **Hemminki E.** Quality of reports of clinical trials submitted by the drug industry to the Finnish and Swedish control authorities. Eur J Clin Pharmacol. 1981;19(3):157-65.
5. **LeBlond RF.** Improving structured abstracts [Letter]. Ann Intern Med. 1989; 111(9):764.
6. **Mosteller F, Gilbert JP, McPeek B.** Reporting Standards and Research Strategies for Controlled Trials. Control Clin Trials. 1980;1:37-58.
7. **Hillman AL, Eisenberg JM, Pauly MV, Bloom BS, Glick H, Kinosian B, Schwartz JS.** Avoiding bias in the conduct and reporting of cost-effectiveness research sponsored by pharmaceutical companies. N Engl J Med. 1991;324(19):1362-5.
8. **Meinert CL, Tonascia S, Higgins K.** Content of reports on clinical trials: a critical review. Control Clin Trials. 1984;5:328-47.
9. **Schoolman HM, Becktel JM, Best WR, Johnson AF.** Statistics in medical research: principles versus practices. J Lab Clin Med. 1968;71(3):357-67.
10. **Journal of the American Medical Association.** Instructions for preparing structured abstracts. JAMA. 1993;271(2): 162-4.
11. **Lionel ND, Herxheimer A.** Assessing reports of therapeutic trials. BMJ. 1970; 3(923):637-40.
12. **Walker AM.** Reporting the results of epidemiological studies. Am J Public Health 1986;76(5):556-8.
13. **Gifford RH, Feinstein AR.** A critique of methodology in studies of anticoagulant therapy for acute myocardial infarction. N Engl J Med. 1969;280(7):351-7.
14. **Mahon WA, Daniel EE.** A method for the assessment of reports of drug trials. Can Med Assoc J. 1964;90:565-9.
15. **Zelen M.** Guidelines for publishing papers on cancer clinical trials: responsibilities of editors and authors. J Clin Oncol. 1983; 1(2):164-9.
16. **Felson DT, Anderson JJ, Meenan RF.** Time for changes in the design, analysis, and reporting of rheumatoid arthritis clinical trials. Arthritis Rheum. 1990;33(1):140-9.
17. **Gotzsche PC.** Methodology and overt and hidden bias in reports of 196 double-blind trials of nonsteroidal antiinflammatory drugs in rheumatoid arthritis. Control Clin Trials. 1989;10(1):31-56. [Erratum. Control Clin Trials. 1989;50(9):356.]
18. **Leis HP Jr, Robbins GF, Greene FL, Cammarata A, Hilfer SE.** Breast cancer statististics: use and misuse. Int Surg. 1986; 71(4):237-43.
19. **Horwitz RI, Feinstein AR.** Methodologic standards and contradictory results in case-control research. Am J Med. 1979;66(4): 556-64.
20. **Goodman SN, Berlin J, Fletcher SW, Fletcher RH.** Manuscript quality before and after peer review and editing at Annals of Internal Medicine. Ann Intern Med. 1994; 121(1):11-21.
21. **Davis NM, Cohen MR.** Medication Errors: Causes and Prevention. Philadelphia: George Stickley Company; 1981.
22. **White SJ.** Statistical errors in papers in the British Journal of Psychiatry. Br J Psychiatry. 1979;135:336-42.
23. **Gross M.** A critique of the methodologies used in clinical studies of hip-joint arthroplasty published in the English-language orthopaedic literature. J Bone Joint Surg [Am]. 1988;70(9):1364-71.

24. **Moskowitz G, Chalmers TC, Sacks HS, Fagerstrom RM, Smith H Jr.** Deficiencies of clinical trials of alcohol withdrawal. Alcohol: Clin Exp Res. 1983;7(1):42-6.
25. **Weiss W, Dambrosia JM.** Common problems in designing therapeutic trials in multiple sclerosis. Arch Neurol. 1983;40:678-80.
26. **Tyson JE, Furzan JA, Reisch JS, Mize SG.** An evaluation of the quality of therapeutic studies in perinatal medicine. J Pediatr. 1983;102(1):10-3.
27. **American Medical Association.** Attributes to Guide the Development of Practice Parameters. Chicago: American Medical Association, 1994:1-11.
28. **Feinstein AR, Spitz H.** The epidemiology of cancer therapy. I. Clinical problems of statistical surveys. Arch Intern Med. 1969; 123(2):171-86.
29. **Ad Hoc Working Group for Critical Appraisal of the Medical Literature.** A proposal for more informative abstracts of clinical articles. Ann Intern Med. 1987; 106(4): 598-604.
30. **Haynes RB.** How to read clinical journals: II. To learn about a diagnostic test. Can Med Assoc J. 1981;124(6):703-10.
31. **Tugwell PX.** How to read clinical journals: III. To learn the clinical course and prognosis of disease. Can Med Assoc J. 1981;124(7): 869-72.
32. **Naylor CD, Guyatt GH.** Users guide to the medical literature. X. How to use an article reporting variations in the outcomes of health services. The Evidence-Based Medicine Working Group. [Editorial]. JAMA. 1996;275(7):554-8.
33. **Schor S.** Statistical proof in inconclusive "negative" trials. Arch Intern Med. 1981; 141(10):1263-4.
34. **Simon R, Wittes RE.** Methodologic guidelines for reports of clinical trials. Cancer Treat Rep. 1985;69(1):1-3.
35. **Sheehan TJ.** The medical literature. Let the reader beware. Arch Intern Med. 1980; 140(4):472-4.
36. **Altman DG, Dore CJ.** Randomisation and baseline comparisons in clinical trials. Lancet. 1990;335(8682):149-53.
37. **Bracken MB.** Reporting observational studies. Br J Obstet Gynaecol. 1989;96(4):383-8.
38. **Begg CB.** Selection of patients for clinical trials. Semin Oncol. 1988;15(5):434-40.
39. **Schultz KF, Chalmers I, Hayes RJ, Altman DG.** Empirical evidence of bias. Dimensions of methodological quality associated with estimates of treatment effects in controlled trials. JAMA. 1995;273(6):408-12.
40. **Schultz KF.** Subverting randomization in controlled trials. JAMA. 1995;274(18): 1457-8.
41. **DerSimonian R, Charette LJ, McPeek B, Mosteller F.** Reporting on methods in clinical trials. N Engl J Med. 1982;306(22):1332-7.
42. **Schultz KF, Chalmers I, Grimes DA, Altman DG.** Assessing the quality of randomization from reports of controlled trials published in Journals of Obstetrics and Gynecology. JAMA. 1994;272(2):125-8.
43. **Bailar JC III, Mosteller F.** Guidelines for statistical reporting in articles for medical journals. Amplifications and explanations. Ann Intern Med. 1988;108(2):266-73.
44. **Committee on Data for Science and Technology.** Biologists' guide for the presentation of numerical data in the primary literature. Paris: International Council of Scientific Unions, Report No. 25; November 1977.
45. **Cooper GS, Zangwill L.** An analysis of the quality of research reports in the Journal of General Internal Medicine. J Gen Intern Med. 1989;4(3):232-6.
46. **Fienberg SE.** Damned lies and statistics: misrepresentations of honest data. In: Council of Biology Editors. Editorial Policy Committee. Ethics and policy in scientific publication. Bethesda, MD: Council of Biology Editors; 1990:202-6.
47. **Evans M, Pollock AV.** Trials on trial. A review of trials of antibiotic prophylaxis. Arch Surg. 1984;119(1):109-13.
48. **Gardner MJ, Machin D, Campbell MJ.** Use of checklists in assessing the statistical content of medical studies. BMJ. 1986;292 (6523):810-2.
49. **Rochon PA, Gurwitz JH, Cheung MC, Hayes JA, Chalmers TC.** Evaluating the

quality of articles published in journal supplements compared with the quality of those published in the parent journal. JAMA. 1994;272(2):108-13.

50. **Chalmers TC, Smith H Jr, Blackburn B, Sliverman B, Schroeder B, Reitman D, Ambroz A.** A method for assessing the quality of a randomized control trial. Control Clin Trials. 1981;2:31-49.
51. **Garcia-Cases C, Duque A, Borja J, Izquierdo I, de la Fuente V, Torrent J, Jane F.** Evaluation of the methodological quality of clinical trial protocols. A preliminary experience in Spain. Eur J Clin Pharmacol. 1993;44(4):401-2.
52. **International Committee of Medical Journal Editors.** Uniform requirements for manuscripts submitted to biomedical journals. N Engl J Med. 1991;324:424-8.
53. **Geller NL, Pocock SJ.** Interim analyses in randomized clinical trials: ramifications and guidelines for practitioners. Biometrics. 1987;43:213-23.
54. **Grant A.** Reporting controlled trials. Br J Obstet Gynaecol. 1989;96:397-400.
55. **Stoto MA.** From data analysis to conclusions: a statistician's view. In: Council of Biology Editors Editorial Policy Committee. Ethics and policy in scientific publication. Bethesda, MD: Council of Biology Editors; 1990:207-18.
56. **Liberati A, Himel HN, Chalmers TC.** A quality assessment of randomized control trials of primary treatment of breast cancer. J Clin Oncol. 1986;4(6):942-51.
57. **Anon [Anonymous].** Methodologic guidelines for reports of clinical trials [Editorial]. Am J Clin Oncol. 1986;9:276.
58. **Lavori PW, Louis TA, Bailar JC, Polanski M.** Designs for experiments—parallel comparisons of treatment. In: Bailar JC, Mosteller F, eds. Medical Uses of Statistics. 2nd ed. Waltham, MA: Massachusetts Medical Society; 1992:61-82.
59. **Bailar JC III.** Science, statistics, and deception. Ann Intern Med. 1986;104:259-60.
60. **Mills JL.** Data torturing [Letter]. N Engl J Med. 1993;329:1196-9.
61. **Altman DG.** Statistics and ethics in medical research. VIII—Improving the quality of statistics in medical journals. BMJ. 1981; 282:44-7.
62. **Marks RG.** Proper statistical analysis and documentation considerations for published research articles. Occup Ther Ment Health. 1987;7(4):51-68.
63. **Vrbos LA, Lorenz MA, Peabody EH, McGregor M.** Clinical methodologies and incidence of appropriate statistical testing in orthopaedic spine literature. Are statistics misleading? Spine. 1993;18(8):1021-9.
64. **Wainer H.** How to display data badly. Am Statistician. 1984;38(2):137-47.
65. **Watts GT.** Statistics in journals [Letter]. Lancet. 1991;337(8738):432.
66. **Simon R.** Confidence intervals for reporting results of clinical trials. Ann Intern Med. 1986;105(3):429-35.
67. **Evans M.** Presentation of manuscripts for publication in the British Journal of Surgery. Br J Surg. 1989;76(12):1311-14.
68. **Ottenbacher KJ.** Statistical conclusion validity and type IV errors in rehabilitation research. Arch Phys Med Rehabil. 1992; 73 (2):121-5.
69. **Haynes RB, Mulrow CD, Huth EJ, Altman DG, Gardner MJ.** More informative abstracts revisited. Ann Intern Med. 1990;113 (1):69-76.
70. **Pocock SJ, Hughes MD, Lee RJ.** Statistical problems in the reporting of clinical trials. A survey of three medical journals. N Engl J Med. 1987;317(7):426-32.
71. **Sackett DL.** How to read clinical journals: V. To distinguish useful from useless or even harmful therapy. Can Med Assoc J. 1981;124(9):1156-62.
72. **Gartland JJ.** Orthopaedic clinical research. Deficiencies in experimental design and determination of outcome. J Bone Joint Surg [Am]. 1988;70(9):1357-64.

Chapter 2

SUMMARIZING DATA

Reporting Data and Descriptive Statistics

...If choosing one summary statistic rather than another can even occasionally affect the clinical judgment of physicians reading a published article, then scrupulous attention must be paid to the use of summary statistics in the medical literature.

L. FORROW, W.C. TAYLOR, AND R.M. ARNOLD (1)

Descriptive statistics are numerical summaries of collections of data. Generating summary statistics is usually the first step in analyzing and presenting the results of a study because they reduce large amounts of data to a few, more manageable numbers. For example, listing the pulse rates of 5000 patients is seldom practical or desirable, but reporting the average pulse rate and perhaps the maximum and minimum pulse rates for the group is both practical and desirable. Here, the average, maximum, and minimum pulse rates are three descriptive statistics that summarize 5000 data points in three numbers.

We present here guidelines for reporting 1) the precision of observations and measurements, 2) percentages, 3) normally and non-normally distributed data, 4) paired data, and 5) transformed data.

NUMERICAL PRECISION

2.1 Report all numbers with the appropriate degree of precision.

False ("spurious") precision is undesirable. Reporting that the patients' mean weight was 67.873 kg adds only the false sense of precision to the fact that for all practical purposes the mean weight was 67.9 kg. The case is made below that numbers should be rounded to two significant digits unless more precision is truly necessary (2). Ehrenberg (2) points out that readers actually can deal effectively only with numbers that contain no more than two significant digits. Compare these three statements (adapted from Ehrenberg (2)):

1. The number of women physicians in training increased from 29 942 to 94 322, and that of men from 13 410 to 36 061.
2. The number of women physicians in training increased from 29 900 to 94 300, and that of men from 13 400 to 36 100.
3. The number of women physicians in training increased from 30 000 to 94 000, and that of men from 13 000 to 36 000.

The three-fold increase in physicians is less apparent in statement 1 because it is difficult to compare two five-digit numbers. Rounding to three significant digits in statement 2 works better, but the third digit still draws attention. In statement 3, however, the numbers have been rounded to two digits, and the approximate three-to-one relationship among them is much clearer.

Numerical data should be rounded when *presented,* not when analyzed (3). Information is lost when numbers are rounded, and this loss can affect the quality of the results. In the example above, the exact numbers of physicians in training may need to be reported for any number of reasons. Rounding helps readers to see the overall pattern of the results but should not be used when more accurate descriptions of data are necessary.

In most clinical and many biological studies, numbers with three or more decimal places should be examined for possible unnecessary precision. Some measurements can be made with a great deal of precision, and such precision is sometimes necessary to report. In biomedical research, however, highly precise measurements may be of little value.

REPORTING PERCENTAGES

2.2 When reporting percentages, always give the numerators and denominators of the calculations.

The advantage of percentages is that they allow groups of different sizes to be compared on a common measure. The disadvantage is that perspective can be lost if only the percentages are given. Thus, a statement that 20% of patients were treated successfully is true for one of five patients, as well as for 1000 of 5000 patients. The numerator and denominator of the percentage can be given in parentheses or vice versa: 25% (650/2598); 33% (30 of 90 patients); 12 of 16 rabbits (75%).

Verify numerators and denominators and recalculate each percentage. A typical problem occurs when percentages are reported not for the entire sample but for subgroups of the sample. For example, "Of 1000 men with heart disease, 800 (80%) had high serum cholesterol levels; of these 800, 250 (31%) were sedentary." The 31% is 250/800, not 250/1000.

2.3 When the sample size is *greater* than 100, report percentages to no more than one decimal place. When sample size is *less* than 100, report percentages in whole numbers. When sample size is less than, say, 20, consider reporting the actual numbers rather than percentages.

The cutpoint of 20 to indicate a small sample is reasonable but arbitrary. Especially in small samples, percentages can be misleading because the size of the percentage can be so much greater than the number it represents: "In this experiment, 33% of the rats lived, 33% died, and the third rat got away."

2.4 When reporting changes in data as percent change, use the following formula:

$$[(\text{Final value} - \text{Initial value})/\text{Initial value}] \times 100\%$$

- If the result is a negative number, the minus sign is removed and the change is called a *decrease*.
- If the result is a positive number, the change is called an *increase*.

EXAMPLES:

- A 10° *increase* in body temperature from 30°C to 40°C is a 33% increase: (40 – 30)/30 = 0.33. The 10° is one third of the 30°.
- A 10° *decrease* in body temperature from 40°C to 30°C is a 25% decrease: (30 – 40)/40 = – 0.25. The 10° is one fourth of the 40°.

SUMMARIZING CATEGORICAL DATA

SAMPLE PRESENTATIONS

Of the 25 tumors, only 5 were malignant.

- The *ratio* of malignant to nonmalignant tumors is 5:20.
- The *proportion* of malignant tumors is 5/25, or 0.2.
- The *percentage* of malignant tumors is (5/25) × 100%, or 20%.
- After 5 years of follow-up on each patient, the tumor was malignant in 5 of the 25 patients, giving a 5-year recurrence rate of 20%. (A *rate* usually is associated with a time factor.)

2.5 Specify the denominators of rates, ratios, proportions, and percentages.

Categorical data (nominal or ordinal data) are counts of the number of participants or observations in each category. Such data are often described with percentages or other ratios. For example, if a sample is divided into four nominal categories on the basis of blood type, the number of patients in each category might be presented as four percentages, which total 100%. Although the numerators of ratios are often easily identified, the denominators may reflect the total group or a subgroup, so it is important to specify which group is being used as the denominator. Blood group AB may constitute 15% of all patients in the sample (say, 15 of 100) but 67% (12 of 18) of 18 patients with a certain condition.

Summarize categorical data in the text unless the number of categories is large enough to justify the use of a bar or column chart. For example, the information in **Figure 2.1** is more efficiently presented in the text than in a figure.

2.6 If continuous data have been separated by "cutpoints" into ordinal categories, give the cutpoints and the rationale for choosing them.

Measures of height for, say, 100 men may be treated as a continuous distribution on a scale of meters, or these measurements may be divided

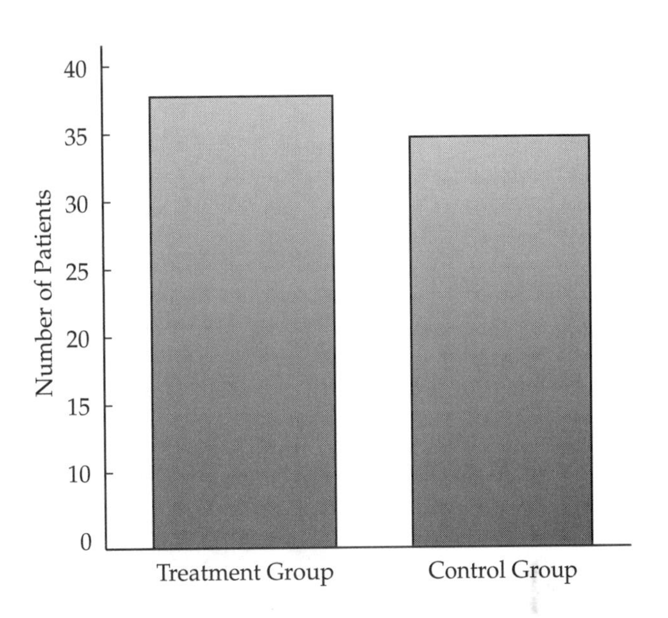

FIGURE 2.1 The value of a chart or graph is that it can present more data more efficiently than text. Here, a great deal of space is required to display only two pieces of information (the number of patients in each group). Such illustrations may be appropriate as overhead transparencies to accompany a talk, but they are inappropriate for publication.

into three ordinal groups: short, medium, and tall men. Because statistically, ordinal data are handled differently than continuous data, it helps to know when and why these categories were used. Dividing continuous data into ordinal categories is usually undesirable because information is lost when individual values are lumped into fewer, more general categories.

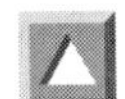

Be cautious when interpreting ordinal data that have been treated as continuous data (4). A common but sometimes questionable practice is to treat a small number of ordinal categories as though they were continuous data. For example, a rating of the severity of disease might use a four-point scale: 1 = absent, 2 = mild disease, 3 = moderate disease, and 4 = severe disease. Scores from several patients might be combined to yield an average severity score of, say, 2.3. But these scores may not be realistic because the conceptual "distance" between the categories is not uniform. The "distance" between no disease and mild disease might be much "greater" than that between moderate and severe disease. Reporting the number of responses for each category, or the category that received the most responses (the **modal** score), may be a better way to summarize these data.

On the other hand, it is sometimes useful to average ordinal scores. For a seven-point scale used to rate satisfaction with a hospital stay, few people would object to an average presented as a fraction, such as 3.2 or 5.3.

SUMMARIZING CONTINUOUS DATA

Sample Presentations

- "Antibody titers ranged from 25 to 347 ng/mL and had a mean (SD) of 110 ng/mL (43 ng/mL)."

If the data are approximately normally distributed, they are appropriately described with the mean and standard deviation.

- "Antibody titers ranged from 25 to 347 ng/mL, with a median (interquartile range) of 110 ng/mL (61 to 159 ng/mL)."

If the data are markedly non-normally distributed, they are appropriately described with the median and interquartile range.

2.7 Provide appropriate measures of central tendency and dispersion when summarizing data that have a continuous distribution.

Continuous data are data that, when graphed, form a distribution of values along a continuum. Such distributions can be summarized by appropriate measures of central tendency and dispersion. **Measures of central tendency,** such as the mean, median, or mode, indicate where on the continuum the data tend to cluster. **Measures of dispersion,** on the other hand, such as the standard deviation, range, or interquartile range, indicate the spread of the data over the continuum.

Distributions that form a "bell-shaped" curve are said to be "approximately normally distributed"; all other distributions are non-normally distributed. Approximately normal distributions can be described with the mean and standard deviation; other distributions may be better described with the median and the range or interquartile range.

Box plots **(Figure 2.2)** and dot charts **(Figure 2.3)** (5) are excellent for presenting either normally or non-normally distributed data (6). Either can show the mean or median, standard deviation or interquartile range, 90% to 10% range, outlying values, and so on.

2.8 Do not summarize continuous data with the mean and the standard error of the mean (SEM).

The standard error of the mean (SEM) is a measure of precision for an estimated population mean, whereas the standard deviation (SD) indi-

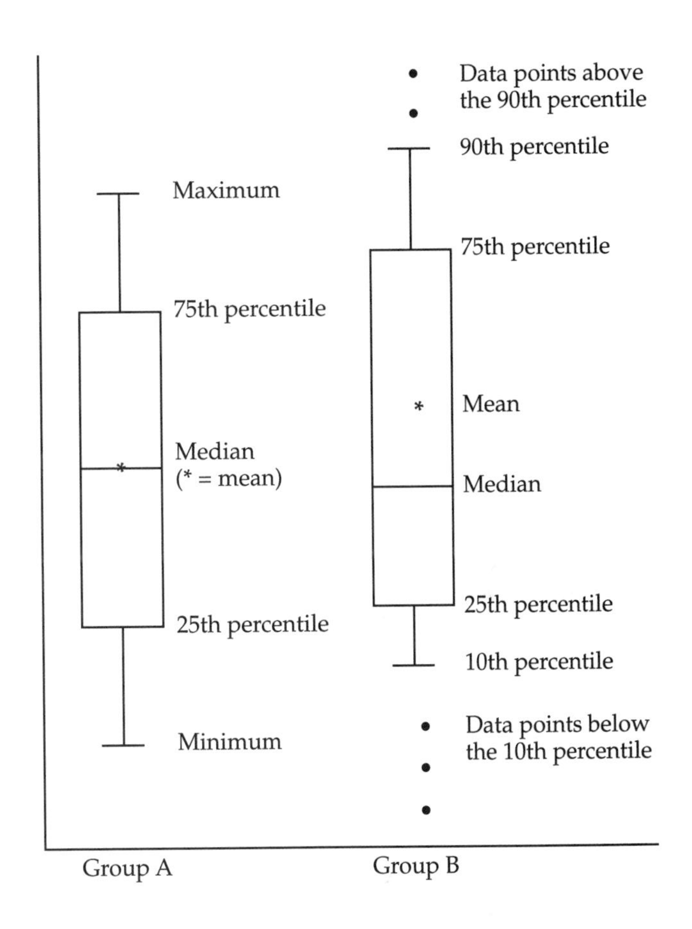

FIGURE 2.2 The box plot can present the distribution of continuous data, whether normally (Group A) or non-normally distributed (Group B).

cates the variability of the actual data around the mean of a single sample of a population. Unlike the standard deviation, the standard error of the mean is not a descriptive statistic and should not be used as such. However, many authors incorrectly use the standard error of the mean as a descriptive statistic to summarize the variability in their data because it is always smaller than the standard deviation, implying, incorrectly, that their measurements are less variable.

The standard error of the mean is correctly used only to indicate the precision of the estimated mean of a population. Even then, however, a 95% confidence interval (that is, the range of values encompassed by about two SEMs above and below the sample mean) is preferred ***(see also Chapter 3).***

EXAMPLES: If the mean weight of a sample of 100 men is 72 kg and the standard deviation is 8 kg, then (assuming a normal distribution), about two thirds of the men (68%) are expected to weigh between 64 and 80 kg. Here, the mean and SD are used correctly to describe this distribution of weight for men.

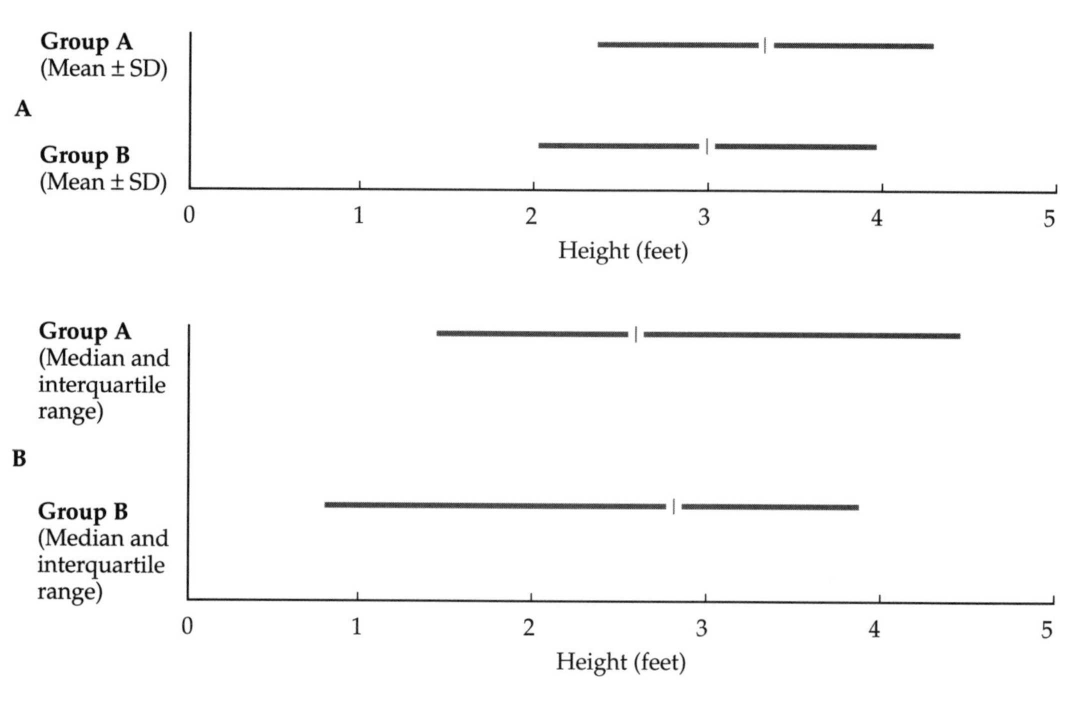

FIGURE 2.3 Dot charts can also present normally **(A)** or non-normally **(B)** distributed data. In addition, dot charts take less space than bar or column charts and can be created with a word-processing program.

However, the mean weight of the sample, 72 kg, is also the best estimate of the mean weight of all men in the population from which the sample was drawn. Using the formula SEM = $SD/\sqrt{n}$, where SD = 8 kg and n = 100, the SEM = 0.8. The interpretation here is that if (random) samples of 100 were repeatedly drawn from the same population of men, about two thirds (68%) of these samples would be expected to have mean values between 71.2 and 72.8 kg (the range of values between one SEM above and below the estimated mean). In this example, the preferred expression for the estimate of the mean and its precision is the mean and the 95% confidence interval (the range of values between two SEMs above and below the mean). Here, the expression would be "The mean weight was 72 kg (95% CI = 70.4 to 73.6 kg)," meaning that if (random) samples of 100 were repeatedly drawn from the same population of men, about 95% of these samples would be expected to have mean values between 70.4 and 73.6 kg.

To summarize, for these data,

- The preferred presentation of the descriptive statistics is: mean ± SD = 72 ± 8 kg.
- The preferred presentation of the estimate and its precision is: mean and 95% CI = 72 kg, 95% CI = 70.4 to 73.6 kg.

Presenting the estimate and its precision as the mean ± SEM is discouraged because it is commonly confused with the mean ± SD.

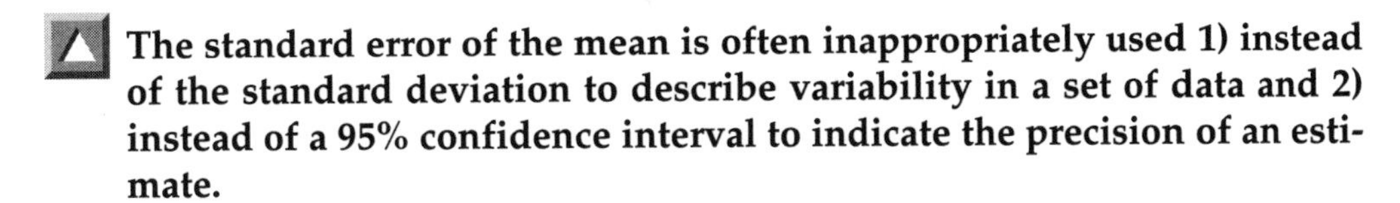
The standard error of the mean is often inappropriately used 1) instead of the standard deviation to describe variability in a set of data and 2) instead of a 95% confidence interval to indicate the precision of an estimate.

SUMMARIZING NORMALLY DISTRIBUTED DATA

2.9 Use the mean and standard deviation (SD) only when describing approximately normally distributed data.

The mean and standard deviation can be computed for any distribution of continuous data. For the average reader of the medical literature, however, the normal (Gaussian) distribution or "bell-shaped" curve is the only easily visualized distribution for which the mean and SD have meaning. That is, most readers know that about 68% of the distribution lies within the mean and plus and minus one SD; that about 95% lies within plus and minus two SDs; and that about 99% lies within plus and minus three SDs.

The mean and standard deviation can be used correctly to describe other known distributions, such as the Poisson and chi-square, but such descriptions do not mean much to nonstatisticians. So, the mean and standard deviation should be used only to describe data that are approximately normally distributed. Markedly non-normal distributions should be described with the median and range or interquartile range.

Guideline 2.12: Non-normally distributed data

Most biological characteristics are not normally distributed (4,7–12). Because most biological characteristics are non-normally distributed, the median and range or interquartile range, not the mean and standard deviation, should probably be the most common descriptive statistics in medical science.

Report mean values to no more than one decimal place more than the data they summarize (3,13–15).

Report standard deviations to no more than two decimal places more than the data they summarize (3,13–15).

Data described with a standard deviation that exceeds one-half the mean are non-normally distributed (assuming that negative values are impossible) and should be described with the median and range or interquartile range (10,11,16–18). "Plasma values were 45 ± 25 mg/dL (mean ± SD)." By definition, 95% of a sample of normally distributed data falls within about two SDs above and two SDs below the mean. Here, 95% of the range would run from –5 to 95 mg/dL, which is not possible [45 – (25 + 25) = –5; 45 + (25 + 25) = 95], indicating that plasma values are not normally distributed.

Subtracting the median from the mean produces a crude estimate of the skewness of the data: the larger the difference, the greater the skewness (19,20). In a normal distribution, the mean and the median values are equal. When the mean is greater than the median, the data are "right-skewed," usually because a few high values increase the mean. In contrast, higher values do not increase the median.

2.10 Use the "±" symbol only when presenting the mean and standard deviation of a distribution and only for approximately normally distributed data. Identify the meaning of the interval (that is, the standard deviation) at first use.

A common source of confusion in the medical literature is uncertainty about the meaning of the interval identified by the "±" symbol. For example, "12 ± 2 mL" may be used to represent the mean and standard deviation (SD), the mean and the standard error of the mean (SEM), or even the estimate and the 95% confidence interval (95% CI) around the estimate.

EXAMPLES:

- Data are presented as means and standard deviations: 12 ± 2 mL.
- The mean (± SD) was 12 mL (± 2 mL).

Because the normal distribution is symmetrical, a single number, such as the standard deviation, can describe the variability of the distribution accurately.

Do not report the standard error of the mean. The 95% confidence interval is the preferred form for describing the precision of an estimate, and its use requires that the upper and lower limits of the interval be given. For example, "The difference was 12 mL (95% CI = 10 to 14 mL)."

Chapter 3. Reporting Estimates and Confidence Intervals

2.11 When comparing the variability of two or more sets of normally distributed data, use the coefficient of variation instead of the standard deviation.

The variability of biological measures typically increases with the magnitude of the measures. For example, the variation in weight at birth is less than the variation of weight at death because as weight increases, so does the range over which it can vary. As a result, examining the variation among samples by comparing their standard deviations may be misleading. The coefficient of variation (CV) is useful because it incorporates both the mean and the standard deviation in a single measure.

The CV is simply the standard deviation expressed as a percentage of the mean. Thus, it gives a measure of dispersion relative to the size of the mean. So, for a mean of 12 and a standard deviation of 3, the CV is 25%.

> **EXAMPLE:** In **Table 2.1**, measure 1 is the most precise; that is, it has the least variation because it has the lowest CV.

The CV is particularly useful for comparing the variability of two or more sets of data with different units of measurement because it is expressed as a percentage rather than in the units measured. For example, one diagnostic test might be reported as the area of an image, measured in square millimeters, and a competing test might measure the uptake

TABLE 2.1 **Illustration of the Coefficient of Variation and the Standard Deviation for Comparing Variability Among Samples. Measure 1 Has the Least Variability.**

Measure	Mean (SD)	Mean (CV)
1	90 mm (15)	90 mm (16.7%)
2	45 mm (15)	45 mm (33.3%)
3	33 mm (13)	33 mm (39.4%)

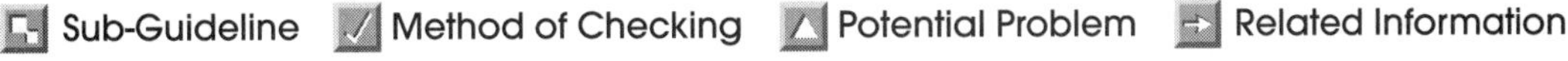
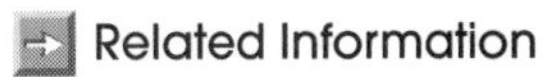

of a radioactive tracer, measured in milliliters per minute. The relative dispersion of these two measurements could be assessed by comparing the CVs.

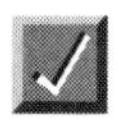 **Check the CV with the following formula:**

$$CV = (SD/mean) \times 100\%$$

SUMMARIZING NON-NORMALLY DISTRIBUTED DATA

The mean and standard deviation are often incorrectly used to summarize all data, irrespective of whether the distribution is approximately normal or not, and even when the sample is too small to determine whether the distribution is normal. When a distribution cannot be said to be approximately normally distributed, it should be summarized with statistics other than the mean and standard deviation, as described below.

Data should be summarized appropriately not only to describe their distribution but for other statistical reasons as well. Approximately normally distributed data can be analyzed with what are called "parametric" statistical tests, but markedly non-normally distributed data should be analyzed with "nonparametric" statistical tests. In some cases, markedly non-normally distributed data can be "transformed" into a more normal distribution and analyzed with parametric tests *(see also Guideline 2.14)*, but both the non-normality of the distribution and the transformation should be reported. Many authors inappropriately use parametric tests on markedly non-normally distributed data.

2.12 Describe markedly non-normally distributed (skewed) data with the median and range or interquartile range (or other interpercentile range).

When data are markedly non-normally distributed, the mean and standard deviation, although they may be mathematically correct, do not allow the reader to picture the distribution accurately. The median (the 50th percentile) and interquartile range (the range of the values between the 25th and 75th percentiles of the distribution) provide a better summary of the distribution because they are not affected by outlying data. Other interpercentile ranges are sometimes used, such as the 10th to the 90th percentile.

EXAMPLES:

- Median weight was 72 kg (interquartile range = 60 to 87 kg).

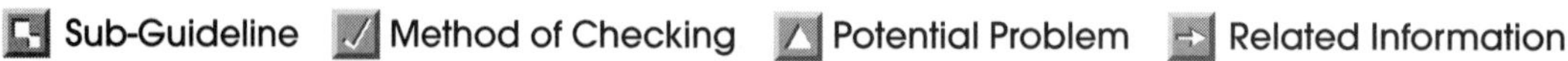

- After 8 weeks, weight (median and interquartile range) was 72 kg (60 to 87 kg).
- Median weight was 72 kg (25th percentile = 60 kg; 75th percentile = 87 kg).

REPORTING PAIRED DATA

2.13 Report paired observations together.

Paired or **matched data** are observations taken from the same participant (such as pre-test and post-test data or data from the right side and left side of the same participant), or from different participants *matched* on certain characteristics to control for the influence of these characteristics on the outcome. Paired observations should be reported together so that the relationship between them is preserved. **Figure 2.4** shows the individual changes that would not be apparent if only group means were presented for the pre- and post-test data. Paired data can be presented in tables, but, if so, the *differences* or *changes in the pairs* should also be presented and summarized. For example, the distribution of the differences should be described with, say, the mean and standard deviation.

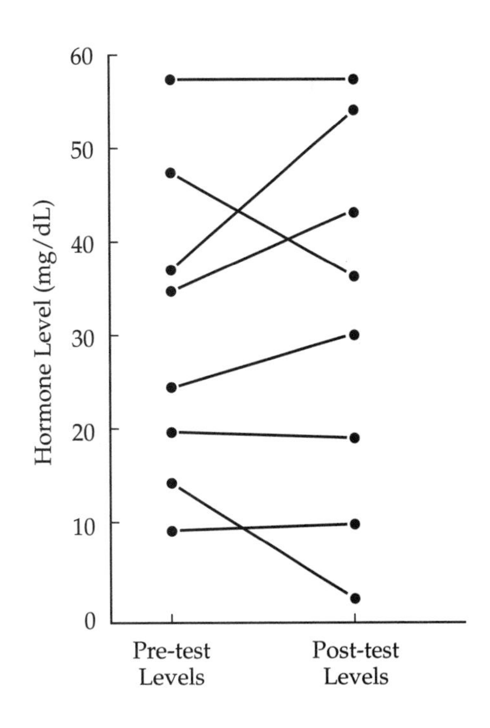

FIGURE 2.4 A graph of paired data showing the changes from pre- to post-test values. Such a graph preserves the relationships for each participant, relationships that would be lost if only group means were reported.

REPORTING TRANSFORMED DATA

2.14 Indicate whether and how markedly non-normally distributed data were transformed into an approximately normal distribution.

A skewed distribution can sometimes be mathematically "transformed" into an approximately normal distribution **(Figure 2.5),** which makes subsequent analysis with "parametric" tests possible. Common transformations in medical science are the

- Logarithmic transformation
- Square-root transformation

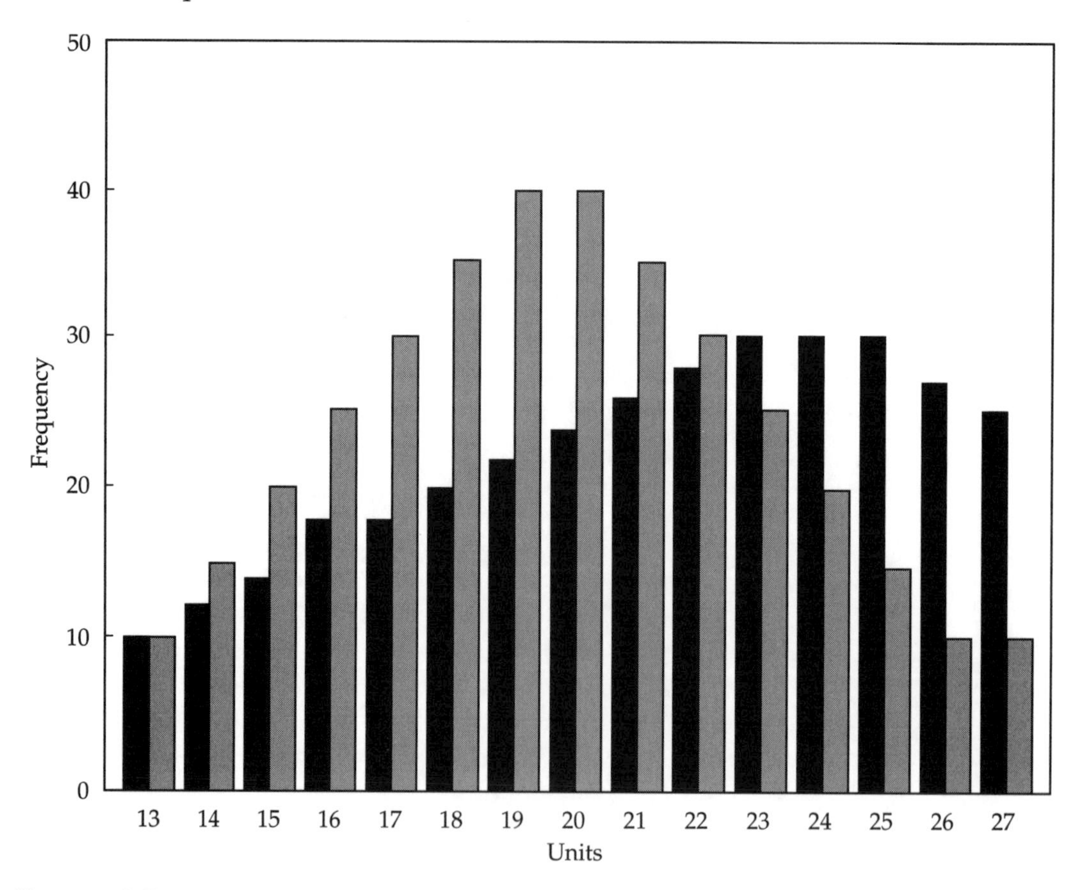

FIGURE 2.5 Examples of non-normally distributed data before (black columns) and after (shaded columns) mathematical transformation. After the analysis is complete, the results should be transformed back into their original scale so that the original units of measurement can be used.

- Exponential transformation
- Reciprocal transformation

2.15 If data have been transformed, convert the units of measurement back to the original units for reporting.

When data are transformed, the unit in which they are expressed changes. For example, in a square-root transformation, "kilogram" becomes "square-root kilogram," which has no real meaning. The results of the analysis, therefore, must be transformed back to be useful; that is, so that they can be correctly expressed in kilograms.

SUMMARIZING DATA FROM SMALL SAMPLES

2.16 If appropriate, present all the data when the number of observations is small or when descriptive statistics would be misleading.

Descriptive statistics are useful because they reduce large amounts of data to a few summary measures. If data do not need to be reduced or summarized, then there is no need to use descriptive statistics.

Standard descriptive statistics (such as the mean and standard deviation) may not adequately summarize small data sets. Not enough data may be available, for example, to determine whether or not the distribution is normal. Means and standard deviations can be computed from as few as two data points, but these statistics mean little under these circumstances.

2.17 Avoid using percentages to summarize small samples.

When percentages are calculated for small samples, they can lose their meaning because only a few percentages are possible. For example, in a study of seven patients, one patient equals 14%, two equal 29%, three equal 43%, and so on. Thus, a table of adverse reactions may show only several entries of 14%, 29%, and 43%, which provides no more information than reporting that 1, 2, or 3 patients were affected.

A cutpoint of 20 to indicate a small sample is reasonable but arbitrary.

Guideline 2.3: Reporting percentages

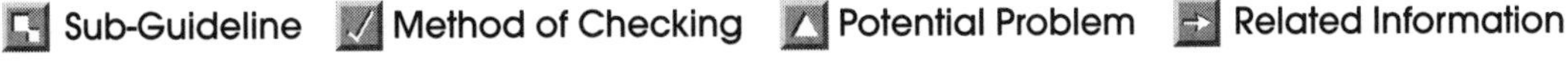

REFERENCES

1. **Forrow L, Taylor WC, Arnold RM.** Absolutely relative: how research results are summarized can affect treatment decisions. Am J Med. 1992;92(2):121-4.
2. **Ehrenberg AS.** The problem of numeracy. Am Statistician. 1981;35(2):67-71.
3. **Altman DG, Gore SM, Gardner MJ, Pocock SJ.** Statistical guidelines for contributors to medical journals. BMJ. 1983;286:1489-93.
4. **Haines SJ.** Six statistical suggestions for surgeons. Neurosurgery. 1981;9(4):414-8.
5. **McGill R, Tukey JW, Larsen WA.** Variation of box plots. Am Statistician. 1978;32(1):12-6.
6. **Simpson RJ, Johnson TA, Amara IA.** The box-plot: an exploratory analysis graph for biomedical publications. Am Heart J. 1988; 116(6 Part 1):1663-5.
7. **Griner PF, Mayewski RJ, Mushlin AI, Greenland P.** Selection and interpretation of diagnostic tests and procedures. Principles and applications. Ann Intern Med. 1981;94(4 part 2):553-600.
8. **Evans M, Pollock AV.** Trials on trial. A review of trials of antibiotic prophylaxis. Arch Surg. 1984;119(1):109-3.
9. **Feinstein AR.** X and ipr_p: an improved summary for scientific communication [editorial]. J Chron Dis. 1987;40(4):283-8.
10. **Hall JC, Hill D, Watts JM.** Misuse of statistical methods in the Australasian surgical literature. Aust N Z J Surg 1982;52(5):541-3.
11. **Hall JC.** The other side of statistical significance: a review of type II errors in the Australian medical literature. Aust N Z Med 1982;12(1):7-9.
12. **Wulff HR, Andersen B, Brandenhoff P, Guttler F.** What do doctors know about statistics? Stat Med. 1987;6(1):3-10.
13. **Sumner D.** Lies, damned lies—or statistics? J Hypertens. 1992;10(1):3-8.
14. **Murray GD.** Statistical guidelines for the *British Journal of Surgery.* Br J Surg. 1991; 78(7):782-4.
15. **Journal of Hypertension.** Statistical guidelines for the *Journal of Hypertension.* J Hypertens. 1992;10(1):6-8.
16. **Brown GW.** Statistics and the medical journal [Editorial]. Am J Dis Child. 1985;139(3): 226-8.
17. **Evans M.** Presentation of manuscripts for publication in the *British Journal of Surgery.* Br J Surg. 1989;76(12):1311-14.
18. **Gardner MJ.** Understanding and presenting variation [Letter]. Lancet. 1975;25(7900): 230-1.
19. **Oliver D, Hall JC.** Usage of statistics in the surgical literature and the 'orphan P' phenomenon. Aust N Z J Surg. 1989;59(6): 449-51.
20. **Gore SM, Jones IG, Rytter EC.** Misuse of statistical methods: critical assessment of articles in BMJ from January to March 1976. BMJ 1977;1(6053):85-7.

Chapter 3

GENERALIZING FROM A SAMPLE TO A POPULATION

Reporting Estimates and Confidence Intervals

The advantage of confidence intervals over significance tests is that confidence intervals shift the interpretation from a qualitative judgment about the role of chance as the first (and sometimes only) interpretive goal to a quantitative estimation of the biologic measure of effect.

K.J. ROTHMAN (1)

Most biomedical research relies on the premise that what is true for a (randomly selected) sample from a population will be true, more or less, for the population from which the sample was drawn. Thus, measurements of the characteristics of a sample are used to *estimate* the same characteristics of the associated population. The accuracy of these estimates depends on the amount of variation associated with the measurement techniques (measurement error), the size and representativeness of the sample (sampling error), and the inherent biological variation in the characteristic (random error). The amount of variation associated with an estimate can be expressed in a confidence interval.

A **confidence interval** is the range of values, consistent with the data, that is believed to encompass the actual or "true" population value. This "true" population value is usually unknowable (unless the study is done on a **census,** which contains all the members of a population), but it does exist and can be estimated from an appropriately drawn sample. Confidence intervals around population estimates provide a sense of how good or precise the estimate is. Wider confidence intervals indicate lesser precision, and narrower intervals indicate greater precision.

When a confidence interval accompanies an estimated value of a population characteristic as described above, it can serve a *descriptive* use. However, confidence intervals are even more useful when they accompany inferences about, for example, estimated differences between groups or estimated changes in the same group over time. These inferences are often those associated with hypothesis testing and *P* values. In this *inferential* use, confidence intervals add useful information to *P* values and aid in interpreting the results.

As described below, the 95% confidence interval is related to statistical significance at the 0.05 level, which means that the interval itself can be used to indicate whether, say, an estimated change is statistically significant at the 0.05 level. The width of the interval also indicates the precision of the estimated change, and precision, in turn, is related to sample size (among other things). Finally, whereas the *P* value is often interpreted as being either statistically significant (a "positive" result) or not (a "negative" result), the confidence interval, by providing a range of values over which the "true" change is believed to occur, allows readers to interpret the implications of the change at either end of the range of values. For example, if one end of the range includes clinically important values but the other does not, the results can be regarded as inconclusive, not simply "positive" or "negative." In addition, whereas *P* values have no units, confidence intervals are typically presented in the units of the response variable, which helps readers to interpret the results. For these reasons, confidence intervals are generally preferred to *P* values, although they are often presented together, especially for primary results.

CONFIDENCE INTERVALS WITH INFERENTIAL FUNCTIONS

Sample Presentation

A comparison of the mean temperatures of the experimental (n = 15) and control groups (n = 15) revealed that the experimental group had a statistically significantly higher mean (± SD) temperature (56 °C ± 3 °C) than the control group (33 °C ± 5 °C). The difference between the means of the groups was 23 °C (95% CI = 19.9 °C to 26.1 °C; Student's $t = 15.3$; df = 28; $P < 0.001$).

Here,

- n is the sample size and is given for each group.
- The means and standard deviations describe the temperature distributions for each group.
- 23 °C is the actual, observed difference between the means of the

Continued

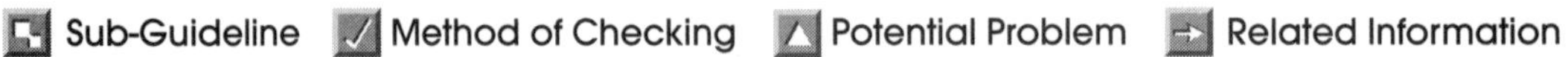
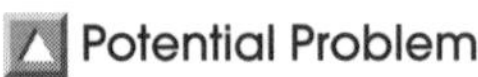

SAMPLE PRESENTATION – *Cont'd.*

experimental and control groups. The difference between the treated and untreated groups that constitute the sample is an *estimate* of the difference expected for treated and untreated groups in the target population. As a single value, this estimate is called a **point estimate.**

- "95% CI" is the **95% confidence interval** around the point estimate. The 95% is the **confidence coefficient.** The confidence interval is a measure of the precision of the point estimate. The "true" difference between the means of the experimental and control groups is believed to fall within this interval in 95 of 100 similar trials.
- The *P* value is the probability of finding a difference as large as 23 °C or larger, assuming that the null hypothesis of no difference between the group means is true.
- Student's *t* test was used to make the comparison; *t* is the test statistic for Student's *t* test, and df is the degrees of freedom for the test.

3.1 Provide confidence intervals for all primary comparisons, whether the results are positive (statistically significant) or negative (statistically nonsignificant).

The results of the primary comparisons should always be reported, whether or not they are statistically significant. Good science depends on accurate answers to good questions, not only on statistically significant results. In addition, the results of any study involving a sample (as opposed to a census) are *estimates:* they are not the "truth" in the absolute sense. Because an estimate is based on only one of many possible samples, it can vary from sample to sample. This variation is reflected in the precision of the estimate and can be expressed as a confidence interval. Confidence intervals around population estimates thus provide a sense of how good or precise the estimate is. Wider confidence intervals indicate lesser precision, and narrower intervals indicate greater precision.

The most common confidence coefficient in medicine is 95%. (The **confidence interval** is the range of values determined from using the selected coefficient.) However, any coefficient can be used: 90% is sometimes used for estimates based on small samples, for example.

To illustrate, suppose that a group of patients had lower diastolic blood pressures after 6 weeks of taking a drug. This result is presented below in several ways, from least to most desirable:

- *The effect of the drug was statistically significant.* This presentation does not reveal the size of the effect, whether the effect is clinically

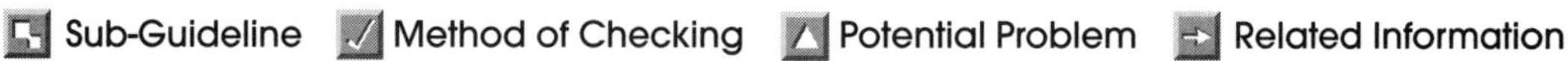

important, or how statistically significant the effect is. Some readers would interpret "statistically significant" in this case to mean that the study endorses the use of the drug.

- *The effect of the drug on lowering diastolic blood pressure was statistically significant ($P < 0.05$).* This presentation includes the direction of the change (the drug lowers blood pressure) and the fact that the *P* value is below the alpha level, which is set by the researcher in advance and defines the threshold of statistical significance. Thus, the *P* value is evidently less than 0.05, but we do not know by how much. A *P* value of 0.049 is technically statistically significant, but it is so close to 0.05 that it should probably be interpreted similarly to a *P* value of 0.051: that the evidence against the null hypothesis is marginal. In addition, there is still no indication of the clinical effectiveness of the drug.
- *The mean diastolic blood pressure of the treatment group dropped from 100 to 92 mm Hg ($P = 0.02$).* This presentation is perhaps the most typical. The pre- and post-test values are given, but readers have to calculate the difference themselves. In addition, because the estimated effect—the 8-mm Hg drop—is not accompanied by a measure of precision, the reader has to guess the variability of the decrease in light of the sample size. If the treatment group consisted of five patients, the decrease would be expected to vary considerably in subsequent similar trials, whereas if the treatment group consisted of 500 patients, the expected variation would be less. A confidence interval would quantify this variation and would take sample size into account.
- *The drug lowered diastolic blood pressure by a mean of 8 mm Hg, from 100 to 92 mm Hg (95% CI = 2 to 14 mm Hg).* Here we are given the average size of the observed effect (a mean decrease of 8 mm Hg), as well as the mean pre- and post-test values from which the effect was calculated. We are also given a range of values believed to encompass the true mean decrease in blood pressure; a range that we can accept with "95% confidence." That is, if the drug were to be tested on 100 samples similar to the one reported, the mean reduction in blood pressure in 95 of those 100 samples would probably be between 2 and 14 mm Hg.

  Knowing the confidence interval allows the clinical significance of the effect to be judged. A decrease of only 2 mm Hg is not apt to be clinically important, but a decrease of 14 mm Hg would be, so although the results are statistically significant, they may not be clinically reliable. When a study produces a confidence interval in which all the values are clinically important, the drug is much more likely to be clinically effective. If none of the values in the interval are clinically important, the drug is likely to be ineffective.

- *The drug lowered diastolic blood pressure by a mean of 8 mm Hg, from 100 to 92 mm Hg (95% CI = 2 to 14 mm Hg; $t = 2.6$; $df = 23$; $P = 0.02$).* This presentation contains all the elements—the pre- and post-test values, the size and direction of the change, the 95% confidence interval, the test statistic, and the actual *P* value—and is the preferred form (assuming that the use of a paired Student's *t* test to analyze the data was reported elsewhere in the text).

Confidence intervals can also be provided for estimated statistics other than differences between group means or mean changes in the same group over time, for example:

- Proportions
- Odds ratios
- Risk ratios

Other common estimates that may be accompanied by confidence intervals include the following:

- Survival rates
- Slopes of regression lines
- Effort-to-yield measures, such as the number needed to treat
- Coefficients in a statistical model (as in **Table 7.1**, p 115)

In general, when the 95% confidence interval for the estimated difference between groups (or in the same group over time) does not include zero, the results are significant at the 0.05 level. In the range of all possible differences between, say, the means of all possible samples of two groups, the most extreme 5% (2.5% on each end of the distribution of differences) are said to be statistically significant at the 0.05 level (assuming what is called a "two-tailed test"; ***see also Guideline 4.7***). The middle 95% of the differences are more likely to occur by chance than differences in the extremes of the range, so a difference in this range is considered to be nonsignificant. When a zero difference is included in this middle 95%, then chance may explain why sometimes the difference would favor one group (the mean of Group A is greater than that of Group B) and sometimes the other (the mean of Group A is less than that of Group B). Only when the zero difference is outside the middle 95% range will the difference favor one group over the other 95% of the time. For example:

- The difference in mean pulmonary function measurements between two groups was 0.51 L/min (95% CI = 0.23 to 0.79 L/min). Here, the difference is statistically significant at the 0.05 level. Zero is not included in the middle 95% of the values over which the observed difference (the estimate) is likely to range; therefore, it must be in the remaining 5%. That is, the likelihood of obtaining a difference of 0 L/min is less than 5 times in 100.

- The difference in mean pulmonary function measurements between two groups was 0.12 L/min (95% CI = –0.16 to 0.40 L/min). Here, the confidence interval includes zero, so the difference is not statistically significant at the 0.05 level. That is, the likelihood of obtaining a difference of 0 L/min is greater than 5 times in 100.

In general, when the 95% confidence interval for an *odds ratio* or a *risk ratio* that compares two groups does not include 1, the results are significant at the 0.05 level. An odds ratio greater than 1 indicates increased risk for one group over the other, a ratio less than 1 indicates decreased risk, and a ratio of 1 indicates no increase or decrease in risk. Only when the odds ratio of 1 is outside of the 95% confidence interval will the risk be increased (or decreased) 95% of the time ***(see also Guideline 7.25).***

- Suppose the odds ratio of the incidence of stroke for smokers and nonsmokers is 4.2 (95% CI = 1.32 to 13.33). That is, on average, smokers were 4.2 times more likely to have a stroke than non-smokers. An odds ratio of 1, meaning that the risk is the same for smokers and nonsmokers, does not appear in the confidence interval, so, assuming the groups have the same risks (that the null hypothesis is true), an odds ratio of 4.2 or greater would be expected by chance less than 5 times in 100; P is less than 0.05.
- Now suppose the odds ratio is 4.2 (95% CI = 0.92 to 18.63). Here, the confidence interval now includes 1, so the difference is not statistically significant at the 0.05 level.

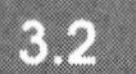

3.2 Report the upper and lower values of the confidence interval. Use the "±" format only in tables to save space and only when the confidence interval is symmetrical.

Providing the upper and lower limits of the confidence interval eliminates the need for readers to calculate the values. In addition, sometimes confidence intervals are not symmetrical and cannot be correctly indicated with the ± sign. For example, the confidence interval given in the example directly above, 0.92 to 18.63, is not symmetrical about the estimated odds ratio of 4.2.

EXAMPLES:

- Poor: In our study, the difference was 28 mg/dL (95% CI = ±3.2 mg/dL).
- Recommended: In our study, the difference was 28 mg/dL (95% CI = 24.8 to 31.2 mg/dL).

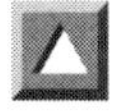

A common source of confusion in the presentation of data is ambiguity about whether "±" notations in the text or the error bars on graphs (Figure 3.1) refer to standard deviations, standard errors (usually the standard error of the mean), or 95% confidence intervals:

- The standard deviation can be thought of as a *descriptive* statistic that indicates the variation among measurements taken from a sample ***(see also Guideline 2.8).***
- The standard error can be thought of as an *inferential* statistic that indicates the precision of an estimate of a population characteristic.
- The 95% confidence interval is the *preferred* inferential statistic for indicating the precision of an estimate of a population characteristic.

If the confidence interval includes both clinically important and clinically unimportant values, the results are probably not precise enough to make a firm conclusion.

CONFIDENCE INTERVALS WITH DESCRIPTIVE FUNCTIONS

Sample Presentation

The mean IGF-I serum level for 138 patients with osteoporosis was 300 ng/mL (95% CI = 273 to 327 ng/mL).

Here,

- The researchers have estimated the mean serum IGF-I level for a population of patients with osteoporosis from a sample of 138 such patients.
- 300 ng/mL is the mean IGF-I level for the sample; it is also a point estimate of the mean IGF-I level for the population.
- The 95% confidence interval—the range of values between 273 and 327 ng/mL—is a measure of the precision of the estimate. It indicates that the "true" population mean is expected to be within this range in 95 of 100 similar studies.

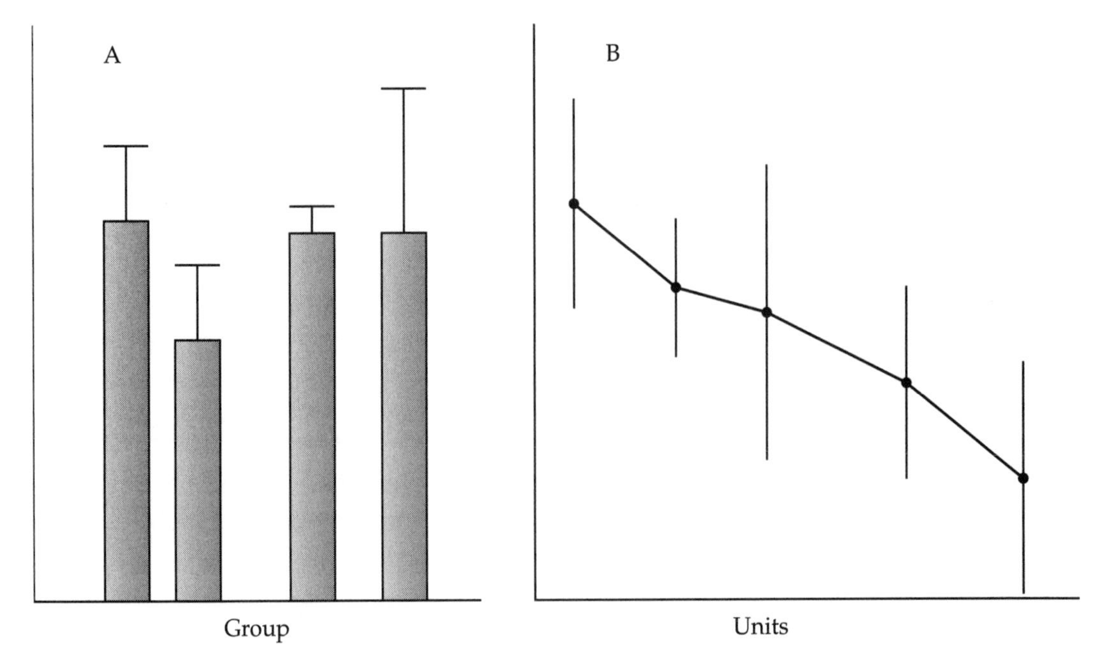

FIGURE 3.1 A common source of confusion in the presentation of data is ambiguity about whether error bars on charts **(A)** or graphs **(B)** refer to standard deviations, standard error of the means (SEMs), or 95% confidence intervals. Error bars should thus be labeled appropriately. The SEM is always smaller than the standard deviation, so it is often used incorrectly to suggest that measurements are more precise than the variability indicated by the standard deviation would imply. The standard deviation is the appropriate descriptive statistic to indicate the dispersion of approximately normally distributed measurements of a *sample.* The range encompassed by the estimate plus or minus one SEM is about a 68% confidence interval, and the range encompassed by the estimate plus or minus two SEMs is about a 95% confidence interval, which is the more conservative and more common measure of precision for estimates of population characteristics. The format shown in **A** is not recommended because it is visually inefficient: a column is not required to indicate a single mean value. In addition, the one-sided error bar visually implies that the variability is in only one direction.

3.3 Report (95%) confidence intervals for all estimates of population characteristics that are of primary interest.

Confidence intervals may accompany the descriptive statistics used to estimate population characteristics. When these estimates are part of the primary outcomes of the study, they should be presented with confidence intervals to indicate their precision. Examples of population characteristics that may be of primary interest include the following:

- Means
- Medians
- Proportions

Do not use the standard error of the mean as a confidence interval (2–7). The mean plus and minus the standard error of the mean (that is, one times the standard error of the mean) is actually about a 68% confidence interval. The more conservative 95% confidence interval (the interval included by the mean plus and minus about two times the standard error of the mean) or the 99% confidence interval (the mean plus and minus about three times the standard error of the mean) are preferred by most authorities. The reason is that 32 of 100 similar studies will likely produce a mean value outside the range identified by a 68% confidence interval, whereas only 5 of 100 similar studies will likely produce a mean value outside the range identified by a 95% confidence interval. *The use of the standard error of the mean as either a descriptive statistic (instead of the standard deviation) or as a confidence interval is discouraged.*

Wide confidence intervals may invalidate the usefulness of the estimate (8). Estimating the average human life span to be 50 years with a 95% confidence interval of 5 to 95 years is possible, but the degree of precision is too low to make the estimate useful. Increasing the sample size should narrow the width of the confidence interval and increase the precision of the estimate.

3.4 Report the upper and lower values of the confidence interval. Use the "±" format only in tables to save space and only when the confidence interval is symmetrical.

Guideline 3.2: Report the upper and lower values of the confidence interval

REFERENCES

1. **Rothman KJ.** Significance questing [Editorial]. Ann Intern Med. 1986;105(3): 445-7.
2. **Gardner MJ, Altman D.** Confidence intervals rather than *P* values: estimation rather than hypothesis testing. BMJ 1986;292: 746-50.
3. **Murray GD.** Statistical guidelines for the British Journal of Surgery. Br J Surg. 1991;78: 782-4.
4. **Wulff HR.** Confidence limits in evaluating controlled therapeutic trials [Letter]. Lancet. 1973;2(835):969-70.
5. **Bulpitt CJ.** Confidence intervals. Lancet. 1987;28(8531):494-7.
6. **Altman DG, Gore SM, Gardner MJ, Pocock SJ.** Statistical guidelines for contributors to medical journals. BMJ. 1983;286: 1489-93.
7. **Feinstein AR.** Clinical biostatistics XXXVII. Demeaned errors, confidence games, nonplussed minuses, inefficient coefficients, and other statistical disruptions of scientific communication. Clin Pharmacol Ther. 1976; 20(5):617-31.
8. **Gore SM, Jones IG, Rytter EC.** Misuse of statistical methods: critical assessment of articles in BMJ from January to March 1976. BMJ. 1977;1(6053):85-7.

Chapter 4

COMPARING GROUPS

I. Reporting *P* Values

We think of tests of significance more as methods of reporting than for making decisions because much more must go into making medical policy than the results of a significance test.

F. MOSTELLER, J.P. GILBERT, AND B. MCPEAK (1)

Although the term *statistically significant* is widely used in the medical literature, its meaning and implications are misunderstood surprisingly often. A probability or *P* value less than 0.05 is often incorrectly regarded as "proof" that a treatment is effective and a *P* value greater than 0.05 is just as often regarded as "proof" that it is not. In fact, a *P* value is not proof of anything.

P values are part of an area of statistics called "hypothesis testing." A **hypothesis** is a tentative but testable statement typically about the relationship between two or more variables—a statement that will be accepted or rejected on the basis of the results of the study. The value of this either-or characteristic is not that it gives a "right" or "wrong" answer, but that it helps guide the interpretation of the results. If one hypothesis can be rejected, another, alternative hypothesis tends to be thought of as more plausible. That is, if a given hypothesis is supported, certain interpretations are more likely, and if the hypothesis is not supported, other alternative interpretations are more likely.

One of the most common hypotheses tested is the **null hypothesis** (that there is no difference in, say, the mean response between two groups), which is posed in contrast to the **alternative hypothesis** (that there is a difference in the mean response between the groups). The null hypothesis is tested by first collecting appropriate data. Then, based on these data, the probability of getting a difference as large or larger than the one observed is calculated, assuming that there is, in fact, no difference between the groups. This probability is called the *P* value. Thus, the ***P* value** is a measure of the strength of the statistical evidence in favor of the null hypothesis. The smaller the *P* value, the stronger the evidence *against* the null hypothesis. The *P* value is compared to a threshold of significance, chosen by the researcher in advance of the study. This threshold is called the **alpha level,** and is commonly set at 0.05. If there is enough evidence against the null hypothesis—if $P < 0.05$—then we conclude that there is a statistically significant difference between groups on the mean response of interest ***(see also Chapter 14).***

The *P* value has no clinical meaning apart from the data, and the alpha level is an arbitrary cutoff point usually set more by tradition than anything else. *P* values that are close to the alpha level on either side can be interpreted similarly; the difference between 0.049 and 0.051 is not black and white. In addition, the clinical importance of the comparison and its results must *always* be considered in interpreting the findings. ***(See also Differences Between Clinical and Statistical Significance,*** p xxiii.) Thus, the result of a hypothesis test should be regarded as a useful tool in interpreting results, not as the "truth."

Sample Presentation

We designed the study to have 90% power to detect a 4-degree difference between the groups in the increased range of elbow flexion. Alpha was set at 0.05. Patients receiving electrical stimulation ($n = 26$) increased their range of elbow flexion by a mean of 16 degrees with a standard deviation of 4.5, whereas patients in the control group ($n = 25$) increased their range of flexion by a mean of only 6.5 degrees with a standard deviation of 3.4. This 9.5-degree difference between means was statistically significant (95% CI = 7.23 to 11.73 degrees; two-tailed Student's *t* test, $t = 8.43$; df = 49; $P < 0.001$).

Here,

- 4 degrees is specified as the minimum difference in increased elbow flexion between the two groups that is considered to be clinically important.
- 90% is the statistical power of the test. That is, given the nature and amount of data collected, there is a 90% chance of detecting at least a 4-degree difference in increased elbow flexion, if such a difference truly exists.
- 0.05 is the alpha level: the threshold of statistical significance set by the researchers.
- The two-tailed (as opposed to the one-tailed) version of the Student's *t* test was used to compare the groups. Student's *t* test uses the *t* statistic and the *t* distribution. The value of the test statistic is 8.43. (Usually, information on whether one- or two-tailed testing was used

Continued

SAMPLE PRESENTATION – *Cont'd.*

is presented in the Statistical Methods subheading of the Materials and Methods section and need not be repeated with each result.)

- The *P* value is the probability of getting a difference as extreme or more extreme than the one observed, assuming that there is, in fact, no difference between the groups. The small *P* value indicates that there is enough evidence ($P < 0.05$) against the null hypothesis of no difference to reject it.
- n indicates the size of each group.
- 9.5 degrees is the actual difference between the means of the groups.
- A 95% confidence interval is also provided to indicate the precision of the estimated 9.5-degree difference. That is, the researchers are 95% confident that the range from 7.23 to 11.73 degrees is the range of plausible values for the true difference that is consistent with the data.

GUIDELINES ADDRESSED IN THE INTRODUCTION

4.1 State the hypothesis being tested.

A hypothesis is a testable statement about a proposed relationship between two or more variables. For example, a hypothesis may say, in effect, that the researcher thinks this drug will work.

In the process of hypothesis testing, two hypotheses are formulated: a null hypothesis and an alternative hypothesis. The null hypothesis is usually the opposite of what the researcher believes to be true. For example, a common null hypothesis is that the mean responses of the groups are the same. The alternative hypothesis is usually what the researcher believes to be true. To continue the example above, the alternative hypothesis is that the mean responses of the groups will *not* be the same. Support for or against the alternative hypothesis comes from first determining the strength of the evidence, from the data, in favor of the null hypothesis. The *P* value provides this evidence. The *P* value is the probability of getting a result as extreme or more extreme than that in the data, assuming that there is, in fact, no difference. The smaller the *P* value, the stronger the evidence against the null hypothesis. In scientific reports of hypothesis testing, the null hypothesis is usually not specified; only the alternative hypothesis is explicitly stated.

EXAMPLES:

- *A null hypothesis:* The mean change in biceps strength in boys enrolled and not enrolled in the exercise program will not differ significantly after 6 weeks.
- *An alternative hypothesis:* After 6 weeks of training, the mean change in biceps strength of boys enrolled in the exercise program will be greater than the mean change in biceps strength of boys not enrolled in the exercise program.

GUIDELINES ADDRESSED IN THE METHODS

The guidelines listed below discuss material usually reported in the Statistical Methods subsection of the Materials and Methods section of an article.

4.2 Specify the minimum difference between the groups that is considered to be clinically important.

Specifying in advance the minimum clinically important difference between groups keeps the analysis focused on clinical issues and helps put statistical issues in perspective. The minimum difference is also a component of the statistical power calculation ***(see also Guideline 4.4),*** which helps determine how large a sample is required to detect this clinically important difference.

4.3 Specify the alpha (α) level: the probability below which findings will be considered to be "statistically significant."

The **alpha level** is the probability chosen by the researcher to be the threshold of statistical significance. The alpha level is an arbitrary value, but by tradition is usually set at 0.05 or 0.01 or, less commonly, 0.001. *P* values less than an alpha level of, say, 0.05, are said to be "significant at the 0.05 level (1)." (Larger alpha levels, such as 0.1, are sometimes used in exploratory analyses to identify promising relationships for later investigation in multivariate or multivariable models.)

The alpha level is actually the probability of committing a **type I error,** or, essentially, of wrongly concluding that a difference exists between the groups.

4.4 If applicable, for primary comparisons, report the details of an a priori power calculation.

Statistical power indicates the ability of a test to detect a difference of a certain size if one truly exists. If no statistically significant difference is found, it may be because there is no true difference or it may be because not enough data were collected to determine whether there was a difference (that is, the sample size may have been too small). A power calculation should be performed before the experiment to determine the sample size needed for the study. This calculation should be reported in the Materials and Methods section. **Table 4.1** illustrates the factors that affect statistical power for a paired *t* test. Most of these factors are included in power calculations for other statistical tests.

Statistical power equals 1 – beta, where beta (β) is the probability of committing a **type II error:** wrongly concluding that there is no difference between the groups. Beta is a probability value between 0 and 1, usually 0.1 (for 90% power) or 0.2 (for 80% power). For example, a study on bone length in which beta is set at 0.2 for a 15-mm difference in treatment effect

TABLE 4.1 Variables* Included in Statistical Power Calculations for a Paired *t* Test and Their Effect on Desired Sample Size.

Variable†	Δ	σ	α	1 – β	n
Two-sided test†	5	20	0.05	0.8	127
One-sided test	5	20	0.05	0.8	100
Increase Δ	**10**	20	0.05	0.8	25
Increase σ	5	**25**	0.05	0.8	155
Decrease α	5	20	**0.01**	0.8	160
Decrease β	5	20	0.05	**0.9**	138

* Values in bold have been varied from the first line to show how changes in each variable affect sample size.

† Two-sided tests are more conservative than one-sided tests in that they require a larger change to obtain statistical significance.

Δ = (delta) the size of the difference or change to be detected—ideally, the smallest difference thought to be clinically important. Specified by the researcher.

σ = (sigma) the standard deviation; the amount of variability in the differences between the paired observations.

α = (alpha) the threshold value below which statistical significance will be declared. Set by the researcher.

1 – β = (one minus beta) the statistical power set by the researcher.

n = (en) the sample size.

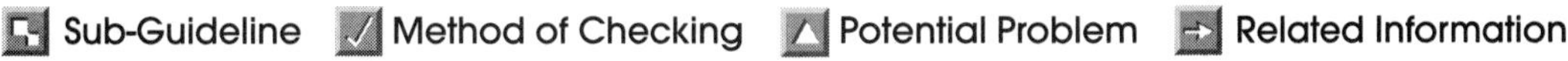

is saying that the researchers are willing to take a 20% chance of missing a 15-mm difference between the treatment and control groups, given the study as designed.

EXAMPLES: When the significance levels of alpha and beta are both set at 5% (that is, a *P* value of less than 0.05 will be considered to be significant and the analysis has 95% power), and the response rate to a drug in a control group is 50%, then, using a *t* test, 5178 subjects would be needed to detect a 5% improvement in the treatment group, 1282 would be needed to detect a 10% improvement, and only 190 would be needed to detect a 25% improvement (2,3).

The statistical power of tests on small samples is often unacceptably low (4–6).

4.5 Identify the statistical test used for each comparison.

There are many, many statistical tests, and several may be appropriate for the comparison in question. Each test is based on several assumptions, however, so it is important to specify which test was used for each analysis. Often, the test cannot be specified until the data have been collected because the data determine which assumptions hold (usually, whether the data are approximately normally distributed and sometimes whether the level of measurement needs to be changed). Thus, the test should be identified in the Statistical Methods subsection of the Materials and Methods section, but it may also be reported in the Results. Tests associated with *P* values given in tables may be identified by footnotes. **Table 4.2** lists several common statistical tests and the circumstances for which they are appropriate.

Using the Guide to Statistical Terms and Tests (p 243), verify that the test is appropriate for the data presented.

4.6 Cite a reference for complex or uncommon statistical tests used to analyze the data.

If others are to verify the analysis, they need to know how the results were determined. Complex or uncommon statistical tests may be appropriate, but readers need to be able to determine that for themselves.

TABLE 4.2. Common Statistical Tests for Comparing Groups of Independent and Paired Samples.*

No. of Groups Compared	Independent Samples	Paired Samples
Groups of Nominal Data		
2 or more	chi-square test	McNemar's test†
Groups of Ordinal Data		
2	Wilcoxon rank-sum test or the Mann-Whitney *U* test†	Wilcoxon signed-rank test†
3 or more	Kruskal-Wallis test†	Friedman one-way ANOVA†
Groups of Continuous Data		
2	Student's *t* test‡ or Wilcoxon rank-sum test or the Mann-Whitney *U* test†	Paired *t* test‡ or Wilcoxon signed-rank test†
3 or more	Analysis of variance (ANOVA or *F* test)‡ or Kruskal-Wallis test†	Repeated-measures ANOVA‡ or Friedman one-way ANOVA†

* Other tests may also be suitable.
† Nonparametric tests.
‡ Parametric tests.

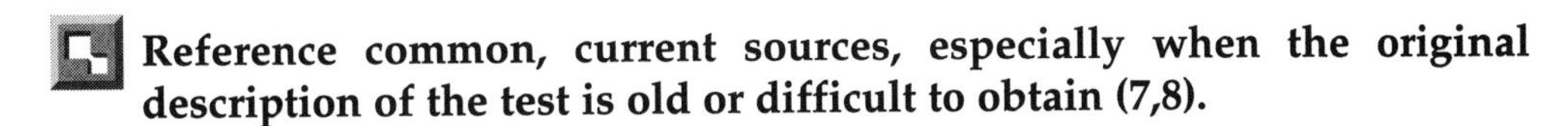

Reference common, current sources, especially when the original description of the test is old or difficult to obtain (7,8).

4.7 If appropriate for the test, specify whether the test is one- or two-tailed. Justify the use of one-tailed tests.

A statistical test is used to calculate the *P* value, which is a measure of the strength of statistical evidence, from the data, in favor of the null hypothesis. The *P* value is compared to the threshold of significance, the alpha level. If the *P* value is less than the alpha level, then the evidence

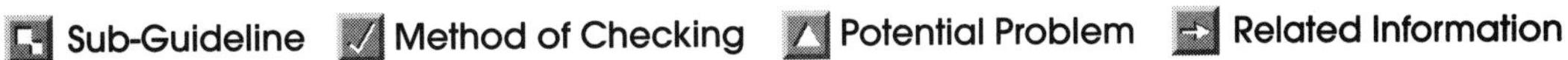

against the null hypothesis is strong enough to reject it. A two-tailed test (based on a symmetrical distribution of probabilities) divides the alpha level, usually 0.05 (5%) into two parts: 2.5% for the cases in which Group A has an endpoint larger than Group B, and 2.5% for the cases in which Group A has an endpoint smaller than Group B. That is, if an intervention may make Group A either better or worse than Group B, a two-tailed test considers both possibilities. A one-tailed test, on the other hand, puts the 5% in only one tail (or direction), if the direction of the result is presumed to be known in advance.

Two-tailed tests require a greater difference to produce the same level of statistical significance (the same *P* value) as one-tailed tests. Two-tailed tests must be used if the direction of the difference is unknown (that is, if the effects of the intervention—either good or bad—are unknown). They are more conservative and are often preferred for this reason.

4.8 Specify whether the test is for unpaired or paired data (that is, whether it is for independent or matched samples).

The statistical tests used to analyze data from paired samples are different from those used to analyze data from independent samples (**Table 4.2**).

> **EXAMPLES:** A study comparing the results of a stop-smoking campaign conducted at two different high schools is comparing two *independent* samples, one from each school. A different study that compares each student's knowledge of the effects of smoking before and after the campaign in a single high school is comparing one sample of *paired data;* that is, the same students are tested twice, and the pairs of test scores constitute the data.

Using the Guide to Statistical Terms and Tests (p 243), verify that the test is appropriate for the data presented.

4.9 Reference the statistical packages or programs used to analyze the data.

Identifying the computer package used in the statistical analysis is important because, although commercial packages generally are validated and updated, privately developed programs may not be. In addition, not all statistical software uses the same algorithms or default options to compute the same statistics. Thus, the results may vary slightly from package to package or from algorithm to algorithm.

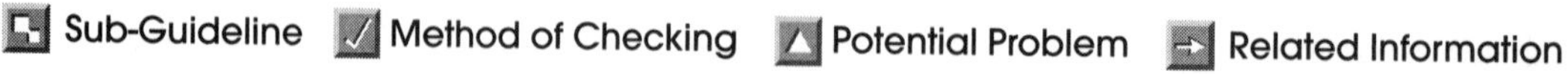

EXAMPLES: Among the more common statistical software packages are

- SAS (Statistical Analysis Systems)
- BMDP
- SPlus
- SPSS (Statistical Package for the Social Sciences)
- StatXact
- StatView
- StatSoft
- InStat
- Statistical Navigator
- SysStat
- Minitab

GUIDELINES ADDRESSED IN THE RESULTS

4.10 Report the results of all primary analyses first.

The focus of a scientific article should be on the primary comparisons that motivated the work. Statistical analysis can and should be exploratory and interpretive to a point, but these secondary explorations should never overshadow the primary analyses. That is, unsupported (statistically nonsignificant) primary analyses should not be neglected for more intriguing (statistically significant) secondary analyses.

Beware of selective reporting. Selective reporting is the practice of presenting only the desirable findings of a study. Such findings are usually those that are statistically significant. The results of all clinically relevant analyses should be reported, whether or not they are statistically significant. It is unethical to suppress contradictory data.

Using the Guide to Statistical Terms and Tests (p 243), verify that the test is reported properly.

In the absence of a statement that the results are from a secondary analysis, the only defense against selective reporting is to determine whether the relationships described make biological sense.

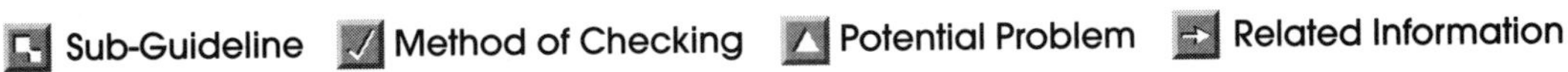
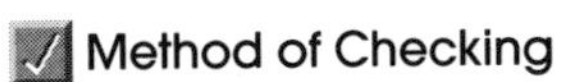
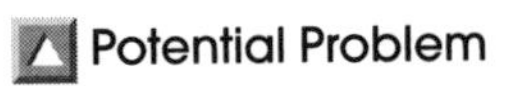

4.11 Report any outlying values and how they were treated in the analysis.

Outliers are extreme values that can occur for any number of legitimate reasons. However, because they are extreme, they can have a disproportionate effect on some statistical analyses. Outliers cannot simply be ignored as inconvenient; they must be acknowledged and must be incorporated appropriately into the analysis. Sometimes, it may be appropriate to report the results with and without outliers to determine their effect on the results.

4.12 Confirm that the assumptions of the test have been met.

Most statistical tests make assumptions about the data. If these assumptions are suspect, the results of the analyses may also be suspect. A statement that the assumptions were verified is all that need be included.

A common assumption is that the data are approximately normally distributed, a characteristic that permits the use of "parametric" tests. This assumption is often violated. When data are markedly non-normally distributed, a mathematical "transformation" may be appropriate to make the distribution more normal, or a "nonparametric" test (which does not require data to be normally distributed) may be used instead. If data have been transformed or analyzed with nonparametric tests, the fact should be reported (see **Table 4.2**).

✓ **For the *t* test and the *F* test (ANOVA), determine whether data are normally distributed within each group, whether group variances are equal, and whether the samples are independent and randomly selected.**

✓ **For the chi-square test, confirm that the *expected* count in each cell (not the observed count) is greater than 5 or that an "exact" testing procedure was used (9–11).** Also, confirm that the test has been performed on categorical data (nominal or ordinal data), not continuous data, from samples that are independent and randomly selected (12).

4.13 Report absolute (and relative, if desirable) changes or differences for all primary endpoints.

Reporting the absolute or actual changes between groups avoids any confusion created by expressing the differences only as relative or percentage changes. For example, if a patient had a final serum cholesterol level of 175 mg/dL and an initial level of 220 mg/dL, the absolute difference is 45 mg/dL. The relative difference, a 20% decrease in serum cholesterol level [([175 – 220]/220) × 100%], could also be described as "a fifth lower than the initial value," which, although accurate, does not include the fact that the actual, observed change was 45 mg/dL.

When there are two groups involved, it is helpful to report differences or changes between the groups in addition to the group means or proportions.

For continuous variables and independent groups, report the group means (or medians, as appropriate) and the absolute difference between the group means (or medians).

For continuous variables and *paired* groups, report the group means (or medians, as appropriate) and the mean (or median) of the *differences* between the members of each pair.

For categorical variables and independent groups, report the group proportions and the absolute difference between the proportions.

For categorical variables and paired groups, report the group proportions.

4.14 Report (95%) confidence intervals for changes or differences in the primary endpoints.

The difference between a treatment and a control group, or between an initial and a final measurement in the same group, is essentially an estimate of the difference that would be expected if the treatment were to be given to the entire target population. The precision of this estimated difference is indicated with a confidence interval. Narrower confidence intervals reflect more precision.

Confidence intervals reflect the influence of sample size and variability, in that larger samples narrow the interval and provide more precise estimates. Less variability in the data also narrows the interval and provides more precise estimates.

> **EXAMPLE:** "The drug slowed clotting time by a mean of 4 min (95% CI = 2.5 to 5.5 min; $P < 0.001$)." The 95% confidence interval indicates that if the drug were to be tested on 100 similar samples, the mean delay in clotting time in 95 of those 100 samples would probably be between 2.5 and 5.5 min. Knowing this confidence interval allows us to judge the clinical significance of the effect. A mean delay in clotting time of even 2.5 min—the

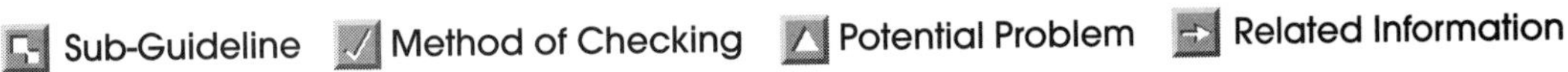
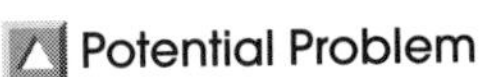
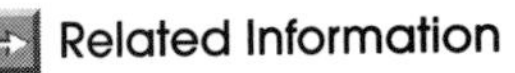

lower boundary of the confidence interval—would be clinically important, so the effect of the drug appears to be both clinically important and statistically significant.

Chapter 3. Reporting Estimates and Confidence Intervals

4.15 Give the actual *P* value, to two significant digits, whether or not the value is statistically significant.

P values less than the alpha level (usually 0.05) are considered to be "statistically significant"; those greater than alpha are not. However, the *P* values of 0.051 and 0.049 are close enough that they should be interpreted similarly, despite the fact that the first would be reported as "not significant" and the second as "significant." Providing the actual *P* value prevents this problem of interpretation. Actual *P* values are also of more value if the study is eventually used in a meta-analysis ***(see Chapter 11).*** In any event, the smallest *P* value that needs to be reported is $P < 0.001$.

***P* values of 1 or 0 are rare and should be questioned if they appear in a scientific article.** Rounding may account for many *P* values of 0 or 1.

If the results are not statistically significant, do not use the phrase "showed a trend toward significance" or "approached significance." The result was simply not statistically significant as defined by the relationship between the *P* value and the alpha level. Comments on the clinical importance of the result are, however, still appropriate.

4.16 Report the value of the test statistic.

In statistical analysis, data are combined mathematically to yield a **test statistic,** a single number that is compared to the appropriate probability distribution to obtain the probability, or *P* value, associated with the statistic. Giving the statistic allows the reader to verify the *P* value.

> **EXAMPLE:** Student's *t* test might be presented as: "$t = 1.34$, 15 df, $P = 0.2$," where 1.34 is the test statistic that is compared to the *t* distribution with 15 degrees of freedom ***(see Guideline 4.17),*** and *P* is the probability value associated with the test statistic: the probability of getting a result as extreme or more extreme than the one observed, assuming that there is no difference between the groups.

4.17 For primary comparisons, specify the degrees of freedom (df) of the test, if applicable.

"Degrees of freedom" is a concept used in several common statistical tests. Computed on the basis of sample size, it is reported so that readers can verify the *P* value by checking the test statistic against the appropriate distribution, each of which has different degrees of freedom. Student's *t* test, ANOVA or the *F* test, and the chi-square test all use the concept of degrees of freedom.

GUIDELINES ADDRESSED IN THE DISCUSSION

4.18 Distinguish between clinical importance and statistical significance.

Gertrude Stein once said: "A difference, to be a difference, must make a difference" (13). A clinically important difference, by definition, is important whether or not it is statistically significant. Further, a statistically significant difference may have no clinical importance. Statistics must be interpreted; they do not provide hard and fast evidence of "truth."

Conclusions should seldom be based exclusively on *P* values. When drawing conclusions from a study, several aspects of the research and results must be kept in mind: the research design, the conduct of the study, the size of the effect, the width of the confidence intervals, biological plausibility, additional confirming evidence, and so on.

> **EXAMPLE:** Small differences between large samples can be statistically significant but clinically unimportant. A 1-week difference in the useful life of a pacemaker after 5 years between two brands may be statistically significant but is probably not clinically important. Also, large differences between small samples scan be clinically important but not statistically significant. Suppose 8 of 16 people received the current treatment and lived, and 12 of 16 others received an experimental treatment and lived. Although the difference in mortality rates may not be statistically significant, the increased survival in the experimental group (by 50%, from 8 to 12) may be clinically important, in which case additional research with a larger sample may be warranted.

"Not statistically different" is not the same as "no difference" (13,14). *(See also Guideline 4.19 and Guideline 5.2.)* Groups that do not differ statistically cannot necessarily be assumed to be clinically equivalent.

4.19 For differences that are *clinically* important but not *statistically* significant, report the observed difference, the (95%) confidence interval for the difference, and the actual *P* value of the comparison.

When authors find a clinically important difference that is not statistically significant, they sometimes report that the difference shows a "trend" toward significance. The belief is that if the sample were larger, and the statistical test had more power, then the result would have been statistically significant as well as clinically important. In fact, if the *P* value could show a "trend" (it cannot), it could just as easily move "away from" the alpha level as "toward" it. The point is that clinically important results should not be overlooked because they are not statistically significant (15).

Results do not "trend toward significance" or "approach significance" (16).

The results of a study with low statistical power and no statistically significant differences are not negative; they are inclusive (5,6,13, 17–30).

Frederick Mosteller once illustrated the concept of low statistical power with this statement: "The increase in infection rate using the new methods was not statistically significant . . . and there was not one chance in ten that we would have detected a 30% increase in rate" (1).

"To observe that nothing happened does not prove that nothing happened" (31,32). Further: "The absence of proof is not proof of absence" (13,33). Studies with low statistical power are common, and the failure to report statistical power is a common error. Freiman and colleagues reported that in 50 of 71 (70%) papers reporting no significant differences between therapies, even a 50% improvement in performance would not have been found (5,34).

Until recently, authors were urged to provide "post hoc power calculations" for nonsignificant differences. That is, if the results of the study were negative, a power calculation was to be performed after the fact to determine the adequacy of the sample size. Confidence intervals also reflect sample size, however, and are more easily interpreted, so the requirement of a post hoc power calculation for nonstatistically significant results has given way to reporting the confidence interval (35) (see **Table 4.1**).

REFERENCES

1. **Mosteller F, Gilbert JP, McPeek B.** Reporting standards and research strategies for controlled trials. Control Clin Trials. 1980;1:37-58.
2. **Walker AM.** Reporting the results of epidemiological studies. Am J Public Health. 1986;76(5): 556-8.
3. **Hall JC.** The other side of statistical significance: a review of type II errors in the Australian medical literature. Aust N Z Med 1982;12:7-9.
4. **Diamond GA, Forrester JS.** Clinical trials and statistical verdicts: probable grounds for appeal. Ann Intern Med. 1983;98:385-94.
5. **Freiman JA, Chalmers TC, Smith H, Kuebler RR.** The importance of beta, the type II error and sample size in the design and interpretation of the randomized control trial. Survey of 71 negative trials. N Engl J Med. 1978;299:690-4.
6. **Glantz SA.** It is all in the numbers [Editorial]. J Am Coll Cardiol. 1993;21(3):835-7.
7. **Bailar JC III, Mosteller F.** Guidelines for statistical reporting in articles for medical journals. Ann Intern Med. 1988;108(2): 266-73.
8. **International Committee of Medical Journal Editors.** Uniform Requirements for Manuscripts Submitted to Biomedical Journals. N Engl J Med. 1991;324(6):424-8.
9. **Avram MJ, Shanks CA, Dykes MH, Ronai AK, Stiers WM.** Statistical methods in anesthesia articles: an evaluation of two American journals during two six-month periods. Anesth Analg. 1985;64(6):607-11.
10. **Shott S.** Statistics in veterinary research. J Am Vet Med Assoc. 1985;187(2):138-41.
11. **White SJ.** Statistical errors in papers in the British Journal of Psychiatry. Br J Psychiatry. 1979;135:336-42.
12. **MacArthur RD, Jackson GG.** An evaluation of the use of statistical methodology in the Journal of Infectious Diseases. J Infect Dis. 1984;149(3):349-54.
13. **Haines SJ.** Six statistical suggestions for surgeons. Neurosurgery. 1981;9(4):414-8.
14. **Evans M.** Presentation of manuscripts for publication in the British Journal of Surgery. Br J Surg. 1989;76(12):1311-5.
15. **Gardner MJ, Altman D.** Confidence intervals rather than *P* values: estimation rather than hypothesis testing. BMJ. 1986;292: 746-50.
16. **Squires BP.** Statistics in biomedical manuscripts: what editors want from authors and peer reviewers [Editorial]. Can Med Assoc J. 1990;142(3):213-4.
17. **Gore SM.** Statistics in question. Assessing methods—confidence intervals. BMJ. 1981; 283:660-2.
18. **Stoto MA.** From data analysis to conclusions: a statistician's view. In: Council of Biology Editors Editorial Policy Committee. Ethics and Policy in Scientific Publication. Bethesda, MD: Council of Biology Editors; 1990:207-18.
19. **Altman DG.** Statistics in medical journals. Stat Med. 1982;1:59-71.
20. **Hujoel PP, Baab DA, De Rouen TA.** The power of tests to detect differences between periodontal treatments in published studies. J Clin Periodontol. 1992;19:779-84.
21. **Gore SM, Jones G, Thompson SG.** The Lancet's statistical review process: areas for improvement by authors. Lancet. 1992;340: 100-2.
22. **Gotzsche PC.** Methodology and overt and hidden bias in reports of 196 double-blind trials of nonsteroidal antiinflammatory drugs in rheumatoid arthritis. Control Clin Trials. 1989;10:31-56.
23. **Hemminki E.** Quality of reports of clinical trials submitted by the drug industry to the Finnish and Swedish control authorities. Eur J Clin Pharmacol. 1981;19(3):157-65.
24. **Mainland D.** Statistical ritual in clinical journals: is there a cure?–I. BMJ. 1984;288: 841-3.
25. **Murray GD.** Confidence intervals [Editorial]. Nuc Med Commun. 1989;10:387-8.
26. **Schoolman HM, Becktel JM, Best WR, Johnson AF.** Statistics in medical research: principles versus practices. J Lab Clin Med. 1968;71(3):357-67.

27. **Schor S, Karten I.** Statistical evaluation of medical journal manuscripts. JAMA. 1966; 195(13):1123-8.
28. **Young MJ, Bresnitz EA, Strom BL.** Sample size nomograms for interpreting negative clinical studies. Ann Intern Med. 1983;99 (2):248-51.
29. **Altman DG.** Statistics in medical journals: developments in the 1980s. Stat Med. 1991; 10:1897-913.
30. **Morris RW.** A statistical study of papers in the Journal of Bone and Joint Surgery [Br] 1984. J Bone Joint Surg [Br]. 1988;70(2): 242-6.
31. **Sheehan TJ.** The medical literature. Let the reader beware. Arch Intern Med. 1980; 140 (4):472-4.
32. **Schor S.** Statistical proof in inconclusive "negative" trials. Arch Intern Med. 1981; 141(10):1263-4.
33. **Wears RL.** What is necessary for proof? Is 95% sure unrealistic? [Letter]. JAMA. 1994; 271(4):272.
34. **DerSimonian R, Charette LJ, McPeek B, Mosteller F.** Reporting on methods in clinical trials. N Engl J Med. 1982;306(22):1332-7.
35. **Goodman SN, Berlin JA.** The use of predicted confidence intervals when planning experiments and the misuse of power when interpreting results. Ann Intern Med. 1994;121:200-6.

Chapter 5

COMPARING GROUPS

II. The Multiple Testing Problem

The more questions asked of a set of data, the more likely it will yield some statistically significant difference even if the treatments are in fact equivalent.

S. YUSUF, J. WITTES, J. PROBSTFIELD, AND H.A. TYROLER (1)

The **multiple testing** (or **"multiple looks"**) problem is that the more hypotheses are tested on the same data, the more likely the chance for a **type I error:** concluding that there is a difference when, in fact, the null hypothesis of no difference is true. For example, assuming that the threshold of statistical significance (alpha) has been set at 0.05 and 100 P values have been calculated from the same data, 5 of these P values are likely to be less than 0.05, even if the null hypothesis of no difference is true. In many instances multiple tests are unavoidable and even desirable, but they must be dealt with carefully to avoid the multiple testing problem (2).

Multiple testing is often encountered when

- *Establishing group equivalence* by testing each of several baseline characteristics or prognostic factors for differences between experimental and control groups (hoping to find none)
- Performing *multiple pairwise comparisons,* which occurs when three or more groups of data are compared two at a time in separate analyses, as is done in analysis of variance (ANOVA) and multiple regression analysis
- Testing *multiple endpoints* or outcomes (response variables) that are influenced by the same set of explanatory variables
- Performing *secondary analyses* of relations observed after the data have been collected and not identified in the original study design
- Performing *subgroup analyses* not planned in the original study design
- Performing *interim analyses of accumulating data* (one endpoint measured at several different times), which is often done in studies potentially involving toxic or harmful effects to avoid putting study participants at risk unnecessarily

- *Comparing groups at multiple time points* with a series of individual group comparisons

Of concern with multiple testing is the phenomenon of **data dredging:** the practice of indiscriminately analyzing any and all relationships and reporting those with statistically significant results (3–17). Historically, great but undue value has been attached to "statistically significant findings" or "positive results." In fact, studies in which the author's hypotheses have been supported are far more common in the literature than studies in which the hypotheses are not supported. Unfortunately, many authors do seem to engage in a "ruthless search for significance" (18) in an attempt to find statistically significant relationships to report.

Multiple testing can be useful, however. Although the formal experiment is designed to produce answers to specific questions, exploring the data with additional analyses (multiple testing) may help to generate better questions (19). However, such exploratory analyses must also be interpreted wisely: "Hypothesis-generating studies (sometimes referred to somewhat contemptuously as "fishing expeditions" [13]) should be identified as such. If the "fishing expedition" catches a boot, the fishermen should throw it back, not claim that they were fishing for boots" (20). To warrant further exploration, findings from such analyses should be biologically plausible. Biological plausibility is even more important if additional studies will be conducted to investigate new or surprising results from exploratory analyses.

Most studies generate several P values, and the decision to adjust for multiple testing is debated among statisticians. The two circumstances in which the requirement is least debated are the multiple pairwise comparisons after an overall group comparison (such as ANOVA; ***see also*** **Sample Presentation, p 129**) and the interim analysis of accumulating data.

Sample Presentation

Differences in the response variable among the six groups were compared with ANOVA. Multiple pairwise comparisons were made with Tukey's procedure, with the overall alpha level set at 0.05.

Here,

- ANOVA is a "group comparison procedure" that essentially determines whether there is a statistically significant difference somewhere among the groups.

Continued

SAMPLE PRESENTATION – *Cont'd.*

- Tukey's procedure is a **multiple pairwise comparisons procedure** used when ANOVA indicates a statistically significant difference among the groups. A multiple pairwise comparisons procedure can be used to compare each group with every other to determine which groups differ significantly. Here, the six groups require 15 pairwise comparisons—15 *P* values—which results in the multiple testing problem. If a multiple comparisons procedure is not used (that is, if 15 Student's *t* tests were used to compare the six groups instead), the chance of erroneously declaring a difference to be statistically significant rises from 5 times in 100 (the overall alpha of 0.05) to 55 times in 100 (an overall alpha of 0.55).
- Alpha is the threshold of statistical significance, set by the researcher before the study, to which the overall *P* value (from, say, ANOVA) is compared when declaring a result to be statistically significant or not.

5.1 Indicate whether any accommodations were made for multiple testing. If so, describe the accommodation.

Statistical significance is declared when a *P* value generated from the data is lower than the alpha level set by the researcher as the threshold of statistical significance. Thus, the alpha level, or sometimes the *P* value, may need to be adjusted to address the multiple testing problem. Typical approaches include:

- Using a stricter criterion for significance, such as an alpha level of 0.01 instead of 0.05 (9,15,21–25)
- Applying Bonferroni's correction, which is a rough measure that compensates for multiple testing by indicating a newer, more restrictive alpha level (21,22,24–29)
- Giving the most credence to the original, a priori hypothesis and less to secondary analyses (8,9,14,20,23,28–34)

✓ **If a large number of *P* values, say, 10 or more, are presented, determine whether the multiple testing problem has been addressed.** Data dredging is often revealed by the reporting of several *P* values (a condition once referred to as "*P*-ing all over the paper") and by reporting *P* values for relationships of dubious clinical value. The rule is, "Don't report *P* values for their own sake" (31).

✓ **Compute Bonferroni's correction for multiple tests (27,29).** One form of Bonferroni's correction is to establish a new alpha level for determining

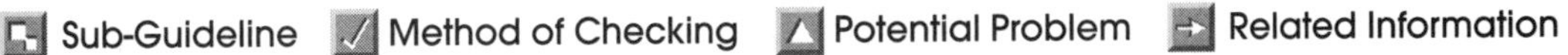
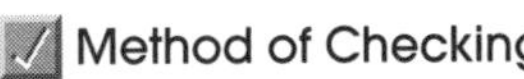
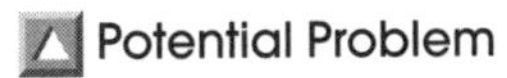

statistical significance. For example, to compensate for multiple Student's *t* tests (two-sided), the new alpha level is computed with the formula: "new alpha" = "old alpha"/*n*, where "new alpha" is the probability that must be achieved to be significant given the number of comparisons, "old alpha" is the level that formerly defined significance, and *n* is the number of comparisons reported in the study. Thus, in a paper reporting 12 comparisons (12 *P* values) with an original alpha level of 0.05, only *P* values less than 0.004 ("new alpha" = 0.05/12) would be considered significant.

However, although Bonferroni's correction is conservative, it does not completely protect against incorrect conclusions. In addition, in studies with many *P* values, the adjusted alpha level or *P* values may be nearly impossible to reach. A study with 30 comparisons and an initial overall alpha level of 0.05 would require that *P* values be less than 0.0017 to be declared significant (29).

ESTABLISHING GROUP EQUIVALENCY

5.2 Report the clinical values used to assess group equivalence at baseline. Do not rely on *P* values to establish equivalence.

Data from the treatment and control groups are usually inspected to see whether the groups were comparable at the beginning of a study. Imbalances between the groups may be indicated by clinically important differences in mean values, for example. Clinically important imbalances should always be identified. (Typically, the effect of the imbalance on the outcome is then assessed with multivariable analysis. *See Chapters 7 and 8*). However, *statistically* comparing, say, two groups on 10 baseline characteristics may result in the multiple testing problem.

In *nonrandomized* trials, baseline characteristics can and often should be compared to determine whether any differences are statistically significant as well as whether these differences are clinically important. Statistically significant differences in baseline variables may indicate systematic bias in assignment. However, nonstatistically significant differences between groups at baseline do not mean that the groups are equivalent *unless there is adequate statistical power to detect a clinically meaningful difference.* Often, such power is lacking.

In *randomized* trials, any clinical or statistical differences found between groups are, by definition, the result of chance. Clinical imbalances, even though the result of chance, are real and need to be incorporated into the multivariable model. Statistical comparisons of baseline characteristics, however, are rarely necessary. Statistically significant differences will be the result of chance, and nonstatistically significant differences do not indicate that the groups are comparable but rather that randomization was effective (35,36). "If randomization has been done fairly, the null hypothesis that the two groups come from the same population is by definition true; so we would expect 5% of such comparisons to be significant at the 5% level. Thus, these tests assess, indirectly, whether randomization was fair, not whether the two groups have similar characteristics" (35).

Altman and Dore (35) studied 80 published randomized controlled trials and found that 46 trials (58%) compared baseline characteristics with hypothesis tests. The median number of baseline characteristics presented was 9; 39% of the trials compared more than 10 characteristics. Overall, some 600 hypothesis tests (*P* values) were included in the 46 trials, an average of 13 per trial.

MULTIPLE PAIRWISE COMPARISONS OF TREATMENT GROUPS

5.3 Specify the multiple comparison procedure used to identify which pairs of groups most influence the overall statistical significance of a group comparison.

When three or more groups of data are compared two at a time in separate analyses, the number of tests soon becomes large enough to encounter the multiple testing problem. For example, if four groups are compared two at a time with Student's *t* tests, six Student's *t* tests are required. If alpha is set at 0.05 for each test, the probability of finding a difference when one does not exist (the probability of a type I error) is no longer 0.05, but 0.3. That is, about one in every three *P* values may be wrongly interpreted.

To prevent this problem, group comparison techniques, such as ANOVA, analyze data from all the groups and determine whether any differences exist among them. If a difference is indicated, a second procedure, called a **multiple comparisons procedure,** is performed to determine which groups most influence the overall difference between groups.

Common multiple comparison procedures associated with analysis of variance include

- Tukey's procedure
- Student-Neuman-Keuls procedure
- Duncan's multiple-range procedure
- Dunnett's procedure
- Scheffe's method
- Fisher's least-significant-difference (LSD) method
- Bonferroni's correction

The most common error in multiple pairwise comparisons is using multiple Student's *t* tests without adjusting the alpha level to locate the significantly different pairs in a group comparison tested with ANOVA (37–39).

Determine how many comparisons are possible with the following formula: k(k – 1)/2, where k is the number of groups available for comparison.

SECONDARY (RETROSPECTIVE OR POST-HOC) ANALYSES

5.4 Differentiate between primary analyses and secondary (retrospective or post-hoc) analyses.

The results of a study may suggest new relationships that were not considered when the study was designed. However, because the study was not designed to test these new relationships, reanalyzing the results according to different criteria may create problems in interpretation.

> EXAMPLE: A study was designed to test for differences in visual acuity between males and females. After seeing the results, researchers decided to reanalyze the data on the basis of age group, rather than by gender. Because the original experimental and control groups were balanced by gender, not by age, such a post hoc analysis should be considered exploratory, no matter how interesting or statistically significant the results.

SUBGROUP ANALYSES

5.5 Specify how the subgroups were identified and the rationale for analyzing them.

Many research projects collect considerable amounts of data that are not related to the primary comparison. For example, demographic data, such as age and sex, are routinely collected because many clinical features vary with these factors. A researcher studying the effects of an antidepressant may find that, overall, the drug does not perform better than a placebo. Continued analysis, however, may show a significant reduction in depression for post-menopausal women; that is, for a subgroup of the original treatment group. Analyzing the great many subgroups possible in a typical study can result in the multiple testing problem.

Results of subgroup analyses can be reported—perhaps the drug in the above example is really affected by hormone levels—but they should be reported as preliminary findings because they are unanticipated by-products of the primary comparison, the overall effectiveness of the drug in treating depression.

An alternative to subgroup analysis is to combine the factors into a single predictive model (an equation), rather than to analyze each subgroup separately. In the above example, the researcher could test for interactions between age, sex, and treatment with the drug on recovery from depression and avoid subgroup analysis (15,21,25). *(See also Chapters 7 and 8.)*

Subgroups defined after the data have been collected may reflect the effects of treatment, and it is then difficult, if not impossible, to interpret any differences resulting from the treatment (40). For example, if all patients who responded well to a drug are placed into a subgroup, it should be easy to prove that the drug was effective in this subgroup. Although this example of circular reasoning is obvious, in other circumstances, such inappropriate subgroup selection may be more subtle.

Subgroup analyses are notoriously unreliable (1,24,28,41–44). The number of participants in a given subgroup can be small, even when the total number of participants in the overall experiment is large. "Because subgroup analyses always include fewer patients than does the overall analysis, they carry a greater risk for making a type II error—falsely concluding that there is no difference" (43).

Is the rationale for subgroup analysis convincing? (1,20). A clear biological mechanism that might explain the difference may make the results more credible. Subgroup analyses are more acceptable when:

- The difference between groups is big enough to be clinically important and statistically significant.
- The subgroup comparison is part of an a priori analysis, not a post-hoc analysis.
- The subgroup comparison was one of a small number of additional hypotheses tested and not the result of "data dredging."
- The difference is based on a comparison within a single study and not with data from different studies.
- The difference is consistent across studies.
- Other indirect evidence supports the existence of a true difference (3,43)

MULTIPLE ENDPOINTS

5.6 Identify the primary endpoints or outcomes of interest before beginning the study.

Analogous to the secondary analysis problem, in which multiple *explanatory* variables are discovered to be significant, is the multiple endpoint problem, in which multiple *response* variables are discovered to be significant ". . . for a trial with five endpoints, the chance under the null hypothesis of at least one treatment difference achieving a significance level of $P < 0.05$ is about 20%, provided that the endpoints are not highly correlated" (21).

> **EXAMPLE:** If a blood pressure drug is coincidentally discovered to stimulate hair growth, the study may be reported as having two endpoints: blood pressure and hair growth. As in the secondary analysis case, the number of effects that can be tested in a typical trial may be large, creating the multiple testing problem. The primary comparison—the effect of the drug on blood pressure—should be the focus of the report, and the serendipitous finding of hair growth should be reported as preliminary.

INTERIM ANALYSES OF ACCUMULATING DATA

5.7 Report all interim analyses of accumulating data and give the rationale for the analyses.

In many studies, especially those that last several months or years, it is sometimes desirable to test the results periodically so that participants are not needlessly put at risk. Such interim analyses are related to what are called "stopping rules" for studies ***(see Guideline 5.8).*** If the interim results indicate that the therapy is statistically either highly effective or obviously inferior or harmful, researchers may be inclined to stop the study. Clearly, if patients are unnecessarily put at risk, the study should be stopped. Interim analyses also allow researchers to verify adherence with the protocol, to confirm the integrity of the data management procedures, and to correct any problems as soon as possible in the course of the study (45).

However, interim analyses increase the number of tests performed and are another example of the multiple testing problem. To take an extreme case, suppose the results of a study were analyzed after each participant completed the protocol; that is, the number of cases analyzed would increase by one for each analysis. By chance, the test may produce a significant result after, say, 23 patients, a nonsignificant result after 27, a significant result after 34, and so on as the data accumulate.

"Unplanned interim analyses present considerable problems of interpretation" (46).

5.8 Report the statistical criteria for stopping the study and indicate whether these criteria were developed before the study began.

One issue in interim analyses is to decide when to stop a study. If the study is stopped too soon (after too few participants have completed the study), its statistical power may be unacceptably low. If it is allowed to continue, it may be putting participants at risk needlessly. Thus, interim analyses should be planned in advance and the criteria for stopping the study specified.

5.9 Identify to whom the results of the interim analyses were reported.

Reporting the results of the interim analysis to the medical community can bias a study. Should one treatment appear to be superior to the other, physicians may not permit their patients to enter the study. Interim results can also create expectations that can bias observations and treatments. In addition, especially in mass media reports, if later results differ from earlier ones, the scientific and general public may lose confidence in the credibility of the study.

Reporting the interim results of clinical trials carries the responsibility for reporting the full and final results (47). Preliminary reports of trials in progress often include the results of interim analyses. Readers need to be aware that the results are preliminary, and the final results need to be published in full. Several studies have found that between 30% and 60% of published abstracts are not followed by the full, published report of the research they represent (48–50).

COMPARING GROUPS AT MULTIPLE TIME POINTS

5.10 If groups were compared at multiple time points, specify the statistical procedure used for the comparisons and what adjustments were made for multiple comparisons.

Some studies compare two or more groups at various time points in the course of a study, which results in multiple *P* values, one for each time point. For example, to determine differences in the onset or duration of anesthesia between two competing anesthetics, measurements may be taken every hour for 12 hours. The two groups could be compared statistically every hour to determine at which point the mean responses differed significantly. In this case, researchers commonly perform multiple individual group comparisons, one at each time point, which creates the multiple testing problem; in this example, 12 *P* values are generated. This approach may be appropriate if the overall alpha level is adjusted for multiple testing (with, say, Bonferroni's correction).

REFERENCES

1. **Yusuf S, Wittes J, Probstfield J, Tyroler HA.** Analysis and interpretation of treatment effects in subgroups of patients in randomized clinical trials. JAMA. 1991;266(1): 93-8.
2. **Chalmers TC, Smith H Jr, Blackburn B, Sliverman B, Schroeder B, Reitman D, Ambroz A.** A method for assessing the quality of a randomized control trial. Cont Clin Trials. 1981;2:31-49.
3. **Guyatt GH, Sackett DL, Cook DJ.** Users' guides to the medical literature. II. How to use an article about therapy or prevention. B. What were the results and will they help me in caring for my patients? The Evidence-Based Medicine Working Group. JAMA. 1994;271(1):59-63.
4. **Bailar JC.** Science, statistics, and deception. Ann Intern Med. 1986;104(2):259-60.
5. **Bailar JC III, Mosteller F.** Guidelines for statistical reporting in articles for medical journals. Amplification and explanations. Ann Intern Med. 1988;108(2):266-73.
6. **Felson DT.** Bias in meta-analytic research. J Clin Epidemiol. 1992;45(8):885-92.
7. **Fienberg SE.** Damned lies and statistics: misrepresentations of honest data. In: Council of Biology Editors. Editorial Policy Committee. Ethics and Policy in Scientific Publication. Bethesda, MD: Council of Biology Editors; 1990:202-6.
8. **Gore SM, Jones G, Thompson SG.** The Lancet's statistical review process: areas for improvement by authors. Lancet. 1992;340 (8811):100-2.
9. **Haines SJ.** Six statistical suggestions for surgeons. Neurosurgery. 1981;9(4):414-8.
10. **MacArthur RD, Jackson GG.** An evaluation of the use of statistical methodology in the Journal of Infectious Diseases. J Infect Dis. 1984;149(3):349-54.
11. **Moskowitz G, Chalmers TC, Sacks HS, Fagerstrom RM, Smith H Jr.** Deficiencies of clinical trials of alcohol withdrawal. Alcohol Clin Exp Res. 1983;7(1):42-6.
12. **Salsburg DS.** The religion of statistics as practiced in medical journals. Am Statistician. 1985:39(3):220-3.
13. **Smith DG, Clemens J, Crede W, Harvey M, Gracely EJ.** Impact of multiple comparisons in randomized clinical trials. Am J Med. 1987;83:545-50.
14. **Stoto MA.** From data analysis to conclusions: a statistician's view. In: Council of Biology Editors. Editorial Policy Committee. Ethics and Policy in Scientific publication. Bethesda, MD: Council of Biology Editors; 1990:207-18.
15. **Sumner D.** Lies, damned lies—or statistics? J Hypertens. 1992;10(1):3-8.
16. **Tyson JE, Furzan JA, Reisch JS, Mize SG.** An evaluation of the quality of therapeutic studies in perinatal medicine. J Pediatr. 1983;102(1):10-3.

17. **Altman DG.** Statistics in medical journals: developments in the 1980s. Stat Med. 1991;10:1897-913.
18. **Morgan PP.** Confidence intervals: from statistical significance to clinical significance [Editorial]. Can Med Assoc J. 1989;141(9): 881-3.
19 **Schoolman HM, Becktel JM, Best WR, Johnson AF.** Statistics in medical research: principles versus practices. J Lab Clin Med. 1968;71(3):357-67.
20. **Mills JL.** Data torturing [Letter]. N Engl J Med. 1993;329(16):1196-9.
21. **Pocock SJ, Hughes MD, Lee RJ.** Statistical problems in the reporting of clinical trials. A survey of three medical journals. N Engl J Med. 1987;317(7):426-32.
22. **Brown GW.** Statistics and the medical journal [Editorial]. Am J Dis Child. 1985;139(3): 226-8.
23. **Altman DG, Gore SM, Gardner MJ, Pocock SJ.** Statistical guidelines for contributors to medical journals. BMJ. 1983;286 (6376):1489-93.
24. **Bulpitt CJ.** Confidence intervals. Lancet. 1987;28(8531):494-7.
25. **Murray GD.** Statistical guidelines for the British Journal of Surgery. Br J Surg. 1991;78 (7):782-4.
26. **Diamond GA, Forrester JS.** Clinical trials and statistical verdicts: probable grounds for appeal. Ann Intern Med. 1983;98(3): 385-94.
27. **Godfrey K.** Comparing the means of several groups. N Engl J Med. 1985;313(23): 1450-6.
28. **Journal of Hypertension.** Statistical Guidelines for the Journal of Hypertension. J Hypertens. 1992;10(1):6-8.
29. **Lee KL, McNeer F, Starmer CF, Harris PJ, Rosati RA.** Clinical judgment and statistics. Lessons from a simulated randomized trial in coronary artery disease. Circulation. 1980;61:508-15.
30. **Altman DG.** Statistics and ethics in medical research. VII—interpreting results. BMJ. 1980;281(6255):1612-4.
31. **Walker AM.** Reporting the results of epidemiological studies. Am J Public Health 1986;76(5): 556-8.
32. **Grant A.** Reporting controlled trials. Br J Obstet Gynaecol. 1989;96(4):397-400.
33. **Gelber RD, Goldhirsch A.** Reporting and interpreting adjuvant therapy clinical trials. Monogr Natl Cancer Inst. 1992;11:59-69.
34. **Bracken MB.** Reporting observational studies. Br J Obstet Gynaecol. 1989;96(4):383-8.
35. **Altman DG, Dore CJ.** Randomisation and baseline comparisons in clinical trials. Lancet. 1990;335(8682):149-53.
36. **Guyatt GH, Sackett DL, Cook DJ.** Users' guides to the medical literature. II. How to use an article about therapy or prevention. A. Are the results of the study valid? The Evidence-Based Medicine Working Group. JAMA. 1993;270(21):2598-601.
37. **Glantz SA.** It is all in the numbers [Editorial]. J Am Coll Cardiol. 1993; 21(3): 835-7.
38. **Glantz SA.** Biostatistics: how to detect, correct and prevent errors in the medical literature. Circulation. 1980;61(1):1-7.
39. **Longnecker DE.** Support versus illumination: trends in medical statistics. Anesthesiology. 1982;57(2):73-4.
40. **Abramson NS, Kelsey SF, Safar P, Sutton-Tyrrell KS.** Simpson's paradox and clinical trials: what you find is not necessarily what you prove. Ann Emerg Med. 1992; 21(12): 1480-2.
41. **Simon R.** Confidence intervals for reporting results of clinical trials. Ann Intern Med. 1986;105(3):429-35.
42. **Murray GD.** Statistical aspects of research methodology. Br J Surg. 1991;78(7):777-81.
43. **Oxman AD, Guyatt GH.** A consumer's guide to subgroup analyses. Ann Intern Med. 1992;116(1):78-84.
44. **Begg CB.** Selection of patients for clinical trials. Semin Oncol. 1988;15(5):434-40.
45. **Ashby D, Machin D.** Stopping rules, interim analyses and data monitoring committees [Editorial]. Br J Cancer. 1993;68(16): 1047-50.
46. **Geller NL, Pocock SJ.** Interim analyses in randomized clinical trials: ramifications and guidelines for practitioners. Biometrics. 1987;43(1):213-23.
47. **Zelen M.** Guidelines for publishing papers on cancer clinical trials: responsibilities of

editors and authors. J Clin Oncol. 1983;1(2): 164-9.

48. **Chalmers I, Adams M, Dickersin K, Hetherington J, Tarnow-Mordi W, Meinert C, Tonascia S, Chalmers TC.** A cohort study of summary reports of controlled trials. JAMA. 1990;263(10):1401-5.

49. **Scherer RW, Dickersin K, Langenberg P.** Full publication of results initially presented in abstracts. A meta-analysis. [Erratum. JAMA. 1994; 272(18):1410] JAMA. 1994; 272(2):158-62.

50. **Garvey WD, Griffith BC.** Scientific communication: its role in the conduct of research and creation of knowledge. Am Psychol. 1971:349-62.

Chapter 6

Testing for Relationships

Reporting Association and Correlation Analyses

Data analysis is largely a search for patterns—that is, for meaningful relations among the various items observed.

K. Godfrey (1)

Association and correlation analyses mathematically identify and describe relationships between variables. In general, two variables are considered to be related when a change in one is likely to be accompanied by a change in the other. In addition, the existence and strength of a proposed association or correlation between variables can be tested with hypothesis tests (*P* values) to determine whether the existence of a relationship or its strength is likely to be real or simply the result of chance.

Although association and correlation are terms with general meanings, in their statistical uses **association** is typically reserved for describing relationships between categorical variables, whereas **correlation** is typically reserved for describing relationships between continuous variables. A measure of association between categorical variables, say, eye color and hair color, may indicate whether participants with a certain eye color also tend to have a certain hair color. In addition, measures of association can be calculated to provide a numerical indicator of the strength of this relationship.

Likewise, a measure of (linear) correlation between two continuous variables, such as heart rate and respiration rate, would indicate whether an increase in one is likely to be accompanied by an increase in the other in, say, a sample of infants. The heart rate and pulse rate for each infant could be graphed in a "scatter plot" **(Figures 6.1** and **6.2)** to show this relationship. The more linear and diagonal the pattern of the scatter plot, the stronger the relationship. In addition, a correlation coefficient can be calculated to provide a numerical indicator of the strength of the relationship.

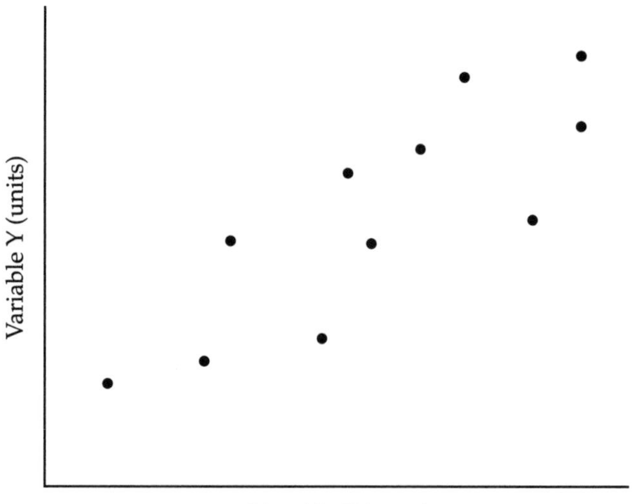

FIGURE 6.1 Hypothetical scatter plot showing a high positive correlation.

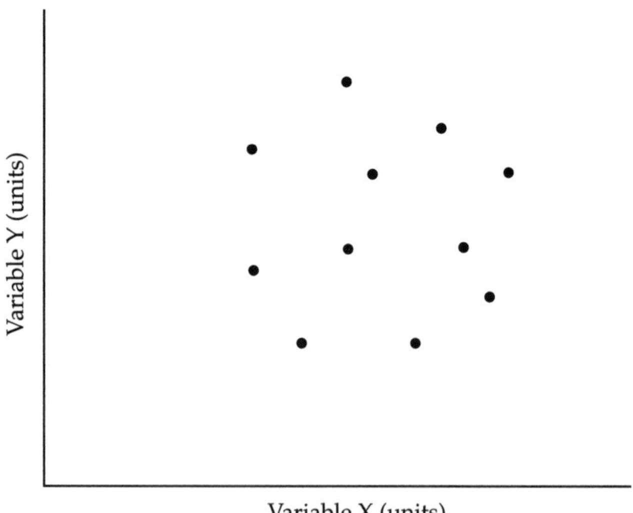

FIGURE 6.2 Hypothetical scatter plot showing a low correlation.

Association and correlation analyses are typically used to describe relationships that occur among characteristics of a sample. The more common measures and tests of association and correlation are described below:

- Relationships between *categorical variables,* such as that between patient satisfaction (satisfied or dissatisfied) and literacy (high or low), are assessed with a *measure of association,* such as the **phi coefficient,** or a *test of association,* usually a form of the **chi-square (χ^2) test.**

- Relationships between a *continuous variable* and a *categorical variable with two levels* (for example, aerobic capacity measured as oxygen uptake and exercise intensity categorized as high or low) can be assessed with the **point biserial correlation coefficient.**
- Relationships between a *continuous variable* and a *categorical variable with three or more levels* (for example, aerobic capacity measured as oxygen uptake and exercise intensity categorized as high, moderate, or low) can be assessed with the **point multiserial correlation coefficient.**
- Relationships between *continuous variables* (for example, the relationship between age and weight) are assessed with **measures** of **correlation**, such as the Pearson product–moment correlation coefficient, *r*, or Spearman's rank-order coefficient, rho.
- Other measures of association include *ratios* that describe the association between, say, exposure and disease or between treatment and an outcome, such as **odds ratios** ***(see Guideline 7.25)*** and **risk** (or **hazard**) **ratios** ***(see Guideline 9.12).***
- Another measure of association that deals specifically with multiple measurements or observations from each study participant is the **kappa statistic,** which is often used to measure agreement or classification accuracy within or between evaluators.

MEASURES AND TESTS OF ASSOCIATION: RELATIONSHIPS BETWEEN TWO CATEGORICAL VARIABLES

Sample Presentation

For the sample of 1760 patients, 542 of the 1106 (49.0%) light-eyed participants and 312 of the 654 (47.7%) dark-eyed participants exhibited the reflex response. The chi-square test revealed that reflex response and eye color were not statistically significantly associated ($\chi^2_{1df} = 0.28$, $P = 0.6$).

Here,

- The frequencies of light- and dark-eyed participants who exhibited the reflex are given. These frequencies were no different than those expected by chance, so there was little or no basis for declaring the two variables to be associated.
- χ^2 identifies the chi-square test that was used to assess whether eye color and the reflex were associated in this sample.

Continued

SAMPLE PRESENTATION – *Cont'd.*

- 0.28 is the chi-square test statistic that is computed from the data and compared to the chi-square distribution that has 1 degree of freedom to determine whether there is a statistically significant association. The chi-square test statistic is difficult to interpret clinically, although it should be reported as the measure of association. (A confidence interval for the statistic could be calculated but it is likewise difficult to interpret clinically and is almost never reported.)
- *P* is the probability of getting a chi-square test statistic as large or larger if, in fact, there is no association between eye color and reflex response. Thus, a large *P* value (*greater* than 0.05) is evidence in favor of the null hypothesis of no association.

6.1 Describe the association of interest.

The purpose of the test should be clearly stated. Testing for an association is not the same as comparing the proportions of two or more groups, although chi-square tests, for example, can be used to perform either analysis. In the case of association, the purpose of the analysis is to describe relationships between variables in a single sample. In the case of comparing group proportions, the purpose of the analysis is to determine whether two groups from the same sample differ significantly.

For example, in the sample presentation above, the chi-square test was used to assess association by *considering the mix of frequencies* among the four possible combinations:

1. People with light-colored eyes and the reflex response
2. People with light-colored eyes and without the reflex response
3. People with dark-colored eyes and the reflex response
4. People with dark-colored eyes and without the reflex response

This mix was compared with the mix of frequencies that could be expected to occur by chance. When the observed frequencies did not differ significantly from those expected by chance, the conclusion was that the two variables were not associated.

Alternatively, the same chi-square test could have been used to *compare the proportions* of light- and dark-eyed participants who expressed the reflex response. In this case, the chi-square test could have compared the differences between the two proportions to determine whether the difference was significantly different from zero. (**Chapter 4** provides guidelines for statistical comparisons of groups.)

6.2 Identify the variables used in the association and summarize each with descriptive statistics.

Tests of association are used to analyze categorical (nominal or ordinal) data. Naming the variables and giving either the *frequency counts* for each (for example, 20 443 inoculated children or 40 000 students) or the *percentage of observations* for each variable (for example, 34% of the 350 hospitals surveyed) makes the comparison explicit.

When using percentages, give the numbers from which they were calculated so that they do not mask small samples.

> **EXAMPLE: Table 6.1** is an example of a "contingency table" used in chi-square analysis. "Hospital type" is reported as one of four nominal categories, and "specialty" as one of three nominal categories. The cells contain the data (frequency counts) with which the analysis is conducted.

6.3 Identify the test of association used.

Many statistical tests are based on any of several "probability distributions," such as the *t* distribution, the *F* distribution, the Poisson distribution, and so on—there are many distributions. Several tests for association are based on the chi-square probability distribution. Chi-square tests are versatile and widely used because they can be applied to many types of analyses of categorical data:

- The **chi-square test of independence** (also called the **chi-square test of association** or **Pearson's chi-square test**) assesses two categorical variables to determine whether they are associated or "independent" (not associated). Such a test would help determine whether, say, skin lesions and respiratory problems occurred together, which may indicate a common cause, or whether they were "independent," that is, that their appearance in the same patient may be coincidental.
- The **chi-square test for goodness-of-fit** compares the results of a study of categorical data with known or standardized results to determine whether the results are typical. For example, the proportions of the four blood types (A, B, AB, and O) observed in a sample can be compared to the known proportions for the population as a whole to determine whether the proportions are similar to those of the population.
- The **exact tests** (tests that have the word *exact* in their names, such as the *exact chi-square test* or *Fisher's exact test*) are used for some of the above purposes when testing small samples. (Here, a "small sample"

TABLE 6.1 **Contingency Table for Assessing the Association between Hospital Type and Three Surgical Specialties.**

Surgical Specialty	Hospital Type 1	2	3	4	Total*
A	56	32	20	14	122
B	13	47	45	34	99
C	27	29	33	45	134
Total*	96	108	98	93	355

* Row and column totals are referred to as "marginals" or "marginal totals." A chi-square test based on this table would yield a test statistic of 60.95, with six degrees of freedom (computed as [the number of rows – 1] times [the number of columns – 1]; in this case, 2 × 3 = 6), and a *P* value of < 0.001. This result would lead to the conclusion that medical specialty and hospital type are associated; that is, that different types of hospitals tend to offer different surgical specialties. The nature of the association is then determined by inspecting the data. One observation can be summarized as follows: Type 1 hospitals tend to offer specialty A more frequently than other types, whereas Type 4 hospitals tend to offer specialty C more frequently than other types, and Types 2 and 3 tend to offer specialty B more frequently than other types.

usually means that the number of observations expected by chance in each cell of the contingency table is less than 5.)

- Although not based on the chi-square distribution, the **phi coefficient** (pronounced "fee" and indicated by the symbol ϕ) is another measure used to indicate the association between two categorical variables. The coefficient ranges from –1 to +1, where –1 and +1 represent perfect inverse and direct associations, respectively, and 0 indicates no association. (This scale is the same as that used in the more common correlation analysis, which describes the relationship between two continuous variables; *see Guideline 6.12*). A *P* value can be computed for the phi coefficient to determine whether it differs significantly from zero.
- The **chi-square test of proportions** is for group comparisons (*see Chapter 4*).

Guideline 6.1: The association of interest

6.4 Indicate whether the test was one- or two-tailed. Justify the use of one-tailed tests.

Two-tailed tests are more conservative and are preferred in the absence of a specific justification to use a one-tailed test.

Guideline 4.7: One- and two-tailed tests

6.5 State that the assumptions of the test have been met.

A statement that the assumptions were verified is all that need be included.

Many tests of association are based on the assumptions that

- The data are categorical and are not, for example, the mean values of continuous data. If continuous data are available, they should be analyzed with the appropriate class of tests.
- The sample was randomly selected.
- Every cell in the contingency table (see **Table 6.1**) has a sufficient number of expected counts. If any of the cells have fewer than, say, five expected counts, "exact" testing should be carried out, and the name of the test specified.

6.6 Report the actual *P* value of the test.

Actual *P* values ($P =$) are preferred to more-than ($P >$) or less-than ($P <$) statements, to abbreviations like NS (for "not significant"), or to cutpoints, such as "significant at the 0.05 level."

Guideline 4.15: Actual *P* Values

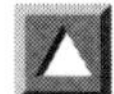

Association is not causation (2). A common error in interpreting an association is to conclude that one variable *causes* the other. For example, highly associated variables may actually be caused by a third variable. To illustrate: the association between death and respiratory disease is significantly greater in the southwestern states, despite the fact that the dry climate is often beneficial for these patients. The climate does not cause the deaths; it simply attracts a disproportionate number of people with respiratory diseases into these states. When these people die, the death rates show an unusually high proportion of deaths among people with respiratory disease.

6.7 For associations of primary interest, report the value of the test statistic and the degrees of freedom.

From the data for the comparison of interest, statistical testing results in the calculation of a single number called a **test statistic.** The test statistic is then compared to the appropriate probability distribution (such as the chi-square distribution), and the probability (the *P* value) associated with that statistic is calculated. The *P* value indicates the probability that a test statistic as extreme or more extreme than the one obtained in the study would occur if there is no association.

The degrees of freedom is a mathematical concept that helps determine which probability distribution is used. For example, there are several chi-square distributions, each of which differs from the others by having different degrees of freedom.

Reporting the test statistic and the degrees of freedom allows readers to verify that the analysis was done correctly. In practice, however, the full reporting of the statistical analysis is cumbersome and only associations of primary interest need be reported in detail.

CORRELATION ANALYSIS: (LINEAR) RELATIONSHIPS BETWEEN TWO CONTINUOUS VARIABLES

Sample Presentation

Dentene lead levels correlated well and inversely with family income, indicating that poorer children have higher levels of lead in their systems (n = 39; Pearson's $r = -0.62$; $P = 0.001$).

Here,

- Pearson's r identifies the correlation coefficient as the Pearson product-moment correlation coefficient.
- r is the coefficient that, here, reports a correlation of –0.62. The minus sign indicates an inverse correlation: one variable increases as the other decreases.
- P is the probability that a correlation this large or larger (irrespective of the positive or negative sign) would occur by chance if, in fact, the two variables were not correlated.

6.8 Describe the relationship of interest.

Correlation analysis describes the linear association between two continuous variables that are thought to vary together over their respective range of values. For example, stride length and height are highly and positively (or directly) correlated: taller people take larger steps than do shorter people.

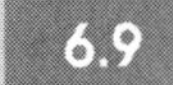

6.9 Identify the variables used in the comparison and summarize each with descriptive statistics.

In correlation analysis, both variables must be continuous, so each can be summarized with a measure of center and a measure of dispersion, such as the mean and standard deviation or the median and interquartile range. These descriptive statistics should be presented, especially for primary comparisons.

Chapter 2. Reporting Descriptive Statistics

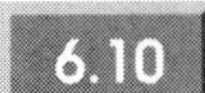

6.10 Identify the correlation coefficient used.

Some common correlation coefficients are:

- **Pearson's product-moment correlation coefficient, *r*,** which is used to assess the relationship between two approximately normally distributed, continuous variables. (Actually, the variables should vary together in a "bivariate normal distribution.")
- **Spearman's rank-order correlation coefficient, rho (ρ),** which is used to assess the relationship between two continuous variables, at least one of which is not normally distributed.
- **Kendall's rank-correlation coefficient, tau (τ),** which is used to assess the relationship between two ordinal variables, or between one ordinal and one continuous variable.
- **The point biserial correlation coefficient,** or simply, biserial correlation, which is used to assess relationships between a continuous variable and a categorical variable with two levels.
- **The point multiserial correlation coefficient,** which is used to assess relationships between a continuous variable and a categorical variable with three or more levels.
- Other measures of association that deal specifically with multiple measurements or observations from each study participant include the **intraclass** and **interclass correlation coefficients,** which indicate the degree of correlation within or between evaluators, respectively.

6.11 State that the assumptions of the test have been met.

EXAMPLE: A statement that the assumptions were verified is all that need be included.

Pearson's product-moment correlation assumes that both data points from each study participant, when considered together, are more or less normally distributed. (That is, that the two variables have a "bivariate normal distribution.") Spearman's rank-order correlation and Kendall's rank-correlation do not.

6.12 Report the value of the correlation coefficient.

A correlation coefficient indicates the strength and direction of the relationship between two variables. Correlation coefficients range from –1 to +1, where 1 is a perfect correlation and 0 is no correlation. A negative coefficient (–1) means that one variable tends to increase as the other decreases (that is, that the relationship is *inversely proportional*), and a positive coefficient (+1) means that both variables tend to increase or decrease together (a *proportional* relationship).

Correlation analysis is often depicted graphically with a "scatter plot" of the data (**Figures 6.1** and **6.2**). A scatter plot that is roughly circular indicates little or no linear correlation. As the scatter plot becomes more linear, the correlation becomes stronger. Sometimes, correlations are assessed for several pairs of variables. In this case, the coefficients can be presented in a correlation matrix **(Table 6.2).**

Correlation is a matter of degree. Although it is common to speak of two variables as being "correlated," there is no point or r value at which they "become" correlated. It is probably better to use phrases such as "the variables were moderately (or poorly or highly) correlated" than to say that they either "are" or "are not" correlated.

How the result is interpreted also depends on the nature of the study. An r of 0.7 between birth weight and retirement income 65 years later would be unusually high because the relationship between these variables is obviously much more complex than suggested. On the other hand, an r of 0.7 between two laboratory tests for the same sample may be low.

Correlation is not causation (3,4). Handwriting quality and shoe size are highly correlated, but one obviously does not cause the other. Both change with age; maturation is probably the real "cause" of both improvements in handwriting and increases in shoe size. Correlation analysis does not test for causal relationships, only whether there is a relationship and to some extent the strength of this relationship.

6.13 Report the actual *P* value of the correlation.

Report all P values to two significant digits. Avoid "P is less than or greater than" statements. A P value for a correlation coefficient results

TABLE 6.2. Sample Correlation Matrix.*

	Variables				
	1	**2**	**3**	**4**	**5**
	r *P* n	*r* *P* n	*r* *P* n	*r* *P* n	*r* *P* n
Variable 1	—	–0.243† 0.20 29	–0.177 0.37 27	0.013 0.94 30	0.009 0.96 30
Variable 2	—	—	–0.226 0.24 28	–0.383 0.03 31	0.038 0.83 31
Variable 3	—	—	—	0.327 0.08 29	–0.119 0.53 29
Variable 4	—	—	—	—	0.289 0.10 32
Variable 5	—	—	—	—	—

*Duplicate cells are usually left blank (indicated by the dashes) to simplify the presentation.
†Here, the correlation for variable 1 and variable 2 is $r = 0.243$ (**P** = 0.20) for the 29 subjects who expressed both variables.
r = correlation coefficient
P = probability value
n = sample size

from testing the null hypothesis that the "true"coefficient is equal to zero; that is, that there is no linear relationship between the two variables. The P value says nothing about the clinical importance or strength of the relationship (5). In significance testing, the r value is usually compared to zero, but it is possible to compute the likelihood that r differs from any value between +1 and –1.

6.14 For primary comparisons, report the (95%) confidence interval for the correlation coefficient, whether or not the coefficient is statistically significant.

Correlation coefficients that are not statistically significant must be interpreted in light of the statistical power of the test to detect a clinically important r value. Confidence intervals are useful because they are related to the adequacy of the sample size, in that studies with larger samples tend to result in narrower confidence intervals.

Guideline 3.1: Reporting confidence intervals

6.15 For primary comparisons, include a scatter plot of the data.

Presenting a graph of the relationship between two variables often makes the relationship easier to understand. **Figure 6.1** shows two highly (linearly) correlated variables; **Figure 6.2** shows two poorly (linearly) correlated variables.

Illustrations take up valuable page space and are more expensive to print than text, so they should be used wisely. Thus, only primary comparisons should be illustrated with scatter plots.

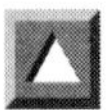

Correlation should be assessed mathematically, not visually (6).

REFERENCES

1. **Godfrey K.** Simple linear regression in medical research. In: Bailar JC, Mosteller F, eds. Medical Uses of Statistics, 2nd edition. Boston: NEJM Books, 1992:201-32.
2. **Murray GD.** Statistical guidelines for the British Journal of Surgery. Br J Surg. 1991;78: 782-4.
3. **Altman DG, Gore SM, Gardner MJ, Pocock SJ.** Statistical guidelines for contributors to medical journals. BMJ. 1983;286: 1489-93.
4. **Schoolman HM, Becktel JM, Best WR, Johnson AF.** Statistics in medical research: principles versus practices. J Lab Clin Med. 1968;71(3):357-67.
5. **Sheehan TJ.** The medical literature. Let the reader beware. Arch Intern Med. 1980;140 (4):472-4.
6. **Badgley RF.** An assessment of research methods reported in 103 scientific articles from two Canadian medical journals. Can Med Assoc J. 1961;85:246-50.

Chapter 7

ANALYZING MULTIPLE VARIABLES

I. Reporting Regression Analyses

. . . a linear regression coefficient indicates the impact of each independent variable on the outcome in the context of (or "adjusting for") all other variables.

J. CONCATO, A.R. FEINSTEIN, AND T.R. HOLFORD (1)

Regression analysis is an area of statistics that attempts to predict or estimate the value of a response variable from the known values of one or more explanatory variables. When the analysis uses a single explanatory variable, the procedure is called **simple regression;** when it uses a combination of explanatory variables, it is called **multiple regression.** When the response variable is a binary categorical variable (such as diseased or not diseased) the procedure is called **logistic regression,** which may also be either simple or multiple, as described.

Typically, a researcher will collect data on several potential explanatory variables, determine which variables are most strongly associated with the response variable, and then incorporate these variables into a mathematical model (a regression equation). In other words, a model is "fit" to the data. The purpose of multiple regression analysis, then, is essentially to identify which combination of variables best predicts the response variable.

Regression models are closely related to another class of statistical models called **analysis of variance (ANOVA)** models. In general, multiple regression analysis is used to analyze explanatory variables that are *continuous,* whereas ANOVA is used to analyze explanatory variables that are *categorical.* When a study includes both continuous *and* categorical explanatory variables, the analysis is typically called multiple regression or sometimes **analysis of covariance (ANCOVA).** ANCOVA generally is used where the primary interest is on a categorical explanatory variable and it is necessary to control for the influence of confounding variables, which are either categorical or continuous. Guidelines for reporting ANOVA are given in **Chapter 8.**

There are several types of regression analyses:

- **Simple linear regression** is used to assess the relationship between a *single* continuous explanatory variable and a *single* continuous response variable that varies linearly over a range of values ***(see Guidelines 7.1 to 7.10).***
- **Multiple linear regression** is used to assess the linear relationship between *two or more* continuous or categorical explanatory variables and a *single* continuous response variable ***(see Guidelines 7.11 to 7.21).***
- **Simple logistic regression** is used to assess the relationship between a *single* continuous or categorical explanatory variable and a *single* categorical response variable, usually a binary variable, such as whether or not a heart attack has occurred ***(see Guidelines 7.22 to 7.28).***
- **Multiple logistic regression** is used to assess the relationship between *two or more* continuous or categorical explanatory variables and a *single* categorical response variable ***(see Guidelines 7.29 to 7.38).***
- **Nonlinear regression** is used to assess variables that are not linearly related and that cannot be transformed into a linear relationship. These equations model more complex relationships than the other forms of regression analysis.
- **Polynomial regression** can be used for any of the above combinations of explanatory and response variables when the relationship among the variables is curvilinear, which requires, say, squaring or cubing one or more explanatory variables in the model.
- **Cox proportional hazards regression,** an aspect of time-to-event (survival) analysis, is used to assess the relationship between two or more continuous or categorical explanatory variables and a single response variable (the time to the event). Typically, the event (usually death) has not yet occurred for all participants in the sample, which creates **censored** observations ***(see Chapter 9).***

Here, we present guidelines for reporting the first four types of regression analysis described above, which are by far the most common types used in medicine. Some of the guidelines apply to more than one type; we have duplicated these where necessary to make each set of guidelines self-sufficient. Explanations and reporting guidelines for nonlinear and polynomial regression analyses are beyond the scope of this book. Cox proportional hazards regression is common in medical research and is described separately in Chapter 9 because it involves a different type of response variable.

SIMPLE LINEAR REGRESSION ANALYSIS: PREDICTING ONE CONTINUOUS RESPONSE VARIABLE FROM ONE CONTINUOUS EXPLANATORY VARIABLE

Sample Presentation

From our 453 participants, we attempted to predict serum levels from weight using simple linear regression analysis. The slope of the regression line was significantly greater than zero, indicating that serum level tends to increase as weight increases (slope = 0.25; 95% CI = 0.19 to 0.31; $t_{451} = 8.3$; $P < 0.001$; Y = 12.6 + 0.25X; $r^2 = 0.67$).

Here,

- 453 is the sample size.
- 0.25 is the slope of the regression line; it also appears in the regression equation as the coefficient of the explanatory variable, X, or weight. A coefficient of 0.25 for weight implies that for every additional 1 kg of weight, mean serum level increases by 0.25 mg/dL.
- The 95% confidence interval estimates the range over which the slopes are likely to be found in 95 of 100 similar studies. The interval does not contain zero, indicating that the results are statistically significant at the 0.05 level.
- 8.3 is the value of the test statistic from the *t* distribution with 451 degrees of freedom that was used to determine the *P* value.
- *P* is the probability of finding a slope as extreme or more extreme than the one observed if there was, in fact, no linear relationship between the variables. Therefore the small *P* value (which is less than 0.05) is evidence against the null hypothesis of a slope of zero.
- The equation describes the regression line, where Y is the predicted value for a given X within the range of X studied; 12.6 is the point at which the line would cross the Y axis (the Y intercept point) if X = 0 kg was in the range of the data; 0.25 is the slope of the regression line; and X is the value from which a prediction is to be made. The numbers 12.6 and 0.25 are called *regression coefficients.* Most statistical testing concerns the regression coefficient for the explanatory variable, the slope of the regression line. As noted above, a coefficient of 0.25 for weight implies that for every additional 1 kg of weight, mean serum level increases by 0.25 mg/dL.
- r^2 is the coefficient of determination, which indicates that 67% of the variance in serum levels is likely to be explained by its relationship with weight.

7.1 Describe the relationship of interest or the purpose of the analysis.

Simple linear regression analysis is used to examine the linear relationship between one explanatory and one response variable, or the tendency of one variable to change with the other. Simple linear regression analysis can also be used to *predict* the response variable from the explanatory variable. For example, simple regression analysis could be used to assess the relationship between age and cholesterol level and to predict cholesterol level from age.

7.2 Identify the variables used in the comparison and summarize each with descriptive statistics.

Simple linear regression analysis requires two continuous variables. One should be identified as the explanatory variable and one as the response variable. The distribution of each variable should be summarized with a measure of center (for example, the mean) and a measure of dispersion (for example, the standard deviation).

7.3 Confirm that the assumptions of simple linear regression analysis were met and state how each was checked.

A statement that the assumptions were verified is all that need be included.

The assumptions of simple linear regression are that

- The relationship between X and Y is linear over the range of values studied.
- The distributions of Y have equal variances (or standard deviations) at each value of X; that is, the standard deviation of Y is the same, no matter what the value of X.
- Each value of Y is independent of the other values of Y.
- The response variable, Y, has a normal distribution at each value of the explanatory variable, X.

There are both formal checks (for example, hypothesis tests) and informal checks (for example, inspection of graphs of residuals) for these assumptions. Sometimes, data that violate the assumptions can be adjusted (for example, with data transformations) to meet the assumptions. If such adjustments were made, they should be identified.

7.4 Report the linear regression equation.

The regression line is described by the equation (or "model") for a line:

$$Y = a + bX$$

where
- Y = the value of the response variable to be predicted
- a = the point at which the regression line crosses the Y axis (the Y intercept point)
- b = the slope of the regression line
- X = the explanatory variable used to predict the value of Y.

Given a value for the explanatory variable, X, the corresponding value of Y can be computed. Thus, Y can be predicted for any value of X within the range of X studied.

Whereas the correlation coefficient, *r*, indicates the direction and strength of the relationship between two variables, the regression coefficient for the explanatory variable (the slope of the regression line, or "b" in the regression equation; **Figure 7.1**) indicates *how much* the average value of the response variable, Y, varies with each unit change in the explanatory variable, X.

The equation can be reported in the text or in a scatter plot of the data ***(see also Guideline 7.9).***

7.5 Report the actual *P* value and the (95%) confidence interval for the regression coefficient of the explanatory variable.

In simple linear regression, the regression coefficient of the explanatory variable (the slope of the regression line) is a measure of the relationship between the two variables. A regression line with a slope of zero—a horizontal line when graphed—means that there is no linear relationship between the variables: the value of the response variable, Y, is the same for any value of the explanatory variable, X. So, a slope of zero becomes the null hypothesis to be tested. That is, the *P* value indicates the probability of finding a slope as extreme or more extreme than the one found if, in fact, there was no linear relationship between the variables. Also, the slope of the regression line is just an estimate, and the precision of this estimate should be indicated with a confidence interval ***(see also Chapter 3).***

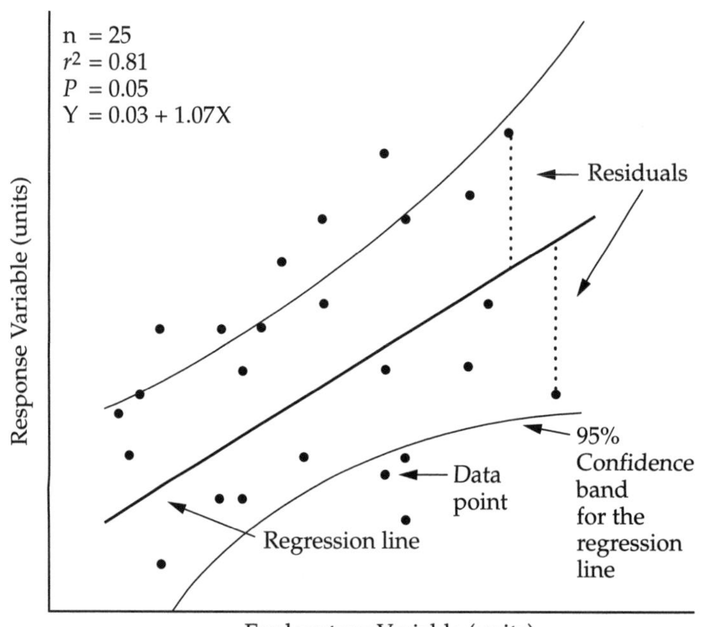

FIGURE 7.1 Hypothetical scatter plot showing the components of the graphed regression analysis. The 95% confidence interval around a regression line (the confidence band) indicates the appropriateness of the given model. These bands are not appropriate for predicting individual or mean responses, rather they are to show the precision of the regression line (8). The confidence bands flare at the ends of the line because there are usually fewer data points at the ends of the range of values measured, which decreases the precision of these estimates at either end of the range. The components of the mathematical regression analysis are also given in the upper left corner of the graph: n is the sample size, r^2 is the coefficient of determination, P is the probability value from testing whether the slope is equal to zero, and Y is the value of the response variable predicted from the regression equation, as shown.

7.6 Report the coefficient of determination (r^2).

Simple linear regression analysis can be thought of as an extension of correlation analysis, except that now one variable is being used to predict the other. As in correlation analysis (**Chapter 6**) scatter plots can be useful for showing this relationship (see **Figure 7.1**). The correlation associated with the scatter plot is also useful, in the form of the coefficient of determination (r^2). The **coefficient of determination** indicates how much of the variability in one variable is explained by knowing the value of the other. If the correlation between blood levels of hormone X and hormone Y is $r = 0.4$, for example, then $r^2 = 0.16$, or 16%. That is, 16% of the variability in hormone Y can be accounted for by the level of hormone X. An r^2 of 1 implies that all data points fall on the regression line, whereas an r^2 of 0 implies that the explanatory variable, X, is not linearly related to the response variable, Y.

Even a correlation of 0.7 explains only about half ($r^2 = 0.7 \times 0.7 = 0.49 =$ 49%) of the variance of interest. So, correlations of, say, 0.3 or below may not be clinically useful because a single variable explains too little of the variation (here, $r^2 = 9\%$). In other circumstances, a single variable explaining 9% of the variation in another may be a breakthrough.

The *coefficient of determination, r^2*, used in simple regression analysis, is analogous to, but different from, the *coefficient of multiple determination, R^2*, used in multiple regression analysis. A lower-case r indicates only two variables (one explanatory and one response variable); an upper-case R indicates more than two (more than one explanatory and one response variable).

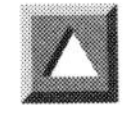

The correlation coefficient and the coefficient of determination in regression analysis describe the effect of the explanatory variable (X) on the response variable (Y); they do not describe the effect of Y on X (2,3).

7.7 Specify whether the model was validated.

Regression models can be "validated" or tested against a similar set of data to show that they explain what they seek to explain.

- One method of validation used when the sample is large is to develop the model on, say, 75% of the data and then to create another model on the remaining 25% and determine whether the models are similar.
- Another method involves removing the data from one subject at a time and recalculating the model. The coefficients and the predictive validity of all the models can then be assessed. Such methods are called **jack-knife** procedures.

- A third method involves developing another model on a different set of comparable data and determining whether the models are similar.

7.8 Report how any outlying data were treated in the analysis.

Outliers are extreme values that appear to be anomalies. Outliers cannot be ignored; in fact, they can indicate special cases that open new areas of research. But they can have a disproportionate effect on the results of a regression analysis. All outliers must be reported, but it is sometimes permissible to analyze the data without them, if they can be legitimately ignored. The practice must be reported, however, and the reasons for ignoring the outlying values should be given (for example, observations from contaminated samples or uncalibrated equipment). If the outliers cannot be legitimately ignored, it is permissible to report the results with and without the outliers to indicate their effect on the results.

△ **"Even a single outlier can have a profound effect on the relationship derived from the regression line" (2,4).**

7.9 For primary comparisons, include a scatter plot of the data, the regression line, and the (95%) confidence interval (or prediction bands) of the regression line.

In simple linear regression, data may be graphed as a scatter plot, as in correlation analysis (**Figures 6.1** and **6.2**, p 94), with the regression line drawn through them (see **Figure 7.1**). Such a graph will show the following:

- The presence of outlying values
- Whether the relationship is, in fact, linear
- The width of the (95%) confidence bands around the regression line, which indicates the appropriateness of the fit.

△ **Do not extend the regression line beyond the data (5–7).** The regression line is valid only over the range of the data from which it is calculated. Because many relationships are linear only within certain ranges, it is unwise to assume that the regression line will remain unchanged at lower or higher values of the explanatory variable **(Figure 7.2).**

√ **Because the regression line should not be extended beyond the data, it should not pass through the Y axis unless X can have a value of 0.** When graphing income versus height, for example, height will never be 0, so the line should not cross the Y axis, despite the fact that there is a Y intercept point for every simple linear regression equation (see **Figure 7.2**).

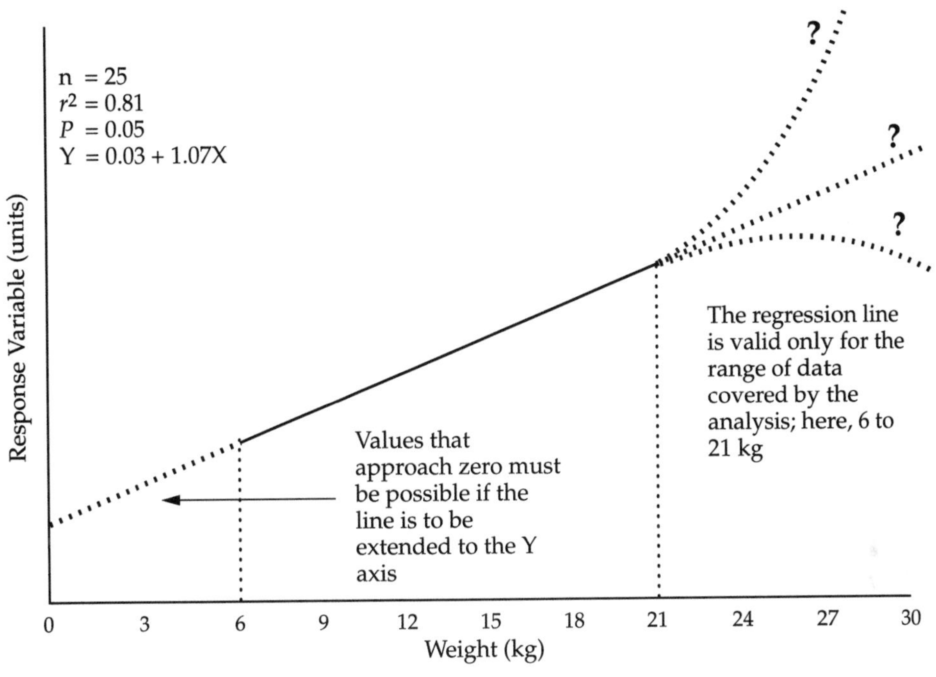

FIGURE 7.2 Hypothetical regression line showing inappropriate extensions beyond the data in both directions. Weight, for example, can never be 0 kg, so the left end of the line should not cross the Y axis, and the relationship may become nonlinear at higher weights, so the right end of the line should not be extended beyond the range of the data.

✓ **Confirm that the number of data points on the graph corresponds with the number of reported observations.** In addition to a simple accuracy check, counting the number of graphed values may reveal whether outliers may have been omitted.

7.10 Name the statistical package or program used in the analysis.

Identifying the computer package used in the statistical analysis is important because, although commercial packages generally are validated and updated, privately developed programs may not be. In addition, not all statistical software uses the same algorithms or default options to compute the same statistics. As a result, the results may vary from package to package or from algorithm to algorithm.

EXAMPLES: Among the more common packages are

- SAS (Statistical Analysis Systems)
- BMDP

- SPSS (Statistical Package for the Social Sciences)
- StatXact
- StatView
- StatSoft
- InStat
- Statistical Navigator
- SysStat
- Minitab
- LISREL
- EQS

MULTIPLE LINEAR REGRESSION ANALYSIS: PREDICTING ONE CONTINUOUS RESPONSE VARIABLE FROM TWO OR MORE EXPLANATORY VARIABLES

SAMPLE PRESENTATION

We developed a model to predict a score of overall function, Y, for patients with multiple sclerosis based on disease severity, X_1 (level 1 being least severe and level 15 being most severe); ambulatory ability (measured as the rate of walking in laps per minute), X_2; and number of lesions, X_3:

$$Y = 40.8 + 3.98X_1 + 1.22X_2 - 2.09X_3$$

Here,

- Y is the response variable, the overall function score.
- X_1, X_2, and X_3 are explanatory variables(sometimes called risk factors)
- The numbers in front of the X's are called regression *coefficients* or *beta weights*. Coefficients are interpreted as follows: if X_1 and X_3 are held constant (or "controlling for" disease severity and number of lesions), then mean functional score increases by about one and one-quarter times (1.22, the coefficient for X_2) for each additional lap per minute (**Table 7.1**).

TABLE 7.1 **Sample Table for Reporting a Multiple Linear Regression Model with Three Explanatory Variables.**

Variable	Coefficient (β)	Standard Error	95% CI	Wald χ^2	*P*
Intercept	40.79	2.55	—	—	—
X_1	3.98	2.37	−0.67 to 8.63	1.68	0.10
X_2	1.23	0.29	0.66 to 1.80	4.20	<0.001
X_3	−2.09	0.28	−2.64 to −1.54	−7.34	<0.001

where
- intercept = a mathematical constant; no clinical interpretation
- X_1 to X_3 = the three explanatory variables
- coefficient = the mathematical weightings of the explanatory variables in the equation
- standard error = estimated precision of the coefficients
- 95% CI = 95% confidence intervals for the coefficients
- Wald χ^2 = the Wald test statistic calculated from the data to be compared with the chi-square distribution with 1 degree of freedom
- *P* value = variables 2 and 3 are statistically significant predictors of the response variable

7.11 Describe the relationships of interest or the purpose of the analysis.

Multiple linear regression analysis can be used for at least four purposes (1):

- *To verify the association between a single explanatory variable and the response variable when controlling for one or more other explanatory variables.* If the explanatory variable continues to be highly associated with the response variable when included in a model with other explanatory variables, it is likely to be an important independent predictor of the response variable. If its association is strengthened or weakened as a result of its relationship with another variable or variables, these relationships can be investigated.
- *To confirm other analyses.* For example, cross-stratification is performed by stratifying one or more of the explanatory variables into smaller, more homogeneous groups, such as when age and gender are divided into, say, women younger than 45 years and men older than 65 years. Age and gender can then be examined to determine which combination of these variables better predicts the response variable.
- *To reduce a large number of variables to a "best" subset of variables of manageable size.* Large clinical registries or administrative databases may contain data for hundreds of explanatory variables. Instead of testing the association between each explanatory variable and the response variable

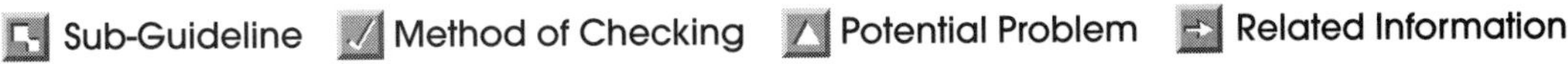
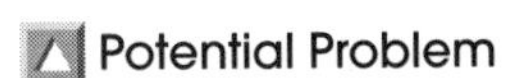

separately, variable-selection techniques, such as *forward, backward, stepwise,* and *best-subset* techniques, can be used to reduce the number of variables included in the final regression model by identifying those that meet specified statistical thresholds. (Investigators must still assess the correlation among the potential explanatory variables and identify which variables are clinically important, however.)

- *To create risk scores.* A **risk score** combines several variables into a single score that is associated with a particular outcome or a particular likelihood of disease. For example, one surgical risk score assigns weights to 13 clinical variables. The weights are then summed to create a score. The scores are then divided into one of nine categories, each of which is associated with a risk of complications after surgery.

7.12 Identify the variables used in the comparison and summarize each with descriptive statistics.

The response variable is continuous and the explanatory variables can be either categorical or continuous.

7.13 Confirm that the assumptions of multiple linear regression analysis have been met and state how each was checked.

A statement that the assumptions were verified is all that need be included.

The assumptions of multiple linear regression are extensions of those of simple linear regression:

- The relationship between *each* X and Y is linear over the range of values studied.
- The distributions of Y have equal variances (or standard deviations) at *each* value of *each* X; that is, the standard deviation of Y is the same, no matter what the value of X.
- Each of the values of Y is independent of one another for *each* value of *each* X.
- The response variable, Y, has a normal distribution at *each* value of *each* explanatory variable, X_1, X_2, X_3, and so on.

7.14 Specify how the explanatory variables that appear in the final model were chosen.

The "model building" of regression analysis is a process of selecting the best combination of explanatory variables to predict the response variable.

Common techniques include stepwise, forward, backward, and best-subset selection techniques ***(see also Guideline 7.11).***

One of the first steps in building a regression model is to identify the explanatory variables that are significantly related to the response variable. Several dozens of variables may be considered one at a time in this process of "univariate analysis." When the model is the focus of the article, it may be useful to report the results of the univariate analyses. Variables can be listed in a table, along with the appropriate descriptive statistics (that is, mean and standard deviation or median and interquartile range) and the P values for their relationship with the response variable. Those variables identified by the univariate analyses are then considered for inclusion in the model.

7.15 Specify whether all potential explanatory variables were assessed for colinearity (nonindependence).

The explanatory variables in a multiple linear regression equation should be independent of one another. If two or more explanatory variables are correlated, that is, if their regression lines are parallel or "colinear," then they are not independent. The variable with the strongest relationship with the response variable should be considered for inclusion in the model.

Failure to identify correlated variables may invalidate the results of the analysis.

7.16 Specify whether the explanatory variables were tested for interaction.

Two explanatory variables are said to interact if the effect of one explanatory variable on the response variable depends on the level of the second explanatory variable. **Figure 7.3** shows an example of this graphically. Interaction implies that the variables should be considered together, not separately.

7.17 Report the multiple linear regression equation or summarize the equation in a table. Include the number of observations in the analysis and the associated standard error, *P* value, and (95%) confidence interval for each coefficient in the equation.

EXAMPLE: **See Table 7.1.**

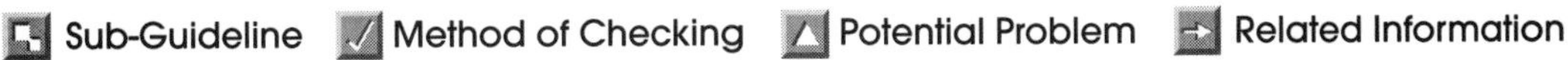

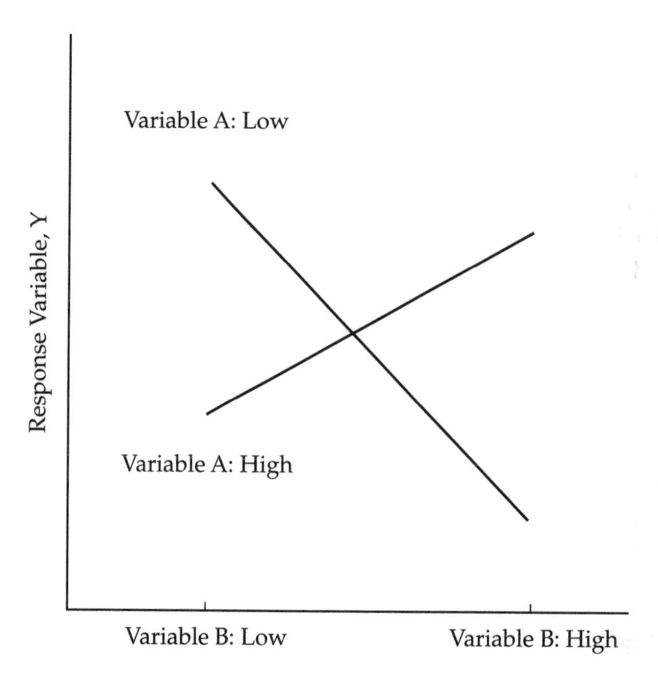

FIGURE 7.3 An example of interaction between two categorical explanatory variables, A and B, on a response variable, Y. The graph shows the mean value of Y on the vertical axis. The lines represent the mean values of Y for high and low values of A at high and low values of B. The effect of B on Y cannot be assessed unless the level of A is also known. Thus, A and B interact and cannot be considered separately in the analysis. Because A and B interact, the *main effects* of A on Y or B on Y are not of interest, but the *interactive* effect is.

7.18 Give the coefficient of multiple determination (R^2).

The coefficient of multiple determination (R^2) indicates how much of the variation in the response variable is accounted for by the explanatory variables included in the model. Higher percentages indicate better models, when compared to competing models with the same number of explanatory variables.

7.19 Specify whether the model was validated.

→ **Guideline 7.7: Validating regression models**

7.20 Report how any outlying data were treated in the analyses.

→ **Guideline 7.8: Treating outlying data**

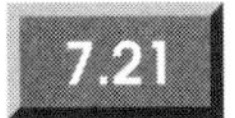

7.21 Name the statistical package or program used in the analysis.

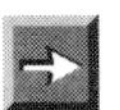

Guideline 7.10: Reporting statistical packages and programs

SIMPLE LOGISTIC REGRESSION ANALYSIS: PREDICTING ONE (BINARY) CATEGORICAL RESPONSE VARIABLE FROM ONE EXPLANATORY VARIABLE

SAMPLE PRESENTATION

Among 453 patients with either high serum levels (>220 mg/dL) or low serum levels (<220 mg/dL), weight proved to be a significant predictor for serum levels (weight coefficient = 0.44; SE = 0.11; $\chi^2_{df=1} = 16.0$; $P < 0.001$, odds ratio = 1.55; 95% CI = 1.25 to 1.93).

Here,

- 453 is the number of participants in the study.
- 0.44 is the regression coefficient for the explanatory variable, weight.
- 0.11 is the standard error of the regression coefficient, indicating the precision of the estimated coefficient.
- 16.0 is the value of the test statistic computed from the sample and that is compared to the chi-square distribution with 1 degree of freedom. The test statistic is used to determine the *P* value.
- *P* is the probability of getting an odds ratio as extreme or more extreme than the one observed if, in fact, the odds ratio is 1. Here, because the *P* value is small (less than 0.05) there is evidence against the null hypothesis of an odds ratio of 1, implying that weight does affect serum levels.
- 1.55 is the odds ratio for weight, indicating that for every additional kilogram of weight there is a 1.55 times higher risk of having high serum levels as defined.
- The 95% confidence interval for the odds ratio indicates that the odds ratio from 95 of 100 similar studies would be expected to fall between 1.25 and 1.93.
- **Table 7.2** is an alternative summary of the analysis.

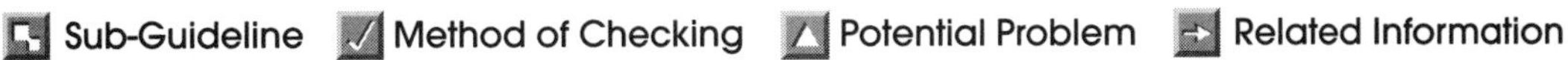

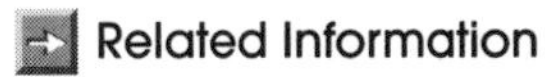

TABLE 7.2 Sample Table for Reporting a Simple Logistic Regression Model Analyzing the Relationship between Weight and High or Low Serum Levels.

Variable	Coefficient (β)	Standard Error	Wald χ^2	*P* Value	Odds Ratio	95% CI
Intercept	–1.89	0.48	—	—	—	—
Weight	0.44	0.11	16.00	<0.001	1.55	1.25 to 1.93

where
- intercept = a mathematical constant; no clinical interpretation
- weight = the explanatory variable (X_1)
- coefficient = the mathematical weighting of the explanatory variable in the equation
- standard error = estimated precision of the coefficient for weight
- Wald χ^2 = the Wald test statistic calculated from the data to be compared to the chi-square distribution with 1 degree of freedom
- *P* value = weight is a statistically significant predictor of high serum levels
- odds ratio = for every unit increase in weight, the odds of high serum levels increase by 1.55
- 95% CI = the "true" odds ratio is likely to fall between 1.25 and 1.93

7.22 Describe the relationship of interest or the purpose of the analysis.

Simple logistic regression analysis is most often used when the response variable has two values (but sometimes three or more). As in simple linear regression analysis, a single continuous explanatory variable is used to predict the response variable.

7.23 Identify the variables used in the comparison and summarize each with descriptive statistics.

The explanatory variable will be continuous or categorical and the response variable will be binary. The particular measurement or coding scheme can have substantial effects on the numerical values and interpretation of the regression coefficients (1). For example, the effect of age differs when coded in 1-year increments, 10-year increments, or binary categories (younger or older than age 65 years).

7.24 Confirm that the assumptions of simple logistic regression analysis were met and state how each was checked.

A statement that the assumptions were verified is all that needs to be included.

The assumptions of simple (and multiple) logistic regression analysis are beyond the scope of this book, but as in all regression analyses, some assurance should be given that the assumptions were met, and some indication should be given as to how the assumptions were checked. As before *(see Guideline 7.3)*, there are both formal testing procedures and informal (graphical) checks. Sometimes, data that violate the assumptions can be adjusted to meet the assumptions. If such adjustments were made, they should be identified.

7.25 Summarize the logistic regression equation in a table. Include the number of observations in the analysis, the coefficient of the explanatory variable and the associated standard error, odds ratio, the (95%) confidence interval of the odds ratio, and the *P* value.

Logistic regression equations, like that shown below, are seldom reported because they are difficult to interpret. Instead, the equation is summarized in a table (see **Table 7.2**).

$$\text{Probability of outcome} = \frac{1}{1 + e^{-(b_0 + b_1 X)}}$$

where

e = a mathematical constant (fixed at approximately 2.72)

b_0 = a constant for each model

b_1 = the coefficient for the explanatory variable X

Odds ratios are widely used in logistic regression analysis. For a binary explanatory variable, the odds ratio is the ratio of the odds that an event will occur in one group to the odds that the event will occur in the other group.

For example, suppose that smoking is studied to determine whether it is a risk factor for heart attack. As a binary explanatory variable, smoking might be expressed as present (smokers) or absent (nonsmokers). The response variable, heart attack, would be determined from a chart review in a sample of patients with a history of heart attack or without such a history. The data might be summarized as:

	Heart Attack		
Group	**Yes**	**No**	**Total**
Smokers	14	22	36
Nonsmokers	5	33	38
Total	19	55	74

For the smokers, the odds of having a heart attack are 14/22 = 0.636, whereas the odds for the nonsmokers are 5/33 = 0.152. The **odds ratio** is the ratio of these two odds: 0.636/0.152 = 4.2, meaning that the smokers

are 4.2 times more likely to have a heart attack than nonsmokers.

The odds ratio is sometimes called a *cross-product ratio* because it can be computed by multiplying the counts in the diagonal cells and dividing as follows:

$$(14 \times 33) \; / \; (5 \times 22) = 4.2$$

An odds ratio of 1 means that both groups have a similar likelihood of having a heart attack. The larger the odds ratio, the more likely the event is expected to occur in the group used in the numerator.

An odds ratio is an estimate, and the precision of the estimate can therefore be described with a confidence interval. In the above example, the results might be reported as: "Smokers were 4.2 times as likely to have a heart attack as nonsmokers (95% CI = 1.32 to 13.33; $P = 0.03$)."

7.26 Specify whether the model was validated.

→ **Guideline 7.7: Validating regression models**

7.27 Report how any outlying data were treated in the analysis.

→ **Guideline 7.8: Treating outlying data**

7.28 Name the statistical package or program used in the analysis.

→ **Guideline 7.10: Reporting statistical packages and programs**

MULTIPLE LOGISTIC REGRESSION ANALYSIS: PREDICTING ONE (BINARY) CATEGORICAL RESPONSE VARIABLE FROM TWO OR MORE EXPLANATORY VARIABLES

SAMPLE PRESENTATION

Our results were used to construct a model to predict the occurrence of stroke, Y, based on smoking, X_1, weight, X_2, age, X_3, and gender, X_4 (**Table 7.3**). Here,

- Y is the response variable: the presence or absence of stroke.

Continued

SAMPLE PRESENTATION – *Cont'd.*

- X_1, X_2, X_3, and X_4 are explanatory variables (sometimes called *risk factors*).
- The numbers in front of the X's are called *coefficients* or *beta weights.*
- **Table 7.3** shows the results of this hypothetical analysis.

7.29 Describe the relationships of interest or the purpose of the analysis.

Guideline 7.11: Purpose of regression analysis

In addition to the purposes outlined in Guideline 7.11 for multiple linear regression, multiple logistic regression is also used:

- *To quantify the risk associated with individual explanatory variables.* In the study of risk factors, it is sometime useful to determine the change in risk associated with an incremental change in an explanatory variable, such as changes in the risk of stroke for every 20-mm Hg decrease in systolic blood pressure. In this application, the regression coefficients are converted to relative risks (with Cox proportional regression analysis (***see also Chapter 9***) or odds ratios (with multiple logistic regression analysis; see below).

7.30 Identify the variables used in the comparison and summarize each with descriptive statistics.

Guideline 7.23: Summarizing variables

7.31 Confirm that the assumptions of multiple logistic regression analysis have been met and state how each was checked.

Guideline 7.24: Assumptions of regression analysis

7.32 Specify how the explanatory variables that appear in the final model were chosen.

Guideline 7.14: Choosing variables for the model

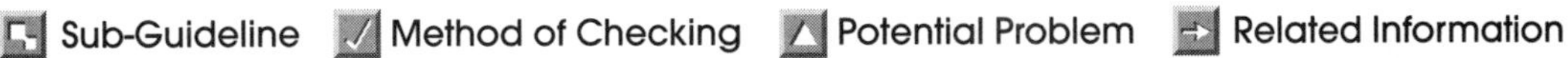

TABLE 7.3 Sample Table for Reporting a Multiple Logistic Regression Model with Four Explanatory Variables.

Variable	Coefficient (β)	Standard Error	Wald χ^2	*P* Value	Odds Ratio	95% CI
Intercept	–1.88	0.48	—	—	—	—
X_1	1.435	0.589	5.93	0.02	4.2	1.32 to 13.33
X_2	–0.847	0.690	1.51	0.22	0.43	0.111 to 1.66
X_3	3.045	1.260	5.84	0.02	21.01	1.78 to 248.29
X_4	2.200	0.990	4.94	0.03	9.03	1.30 to 62.83

where

intercept = a mathematical constant; no clinical interpretation
X_1 to X_4 = four explanatory variables
coefficient (β) = the mathematical weighting of each variable in the model
standard error = the estimated error of the mathematical weighting
Wald χ^2 = the Wald test statistic calculated from the data to be compared with the chi-square distribution with 1 degree of freedom
P value = the probability value indicating that variables 1, 3, and 4 are statistically significantly associated with the response variable
odds ratio = controlling for other variables in the model, for every unit increase in, say, variable 1, the odds of having the event of interest increase by 4.2. Likewise, controlling for other variables in the model, for every unit increase in, say, variable 2, the odds of having the event decrease by 0.43, and so on.
95% CI = the 95% confidence interval for the estimated odds ratio

7.33 Specify whether the potential explanatory variables were assessed for correlation or association.

The explanatory variables in a multiple logistic regression equation should be independent of one another. If two or more are correlated or associated, they are not independent. The variable with the strongest relationship with the response variable should be considered for inclusion in the model.

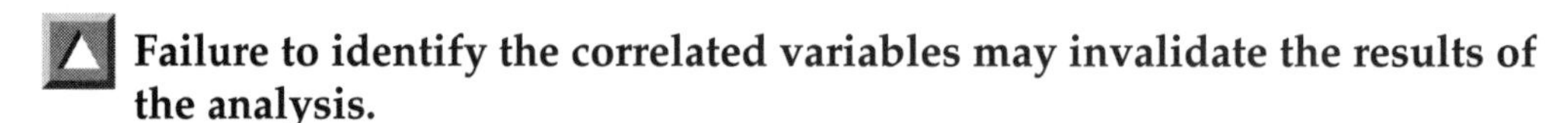

Failure to identify the correlated variables may invalidate the results of the analysis.

7.34 Specify whether the explanatory variables were tested for interaction.

Guideline 7.16: Testing for interaction

7.35 Summarize the multiple logistic regression equation in a table. Include the number of observations in the analysis, the coefficients of the explanatory variables, the associated standard errors, the odds ratios, the (95%) confidence intervals for the odds ratios, and the actual *P* values.

EXAMPLE: See Table 7.3.

➔ Guideline 7.25: Reporting odds ratios

7.36 Specify whether the model was validated.

➔ Guideline 7.7: Validating regression models

7.37 Report how any outlying data were treated in the analysis.

➔ Guideline 7.8: Treating outlying data

7.38 Name the statistical package or program used in the analysis.

➔ Guideline 7.10: Reporting statistical packages and programs

REFERENCES

1. **Concato J, Feinstein AR, Holford TR.** The risk of determining risk with multivariable models. Ann Intern Med. 1993;118(3):201-10.
2. **Godfrey K.** Simple linear regression in medical research. In: Bailar JC, Mosteller F, eds. Medical Uses of Statistics, 2nd edition. Boston: NEJM Books; 1992:201-32.
3. **Altman DG, Gore SM, Gardner MJ, Pocock SJ.** Statistical guidelines for contributors to medical journals. BMJ. 1983a; 286 (6376):1489-93.
4. **Hosmer DW, Taber S, Lemeshow S.** The importance of assessing the fit of logistic regression models: a case study. Am J Public Health. 1991;81(12):1630-5.
5. **Altman DG.** Statistics and ethics in medical research. VI—presentation of results. BMJ. 1980;281(6254):1542-4.
6. **Altman DG.** Statistics in medical journals. Stat Med. 1982;1(1):59-71.
7. **O'Brien PC, Shampo MA.** Statistics for clinicians: 7. Regression. Mayo Clin Proc. 1981;56(7):452-4.
8. **Yancy JM.** Ten rules for reading clinical research reports [Editorial]. Am J Surg. 1990;159(4): 553-9.

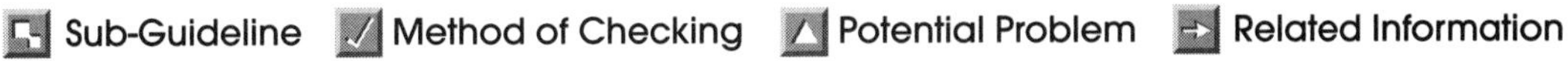

Chapter 8

Analyzing Multiple Variables

II. Reporting Analysis of Variance (ANOVA)

We may speak of testing the equality of treatment means or testing that the treatment effects are zero. The appropriate procedure for testing the equality of means is the analysis of variance.

D.C. Montgomery (1)

Analysis of variance (ANOVA) is a form of hypothesis testing for studies involving two or more variables. It is closely related to another set of techniques called *regression analysis*. In general, ANOVA is used to assess *categorical* explanatory variables, whereas regression analysis is used to assess *continuous* explanatory variables. When a study includes both continuous and categorical explanatory variables, the analysis may be called **multiple regression** *or* **analysis of covariance (ANCOVA).** Guidelines for reporting regression analyses are included in **Chapter 7.** Typically, the term *ANOVA* alone refers to "one-way ANOVA" (see below), but it is also used to refer to any type of ANOVA, just as "regression analysis" can refer to many types of regression analysis. Both types of analyses involve equations or "models" that summarize the relationships between explanatory and response variables.

Briefly, ANOVA separates the variation in all the data into two parts: the variation between each group mean and the overall mean for all the groups (the **between-group variability**) and the variation between each study participant and the participant's group mean (the **within-group variability**). If the between-group variability is much greater than the within-group variability, there are likely to be differences between the group means.

ANOVA is a "**group comparison**" that determines whether a statistically significant difference exists somewhere among the groups studied. If a significant difference is indicated, ANOVA is usually followed by a **multiple comparison procedure** that compares combinations of groups to examine further any differences among them. The most common multiple comparison procedure is the "pairwise comparison," in which each group mean is compared (two at a time) to all other group means to determine which groups differ significantly. Multiple comparisons create the multiple testing problem described in **Chapter 5** and so are performed with procedures designed to address this problem.

The most common ANOVA procedures used in biomedical research are described below. (The example is intended only to help distinguish among the various forms of ANOVA. We do not recommend sequentially expanding an analysis by adding variables one at a time.)

- **One-way ANOVA** assesses the effect of a single (hence the "one-way" designation) categorical explanatory variable (sometimes called a *factor*) on a single continuous response variable. Note, too, that the factor (category) has three or more alternatives (or "levels" or "values"; for example, blood type is A, B, AB, or O). When there are only two alternatives (two groups), this analysis reduces to Student's t test.

  EXAMPLE: Women with osteoporosis have been randomly assigned to one of three groups: a standard treatment, a new treatment, or a placebo. The response variable is the change in bone mineral density, a continuous variable. The explanatory variable is the form of treatment, which distinguishes each group. The results can be analyzed with a one-way ANOVA.

- **Two-way ANOVA** assesses the effect of *two* categorical explanatory variables (again, sometimes called factors) on a single continuous response variable.

  EXAMPLE: To the above example we now add age as a second explanatory variable. Age is coded as one of four ordinal categories: 30 to 40 years old, 41 to 50 years old, 51 to 60 years old, and 61 or more years old. With two categorical variables, treatment (or group) and age, the data can be analyzed with two-way ANOVA.

- **Multiway ANOVA** assesses the effect of three or more categorical explanatory variables (still called factors) on a single continuous response variable.

  EXAMPLE: To the above example, the addition of more categorical explanatory variables, such as diet (vegetarian or not vegetarian) and alcohol consumption (less than 2 ounces of alcohol per day, 2 to 5 ounces per day, or 6 or more ounces per day), would move the analysis from two-way to four-way ANOVA, or simply, multiway ANOVA.

- **Analysis of covariance (ANCOVA)** assesses the effect of one or more categorical explanatory variables while controlling for the effects of some other (possibly continuous) explanatory variables (now called *covariates*) on a single continuous response variable.

  EXAMPLE: To the above example we now may wish to control for the severity of disease. Women with more severe osteoporosis may have different bone mineral densities than women with less severe disease. If we are to study the relationship between treatment and age on bone mineral density, we must control for disease severity. We thus add another (categorical) explanatory variable, disease severity (mild, moderate, and severe). The analysis is now called analysis of covariance (ANCOVA).

- **Repeated-measures ANOVA** is used to assess several, or repeated, measurements of the same participants under different conditions (such as blood pressure measurements taken while the patient is supine, sitting, or standing) or at different points over time (such as muscle strength measured 1, 5, 10, and 20 days after surgery).

  EXAMPLE: Again, building from the above example, suppose we have measurements of bone mineral density for all patients at the onset of symptoms and at 6 months and 12 months after the onset of symptoms. "Time" can now be added to the ANOVA model as an explanatory variable. Here, time is a "repeated measure"; although each woman belongs to a single treatment group and to a single age category, each has bone density measurements at three points in time (0, 6, and 12 months).

Sample Presentation

Sixty-six women with osteoporosis were alternately assigned to one of three treatment groups: Group 1 (n = 22), group 2 (n = 22), and controls (n = 22). After 6 weeks, the change in bone mineral density from baseline was measured. Analysis with one-way ANOVA indicated a statistically significant difference among the groups ($F_{2,63} = 61.07$; $P < 0.001$; **Table 8.1**).

Continued

SAMPLE PRESENTATIONS – *Cont'd.*

Further analysis with Tukey's pairwise comparison procedure to control for multiple testing revealed that the mean change (± SD) of group 2 (1.6 g/cm^2 ± 0.2) was significantly greater than that of group 1 (1.1 g/cm^2 ± 0.2) and that of the controls (1.0 g/cm^2 ± 0.2) with an overall alpha level of 0.05.

Here,

- The size of each group, n, is given.
- Although alternating assignment is not to be preferred to true random assignment, the method of allocating patients to the groups is specified.
- The group comparison is identified as one-way ANOVA, and the results of this comparison are given in **Table 8.1.**
- The follow-up multiple comparisons were made with Tukey's procedure, and the actual mean changes and standard deviations for the groups compared are given.
- The alpha level, or the threshold at which statistical significance is declared, is given as 0.05.
- 61.07 is the *F* test statistic, with 2 degrees of freedom for the numerator and 63 degrees of freedom for the denominator (expressed as the subscript $F_{2,63}$), that is calculated from the data.
- The *P* value is the probability of getting a "group effect," or an effect of treatment on bone mineral density, as extreme or more extreme than the one observed if in fact all group means are equal. Here, patients with different treatments have statistically significantly different responses to the treatment. The small *P* value reflects that there is evidence in the data against the null hypothesis of no difference between the group means.

GUIDELINES ADDRESSED IN THE INTRODUCTION

8.1 Describe the relationships of interest or the purpose of the analysis.

ANOVA is typically used to compare three or more group means on a certain response variable. It can also be expanded to include additional explanatory variables and can assess their simultaneous effects on the response variable. Whereas the purpose of regression analyses is usually to predict the value of the response variable, the purpose of ANOVA is

TABLE 8.1 Sample Table for Reporting the Results of a One-Way ANOVA*: Analyzing the Differences Among Three Treatment Groups of Women with Osteoporosis (n = 66).

Source of Variation	df	Sums of Squares	Mean Square	*F*	*P*
Group	2	4.96	2.48	61.07	<0.001
Error	63	2.56	0.04	—	—

* The "one-way" indicates a single factor, "group," which here has three "levels": treatment groups 1, 2, and controls. See the Sample Presentation on pp 129–130.

Source of variation = identifies the sources of variability in bone mineral density as the factors in the model and as random error (the variability not explained by the factors). Here, group is the only factor

df = the degrees of freedom, a mathematical concept. Here, for three groups, the df is 3 – 1, or 2; for 66 patients, the df for error is [(66 – 1) – (3 – 1)], or 63.

Sum of squares = for group, a measure of the magnitude of the differences *between* groups; for error, a measure of the magnitude of the differences *within* groups

Mean square = the sums of squares divided by the degrees of freedom; essentially, estimates of the variation in the data

F = the test statistic computed from the data and to be compared to the *F* distribution; equals the mean square between groups divided by the mean square within groups

P = the probability value indicating that the group effect, or the effect of treatment on bone mineral density, was larger than would be expected by chance, given that all the group means are equal; that is, the groups had statistically significantly different responses to treatment

usually to compare groups for differences in the means of the response variable.

GUIDELINES ADDRESSED IN THE METHODS

8.2 Identify the variables used in the comparison and summarize each with descriptive statistics.

The explanatory variables will usually be categorical (the group designations). The response variable will be continuous and should be summarized with a measure of center (the mean or median) and a measure of dispersion (the standard deviation or interquartile range), as appropriate.

8.3 Identify the type of analysis used.

The types of ANOVA are listed above. It is important to specify whether repeated-measures ANOVA was used because serial measurements from the same participants must be analyzed differently.

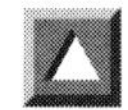

Do not confuse the number of *groups* with the number of *factors* in identifying the type of ANOVA. In ANOVA, *group* is a general term for a single factor that may include three or more specific groups. In one-way ANOVA, only groups are compared, and "group" is the only factor in the analysis. In two-way ANOVA, "group" and a second, additional factor, which itself may include several "levels" or subdivisions, are analyzed. For example, blood type might be the factor, whereas A, B, AB, and O are the levels of this factor. Thus, the type of ANOVA is *not* determined by the number of levels, groups, or categories but by the number of *factors*.

GUIDELINES ADDRESSED IN THE RESULTS

8.4 Confirm that the assumptions of the analysis have been met.

A statement that the assumptions were verified is all that need be included.

The assumptions of ANOVA are as follows:

- The response variable, Y, is approximately normally distributed within each level of each factor (the explanatory variable, X).
- The distributions of Y have equal variances (or standard deviations) within each level of each factor (the explanatory variable, X); that is, the standard deviation of Y is the same, no matter what the value of X.
- Each value of Y is independent of the other values of Y (that is, the values of Y are not paired or correlated). This assumption does not apply to repeated-measures ANOVA because, by definition, repeated measurements on the same participants are correlated. Repeated-measures ANOVA is designed to accommodate this correlation.

8.5 Report the results of the ANOVA in a table.

EXAMPLES: **Tables 8.1** and **8.2** illustrate how the results of ANOVA are commonly presented.

8.6 Specify whether the explanatory variables were tested for interaction and how these interactions were treated.

Two factors (explanatory variables) are said to interact if the effect of one factor on the response variable depends on the level of the second factor. **Figure 7.3** (p 118) shows this concept graphically. Interaction implies that the factors should be considered together, not separately.

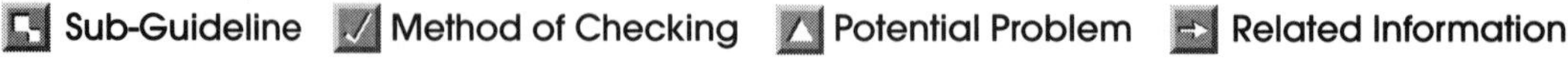

TABLE 8.2 **Sample Table for Presenting the Results of a Two-Way Analysis of Variance for Analyzing Two Factors: Group and Age.***

Source of Variation	df	Sums of Squares	Mean Square	*F*	*P*
Group	1	0.64	0.64	2.24	0.16
Age	3	3.92	1.31	4.57	0.02
Group × age	3	4.91	1.64	5.72	0.01
Error	12	3.43	0.29	—	—

* The analysis includes two factors: group (two levels or categories) and age (four categories or levels). The levels of each category should be stated in the description of the study. Group and age significantly interact and so must be considered together.

Source of variation = identifies the sources of variability in the response variable as the factors in the model (group, age, and the interaction between group and age) and as random error (the variability not explained by the factors)

df = the degrees of freedom, a mathematical concept. Here, for two groups, the df is 2 – 1, or 1. For four age categories, the df is 4 – 1, or 3. For the interaction effect between group and age (group × age) the degrees of freedom for each factor are multiplied: 3 × 1 = 3.

Sums of squares = Unlike one-way ANOVA, the sums of squares in multiway ANOVA are not easily explained and are best regarded as simply steps in the calculation of the mean squares.

Mean square = the sums of squares divided by the degrees of freedom; essentially, estimates of the variation in the data.

F = the test statistic for the *F* distribution; for testing for interaction effects and main effects; equals the mean square for each factor divided by the mean square of the error.

P = the probability values indicating the statistical significance of the effect of each factor on the response variable. Age and group interact ($P = 0.01$) in affecting the response variable and should be further investigated *together.* That is, the "main effect" of group or the "main effect" of age should not be investigated alone.

8.7 Report the actual *P* value for each explanatory variable.

A common null hypothesis tested with ANOVA is that all group means are equal. If a significant *P* value is found, indicating an overall group difference, a multiple comparisons procedure is performed to determine, say, which group means are different from each other. Further, all factors (explanatory variables) significantly associated with the response variable, including interactions among the factors, can be further assessed with multiple comparisons procedures.

8.8 Provide an assessment of the goodness-of-fit of the ANOVA model to the data.

An assessment of goodness-of-fit indicates how well the model expresses the relationships observed in the data. As in regression analysis (*see*

Chapter 7), examining the residuals (the differences between the observed values and those estimated by the model) helps to determine the aptness of the model. The results of the analysis of residuals need not be reported; a statement that the residuals were examined and that the model did or did not fit the data well will suffice.

8.9 Specify whether the model was validated.

ANOVA models can be "validated" or tested against a similar set of data to show that they explain what they seek to explain.

- One method of validation when the sample size is large is to develop the model on, say, 70% of the data and then to develop another model on the remaining 30% to see whether the models are similar.
- Another method involves removing the data from one subject at a time and recalculating the model. The coefficients of all the models (there may be hundreds) can then be compared. Such methods are called **jack-knife** procedures.
- A third method involves developing a new model on a new set of comparable data to determine whether the results are similar.

8.10 Report how any outlying data were treated in the analysis.

Outliers are extreme values that appear to be anomalies (as opposed to data collection or recording errors, which are simply mistakes). True outliers cannot be ignored; in fact, they often indicate special cases that open new areas of research. But they can have a disproportionate effect on the results of an ANOVA. Outliers can also skew the distribution of the data and thus can sometimes be accommodated by transforming the data (*see Guideline 2.14*). All outliers must be reported, but it is sometimes permissible to analyze the data without them, if they can be legitimately ignored. The practice must be reported, however, and the reasons for ignoring the outlying values should be given. If the outliers cannot be legitimately ignored, it is permissible to report the results with and without the outliers to indicate their effect on the results.

8.11 Name the statistical package or program used in the analysis.

Identifying the computer package used in the statistical analysis is important because, although commercial packages generally are validated and updated, privately developed algorithms may not be. In addition, not all statistical software uses the same algorithms or default options to compute the same statistics. As a result, the results may vary from package to package or from algorithm to algorithm.

ANOVA is included in most major statistical packages.

EXAMPLES: Among the more common packages are

- SAS (Statistical Analysis Systems)
- BMDP
- SPSS (Statistical Package for the Social Sciences)
- StatXact
- StatView
- StatSoft
- InStat
- Statistical Navigator
- SysStat
- Minitab
- LISREL
- EQS

REFERENCE

1. **Montgomery DC.** Design and Analysis of Experiments. 2nd ed. New York: John Wiley and Sons, 1984.

Chapter 9

Assessing Time-to-an-Event as an Endpoint

Reporting Survival Analyses

Survival curves provide estimates of the probability of survival as a function of time from entry into the study. They give the most complete picture of how different treatment groups fared over time with respect to survival.

F. Mosteller, J.P. Gilbert, and B.M. McPeek (1)

Time-to-event analysis involves estimating the probability that an event will occur at different points in time. For example, **survival analysis,** the most common application of time-to-event analysis in medicine, estimates the probability of survival as a function of time from a starting point, say, from the date of a diagnosis or of an intervention. In this chapter, we use death as the event of interest, but any event, such as a relapse into disease, equipment failure, or the clearing of symptoms, can be used as the event in such analyses.

The statistical methods described in other chapters of this book cannot be used to analyze survival data because death may not have occurred in all patients when the analysis is performed and, in fact, may never occur during the study period. Data from participants who have not yet died are said to be *censored.* Survival analysis is designed to accommodate these kinds of data.

In survival analysis, the period between the starting time and death (or the date of the last follow-up observation before the analysis if the subject is still alive) is recorded for each subject. The percentage of participants still alive at the end of each specified time period (such as each month, each year, or each 5 years) is used to estimate the probability that a typical subject will be alive at the end of any given period. When graphed, these estimates form a distribution of the probabilities of survival for the different time periods (a survival curve). In addition, two or more survival curves can be compared to determine whether the associated treatments differ statistically in their effectiveness as measured by survival rate. Statistical models can also be created to estimate the risk of death associated with a given characteristic and adjusted for the effects of other characteristics, such as gender or age.

Sample Presentation

As shown in **Figure 9.1**, for our patients with cancer, the Kaplan-Meier estimates of the 5-year survival rate after treatment were 67% (95% CI = 52.9% to 81.1%) for the surgically treated group (n = 55) and 10% (95% CI = 0.6% to 19.4%) for the medically treated group (n = 46). The log-rank test revealed a statistically significant difference between the survival rates over time ($P < 0.001$). Median survival time was 6.3 years for the surgical group but only 3.8 years for the medical group. Surgery was thus more effective in prolonging life than medical therapy. Further investigation with Cox proportional hazards regression analysis, which controlled for the effect of treatment, indicated that patients with metastatic cancer were 6.5 times more likely to die of cancer than those whose cancer had not metastasized (95% CI for the hazard or risk ratio = 2.8 to 15.0; $P < 0.001$).

Here,

- **Figure 9.1** shows the Kaplan-Meier curves for these data.
- The study population is identified as 101 patients receiving treatment for cancer, 55 with surgical and 46 with medical therapy.
- The Kaplan-Meier method of survival analysis estimated that the 5-year survival rates for the surgical and medical groups were 67% and 10%, respectively. The 95% confidence intervals for these estimates are also given.
- An estimated 50% of the surgical patients will die within 6.3 years after surgery; the other 50% will either still be alive or will die more than 6.3 years after surgery. In contrast, half of the medically treated patients will die within 3.8 years of treatment. (These results are the *median survival times.*)
- The log-rank test, used to compare survival curves from the two groups, shows a statistically significant difference between the groups.
- After controlling for group differences (that is, adjusting for the effect of receiving either surgical or medical treatment), the hazard ratio (or risk ratio) for metastatic cancer was 6.5 to 1, meaning that patients with metastatic cancer were 6.5 times as likely to die of cancer as were

Continued

SAMPLE PRESENTATION – *Cont'd.*

patients without metastatic cancer, as determined by Cox proportional hazards regression analysis.

- The 95% confidence interval for the hazards ratio indicates the precision of this estimate.
- The *P* values indicate that, under the null hypothesis, chance is not a likely explanation for the differences in survival times between the two treatment groups or for the risk of death represented by metastatic cancer. Here the small *P* values are evidence against the null hypothesis of no difference.

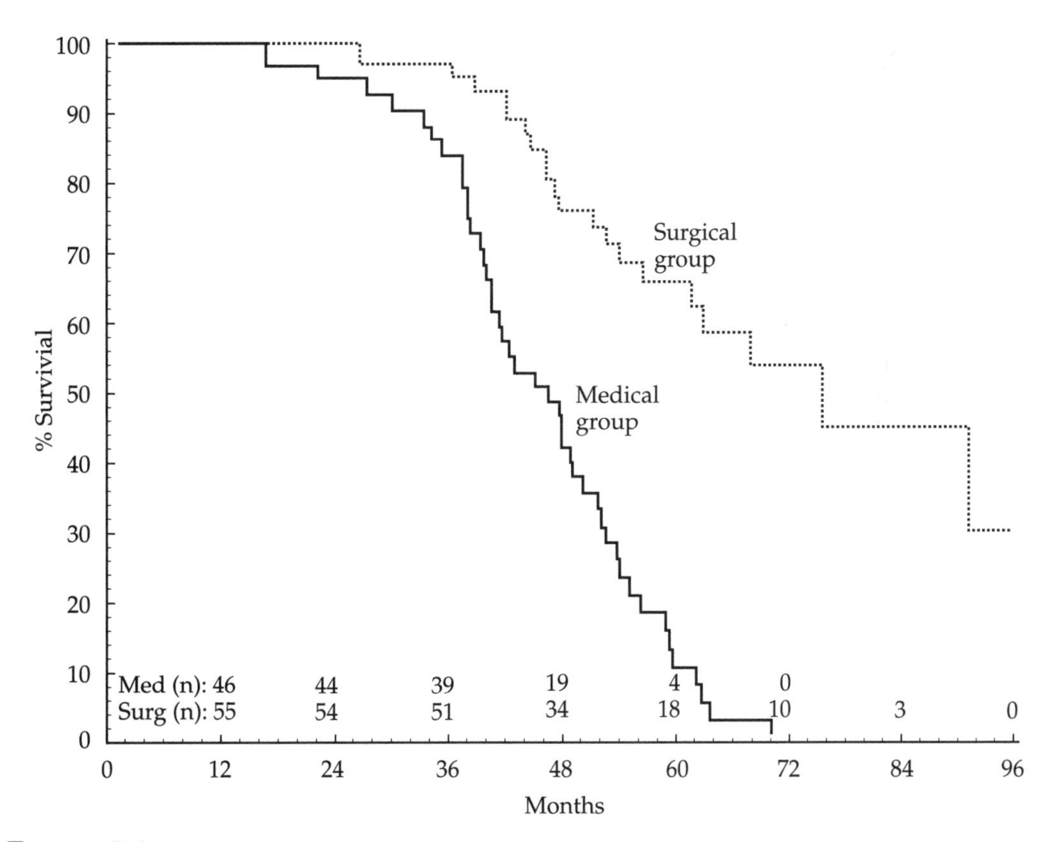

FIGURE 9.1 The Kaplan-Meier curve is a step-function that indicates the estimated percentages of participants alive at various times after the start of the study. The number of patients alive at each major time point and on whom the estimates are based should also be given, as indicated here.

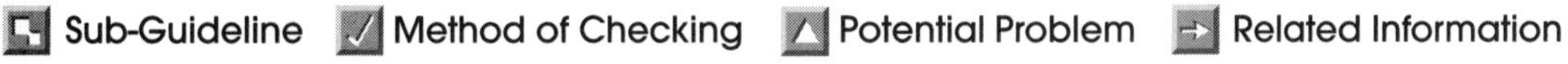

9.1 Describe the relationship to be studied and the reasons for studying it.

Specify the event of interest—although remember that the endpoint or response variable in survival analysis is actually the *time to the event,* not the event itself—and the factors that are believed to be associated with the event or to promote or inhibit its occurrence (the explanatory variables). When the event is something other than death, such as equipment failure or the disappearance of clinical symptoms, the clinical importance of the event and the value of its prediction should also be made clear.

9.2 Describe the clinical characteristics of the population under study.

Patients with the same disease may differ on a number of characteristics that may affect the outcome of interest. At a minimum, describe the relevant:

- **Demographic features:** age, sex, occupation, lifestyle choices (smoking, exercise level, nutrition, and so on)
- **Clinical features:** the nature and duration of signs and symptoms
- **Paraclinical features:** the test and imaging results indicating the stage or progression of disease
- **Co-morbidities:** other conditions that may interact with the disease or treatment under study

9.3 Specify the starting time that marks the beginning of the analysis.

Survival time can be measured from any of several different starting times: onset of symptoms, first abnormal test results, date of diagnosis, date of hospital admission, date of first treatment, date after the passing of the "operative mortality" period, and so on. The starting time must be specified to avoid ambiguity. Studies with different starting points may not be comparable because of **lead-time bias,** in which patients diagnosed earlier in the course of disease have longer median survival times, not necessarily because treatment was better but because they were simply diagnosed earlier.

9.4 Specify the nature of any censored data.

Survival analysis may take into account two types of data: censored and uncensored. **Uncensored data** are "complete data": death has occurred, and the interval between the starting time and death is known (**Figure 9.2**).

In addition, the cause of death is believed to be related to the intervention or diagnosis under study.

Censored data, on the other hand, are "incomplete data" from participants who

- Are still alive; that is, death has not occurred at the time of the analysis, so the survival time is unknown.
- Died of causes unrelated to the disease or treatment. (These deaths may not be recorded as events because they are unrelated to the disease or treatment under study.)
- Are no longer participating in the study, having dropped out of the study or having been lost to follow-up. The disposition of these participants is also important to report if the study used intent-to-treat analysis (*see Guideline 1.26*).

9.5 Specify the statistical methods used to estimate the survival rate.

Several statistical methods are available for analyzing survival data. However, the most common methods are

- The **Kaplan-Meier method** (or the product-limit method), in which

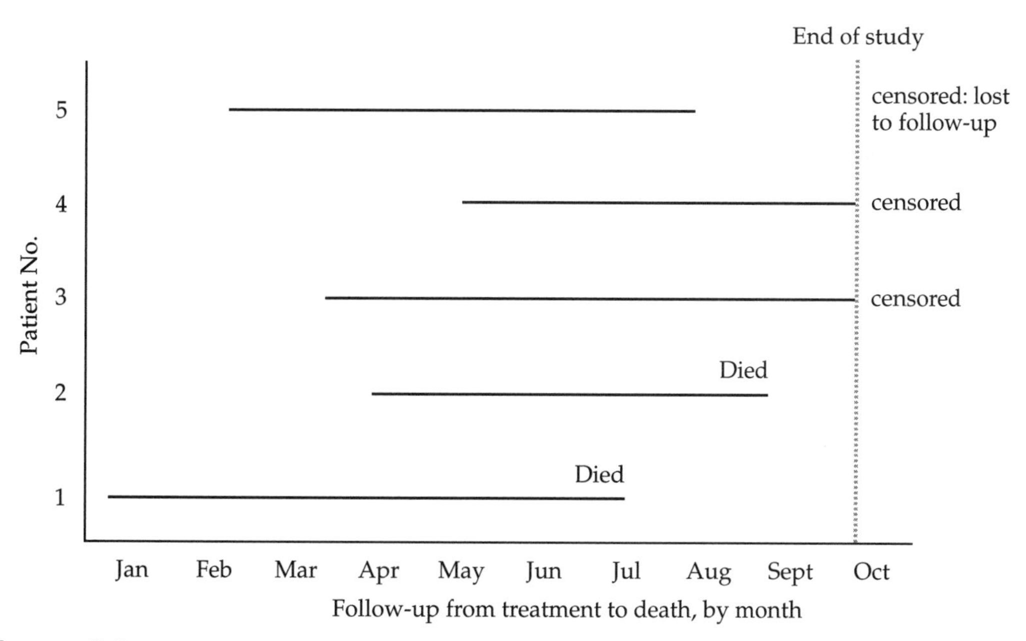

FIGURE 9.2 In most survival analyses, patients enter and leave a study at different times. Thus, at the end of the study, some patients (here, patients 3 and 4) have not experienced the event of interest. Patients 3 and 4, who were still alive at the end of the study, and patient 5, who was lost to follow-up and whose survival status is thus unknown, represent "censored" data.

individual deaths are recorded by exact dates. This method is suitable for both large and small sample sizes.

- The **life table method** (or the Cutler-Ederer or the actuarial or the Berkson-Gage method), in which deaths are recorded by time interval (for example, every month; every year). The life table method is most commonly used for very large samples, such as those in epidemiological studies.

9.6 Confirm that the requirements of survival analysis have been met.

Simply state whether the requirements were met.

The requirements of survival analysis with either the Kaplan-Meier curve or the life table methods are that

- No changes in diagnosis, treatment, or follow-up procedures occurred during the study.
- The risk of consequences did not change over the course of the study.
- Deaths, withdrawals, and patient accrual occurred uniformly over the follow-up interval.
- Patients represented by censored data would have experienced the same distribution of consequences as those remaining under study.

9.7 For each group, give the estimated survival rate at appropriate follow-up times, with confidence intervals, and the number of participants at risk for death at each time.

A survival rate is the *percentage of the participants who were alive at a given time.* Like all estimates, the survival rate should be accompanied by a 95% confidence interval to indicate the precision of the estimate. Giving the number and status (alive or dead) of participants on which each estimate is based also helps to put these estimates in perspective. Estimates should be provided for logical follow-up times (for example, at 1 year, 5 years, 10 years or 3 months, 6 months, 12 months).

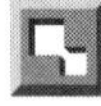

It is sometimes desirable to report the results of survival analysis in terms of the *median survival time,* or the length of time during which the first 50% of the sample died.

The results of survival analysis can also be expressed in terms of *the length of time that the participants survived.* When all the members of the group have died, survival data are uncensored, and the distribution of individual survival times may be described with the median and interquartile range (or with the mean and standard deviation if the data are approximately normally distributed).

However, because participants die at different times, at any given time, some participants may still be alive, and so are considered to be censored. The survival times of censored participants are unknown, so the true shape of the distribution of survival times cannot be assumed to be normal, and the mean is therefore not an appropriate measure of the center of the distribution. The median survival time—the period within which 50% of the participants died and beyond which 50% of the participants were still alive—is thus a better description of central tendency for survival time (2).

9.8 When indicated, present the full results in a graph or table.

In some studies, only a single estimate of survival may be of interest, such as the 5-year survival rate often used in reporting cancer research. Other studies may require that estimates be presented for several times over a long period. The most common graphical presentation of a series of estimates is the Kaplan-Meier curve (**Figure 9.1**). The Kaplan-Meier "curve" is a graph that descends step-like over time and that plots the percentage of the population still alive after a given period. Kaplan-Meier estimates can also be presented in table form (**Table 9.1**). Results of the life table method can also be presented in table form (**Table 9.2**).

9.9 Specify the statistical methods used to compare two or more survival curves.

Two or more survival curves can be compared with hypothesis tests to determine whether they differ statistically. The two most common such methods for comparing survival curves are

- The **log-rank test** (also called the Cox-Mantel test), which is more powerful for detecting late differences in the probabilities of survival.
- **Wilcoxon's test** (or Breslow's generalized Wilcoxon test), which is more powerful for detecting early differences in the probabilities of survival. Given that the requirements for survival analysis hold (*see* ***Guideline 9.6***), either procedure can be used.

9.10 When comparing two or more survival curves with hypothesis tests, report the actual *P* value of the comparison.

The null hypothesis is that the survival distributions are the same. The *P* value indicates the probability of finding a difference between the

TABLE 9.1 Tabular Summary of Kaplan-Meier Estimates for a Sample of 145 Patients.*

Time	% Survival	95% CI† (%)	Number of Deaths	Number Censored	Number at Risk
6 months	97.9	95.5 to 100.0	3	0	142
1 year	97.2	94.5 to 100.0	4	0	141
2 years	95.1	91.6 to 95.1	7	3	135
3 years	85.2	79.7 to 90.7	21	68	56
5 years	77.6	68.0 to 87.2	26	118	1

* Other columns may also be appropriate.
† The standard error is often reported instead of the 95% confidence interval.

Time = the time (or time interval) for which the estimate was computed, measured from the starting time of the analysis; chosen by the researcher

% survival = the percentage of the original sample still alive at a particular time; also called the *survival rate*

95% CI = an indication of the precision of the estimate of the survival rate

Number of deaths = the number of deaths occurring in each time interval

Number censored = number of patients censored at the beginning of the time interval; includes those who have been lost to follow-up, who have died from causes other than that under study, or who were still alive at the end of the last interval

Number at risk = number of patients alive (and therefore at risk for death) at the end of the time period

TABLE 9.2 An Example of a Life Table for 1999 Patients.*

Year After Diagnosis	Patients Lost to Follow-up (n)	Patients Dying (n)	Patients Exposed to Risk (n)	Proportion Survived	Standard Error
0–1	0	300	1999	1.00	—
1–2	35	212	1682	0.85	0.003
2–3	20	150	1443	0.74	0.009
3–4	21	180	1272	0.67	0.011
4–5	25	130	1069	0.58	0.019
5–6	43	89	928	0.50	0.033

* Additional columns may also be appropriate.

Year after diagnosis = intervals for which survival times are estimated

Patients lost to follow-up = number of participants whose survival status is unknown

Patients dying = number of participants who died during the interval

Patients exposed to risk = number of participants alive during the interval and, hence, at risk for death

Proportion survived = proportion of participants alive at the beginning of the interval; sometimes called the *cumulative survival rate*

Standard error = an estimate of the precision of the estimated cumulative survival rate; there is no standard error when the proportion surviving is 1.0

curves as extreme or more extreme than the one observed, assuming that the survival distributions are the same.

9.11 Report the regression model used to assess the associations between explanatory variables and the survival rate.

A common technique for assessing the association between explanatory variables and survival rate is Cox proportional hazards regression analysis (also called Cox regression analysis). This analysis results in an equation, or a model, that can be presented in a table, such as that shown in **Table 9.3**.

9.12 Report a measure of risk for each explanatory variable.

The measure of risk usually provided for each explanatory variable in a Cox regression analysis is the *risk ratio* (also called a *hazard ratio*). For a binary variable, a risk ratio of 1 means that the risk of death is the same, whether a participant has the characteristic or not. A risk ratio greater than

TABLE 9.3 A Tabular Presentation of a Cox Proportional Hazards Model Showing the Effect of Five Variables on the Risk of Death.*

Variable	Coefficient (β)	Standard Error	Wald χ^2	*P* Value	Risk Ratio	95% CI
X_1 Age	0.23	0.07	10.80	0.001	1.26	1.10 to 1.44
X_2 Blood pressure	1.46	0.62	5.55	0.02	4.31	1.28 to 14.52
X_3 Serum cholesterol	0.84	0.43	3.82	0.05	2.32	1.00 to 5.38
X_4 History of smoking	0.27	0.14	3.72	0.05	1.31	1.00 to 1.72
X_5 History of heart disease	1.44	0.27	28.44	<0.001	4.22	2.49 to 7.16

* Data are hypothetical.

Variable = the explanatory variables of interest: X is the symbol for an explanatory variable.

Coefficient = sometimes referred to as parameter estimates, coefficients are the weightings for each variable in the regression equation

Standard error = the variability of each of the estimated coefficients

Wald χ^2 = the test statistic computed from the data and from which *P* values are determined

P values = the probability of observing results as extreme or more extreme than those actually found, if the null hypothesis is true. Here, the *P* values indicate that all variables are significantly associated with the risk of death.

Risk ratio (or hazards ratio) = the degree of risk associated with each variable while controlling for all other variables. For binary variables, a risk ratio of 1 indicates that having the characteristic of the variable neither promotes nor protects against the event. Ratios less than 1 indicate reduced risk, those above 1 indicate increased risk. Here, a patient with a history of heart disease is 4.22 times more likely to die within 5 years than a patient without such a history. In general, the risk ratio is the amount of increased risk for every unit or level increase in the explanatory variable.

95% CI = the precision of the estimated risk ratio. The narrower the confidence intervals, the more precise the estimates.

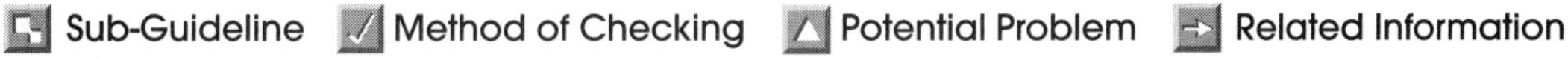

1 indicates an increased risk for those with the characteristic; a ratio less than 1, a decreased risk. Thus, if a high-fat diet has a risk ratio of 5.4 with respect to stroke, then patients who eat a high-fat diet are 5.4 times as likely to experience stroke than patients who eat a low-fat diet. In general, the risk ratio is the amount of increased risk for every unit or level increase in the explanatory variable.

The risk ratio and a 95% confidence interval can be given in the table that reports the Cox regression analysis.

Guideline 9.11 and Table 9.3: Reporting Cox regression models

9.13 Describe the quality of life for survivors.

Survival, by itself, is not necessarily an adequate endpoint in medicine; some technologies do not delay death so much as they prolong suffering. The intelligent use of medical technologies requires an appreciation of their effect on quality of life, as well as their effect on survival.

REFERENCES

1. **Mosteller F, Gilbert JP, McPeek B.** Reporting standards and research strategies for controlled trials. Control Clin Trials. 1980;1: 37-58.

2. **Altman DG, Gore SM, Gardner MJ, Pocock SJ.** Statistical guidelines for contributors to medical journals. BMJ. 1983;286: 1489-93.

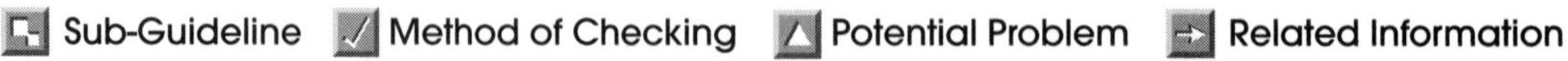
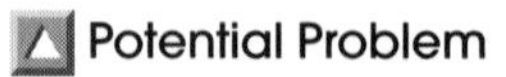

Chapter 10

Determining the Presence or Absence of Disease

Reporting the Characteristics of Diagnostic Tests

The ultimate criterion for the usefulness of a diagnostic test is whether it adds information beyond that otherwise available, and whether this information leads to a change in management that is ultimately beneficial to the patient.

R. Jaeschke, G.H. Guyatt, and D.L. Sackett (1)

Effective medical treatment usually depends on accurately diagnosing a patient's condition. Diagnostic tests can take many forms: observations of the presence or absence of clinical signs and symptoms, a biochemical assay of tissue, a questionnaire, a reading of a radiographic image, changes in electrical potentials, the appearance of cell types, and so on.

The guidelines below are particularly appropriate for describing the development and characteristics of a new diagnostic test. However, most references to diagnostic tests are to their use in a larger study, which reduces the number of guidelines that need to be considered. For reporting clinical trials designed specifically to evaluate a new diagnostic test, also follow the guidelines in **Chapter 1.**

In this chapter, we also briefly describe applications of Bayes' theorem that are sometimes used to characterize diagnostic tests.

Sample Presentation

Hysteroscopy was used to diagnose uterine cancer in premenopausal women. This procedure is 80% sensitive and 90% specific when compared to the criterion standard of pathologic analysis, resulting in a likelihood ratio of 8. In our referral area, the prevalence of uterine cancer is 10%. The

Continued

SAMPLE PRESENTATION – *Cont'd.*

positive predictive value for the test was thus 47.1%. A positive test indicated the presence of a malignancy that should be treated. Inter-rater reliability is about 82%.

Here,

- **Sensitivity** is the ability of the test to correctly identify patients who have a disease. Here, of the women who actually have uterine cancer as determined by pathologic analysis, 80% will have positive hysteroscopy evaluations. Sensitivity is the percentage of "true-positive" results. The remaining 20% of diseased patients are women who have negative hysteroscopy evaluations but nonetheless have cancer. These results are called "false-negative" results.
- **Specificity** is the ability of the test to correctly identify patients who do not have a disease. Here, of the women who do not have uterine cancer as determined by pathologic analysis, 90% will have negative hysteroscopy evaluations. Specificity is the percentage of "true-negative" results. The remaining 10% of nondiseased patients are women who have positive hysteroscopy evaluations but who do not have cancer. These results are called "false-positive" results.
- The **criterion** (gold) **standard** is the standard to which the accuracy of the new "index" test was established. The criterion standard represents the "truth," or as close to the truth as current measurements allow.
- **The likelihood ratio for a positive test** combines sensitivity and specificity into a single number relating the likelihood that a patient with the disease will have a positive test to the likelihood that a patient without the disease will have a positive test. A likelihood ratio of 8 indicates that a positive test result is eight times more likely to occur in patients with the disease than in patients without.
- The **prevalence of disease** is the proportion of the population affected by the disease and is a factor in computing the positive and negative predictive values. If the disease prevalence is 90% rather than 10% as indicated above, the positive predictive value will be 98.6%: almost everyone with a positive test will have the disease. However, if the prevalence is only, say, 1%, the positive predictive value will be only 7.5%.
- The **positive predictive value** is the likelihood that a patient with a positive hysteroscopy evaluation will actually have uterine cancer. It is not the same as sensitivity. Sensitivity is not affected by the prevalence of the disease in the population being tested, whereas the positive predictive value is. A positive predictive value of 47% means

Continued

Sample Presentation – *Cont'd.*

that 47 of 100 women with positive hysteroscopy evaluations will likely have cancer.

- **Inter-rater reliability** is the degree of agreement between the hysteroscopists in their judgments of whether there was malignancy, which in this case is an appropriate measure of the *reliability of the test* because the "result" of the test is a judgment. In this case, 82% of the judgments by multiple hysteroscopists on the same subjects are concordant.

PURPOSE OF THE TEST

10.1 Identify the purpose of the test.

The purpose of a diagnostic test is to perform a specific *function* in a specific *population* that is believed to have a specific *condition.* Each of these components should be described.

The *medical condition* or *diagnosis* that the test is intended to detect, to define, or to differentiate should be given, as well as the stage in the progression of the condition for which the test is appropriate (early cancer or late cancer, for example), if applicable. ***(See also Guideline 10.2.)***

The *population* for which the test is appropriate should also be identified with the necessary demographic and diagnostic characteristics. For example, it is important to know whether the test was intended for infants with anemia, adult burn victims, or pregnant women with a comorbid condition.

Diagnostic tests usually have one of five *functions* (2):

- A **screening test** is performed on apparently healthy, asymptomatic people to identify "those who are at sufficient risk of a specific disorder to justify a subsequent diagnostic test or procedure, or in certain circumstances direct preventive action" (3). Blood pressure measurements offered at health fairs are an example of a screening test. A good screening test has high *sensitivity* because it identifies most of the people who have the disease, and perhaps a few who do not.
- A **routine test** is performed as part of a battery of tests and may result in a "case finding," or a positive test that is unrelated to the presenting condition. The "standard blood panel" of tests routinely ordered by a physician as part of a routine physical examination may reveal anemia, for example.

- A **test used to establish a diagnosis** is ordered specifically either to identify a disorder so that therapy may be begun or to rule it out, as when a biopsy of an intestinal polyp reveals whether it is benign or cancerous. A good diagnostic test has high *specificity* because it identifies most of the people who do not have the disease and perhaps a few who do.
- A **staging test** is performed to characterize the nature or extent of a medical condition, such as the degree of metastasis of a cancerous tumor or the degree of regurgitation in an incompetent mitral valve.
- A **monitoring test** is performed to track a patient's progress over time. The blood sugar test used by patients with insulin-dependent diabetes to adjust their dose of insulin is a monitoring test.

How useful is the test? "Just as a duck is not often confused with a yak even in the absence of chromosomal analysis, the ability of a diagnostic test to distinguish between disorders not commonly confused in the first place is scant endorsement for its widespread application . . . . [T]he key value of a diagnostic test often lies in its ability to distinguish between otherwise commonly confused disorders, especially when their prognoses or therapies differ sharply" (2).

10.2 Specify the stage of the condition (disease) for which the test is appropriate.

Some tests differ in their ability to detect early and late forms of disease. This "spectrum effect" (4) or "case mix" (5,6) of diagnostic tests may be explained by three components, which should be considered in specifying the stage of disease:

- A *pathologic component* of severity or extent of disease: for example, metastatic cancer may be more easily detected than a localized lesion.
- A *clinical component* of severity or chronicity of symptoms: for example, an acute episode of disease may be more easily detected than a slowly progressive, chronic disease.
- A *comorbid component* of other diseases, not directly related to the disease under study, that may affect test results.

Knowing the spectrum of the disease over which a test is accurate is important because the true value of a diagnostic test most likely lies in its ability to distinguish between closely related or equivocal cases (2). Thus, a test that detects cancer at an earlier stage is more useful than one that detects it at a later stage.

If appropriate, identify any subgroups for which the test may be particularly effective (6,7). Some diagnostic tests that perform poorly when tested in a population with the full spectrum of a disease may perform well in certain subgroups, in which the spectrum is much narrower.

10.3 Explain the meaning or clinical meaning of a positive test result.

A positive test result indicates an abnormal or undesirable condition, whereas a negative test result indicates a normal or desirable condition. However, the clinical meaning of either a positive or a negative result depends on how "normal" and "abnormal" are defined (**Figure 10.1**).

- A **diagnostic definition** of normal is the range of measurements over which the condition is absent and beyond which the condition is likely to be present. This diagnostic definition of normal is a sound one and is (or should be) based on evidence of the presence or absence of disease in the normal and abnormal ranges, respectively.
- A **therapeutic definition** of normal specifies the range of measurements over which a therapy is not indicated (because it is ineffective or even harmful) and beyond which therapy is beneficial. Again, this definition, when based on evidence of the efficacy of the therapy, is a clinically useful definition.

Other definitions of normal are perhaps less useful for clinical decision-making, although they are unfortunately common:

- A **risk-factor definition** of normal includes the range of measurements over which the risk of disease is not increased and beyond which the risk is increased. This definition assumes that altering the risk factor alters the actual risk of disease. For example, with rare exceptions, a high serum cholesterol level is not dangerous in its own right; it is the increased risk of heart disease associated with a high cholesterol level that makes the level "abnormal."
- The **Gaussian definition** of normal is based on measurements taken from a disease-free population. The normal range is usually defined as the range of measurements extending two standard deviations above and below the mean; that is, the range that includes the central 95% of all the measurements. However, the highest 2.5% and the lowest 2.5% of the scores—the "abnormal" scores—may have no clinical implications; they are simply uncommon scores (8,9). Most blood tests define normal in this way. This definition usually assumes that the test results are normally distributed (that is, that they follow the Gaussian distri-

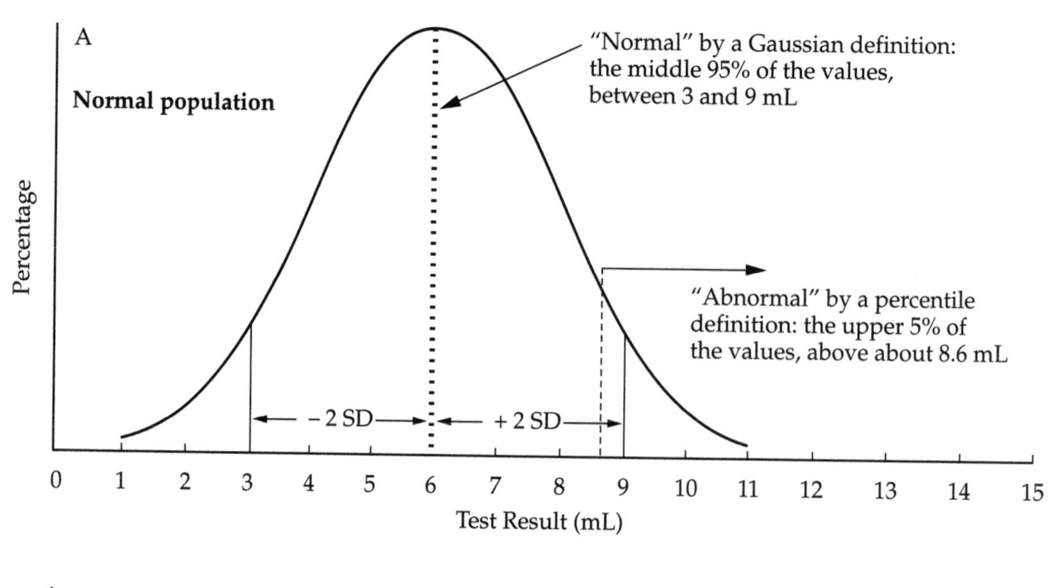

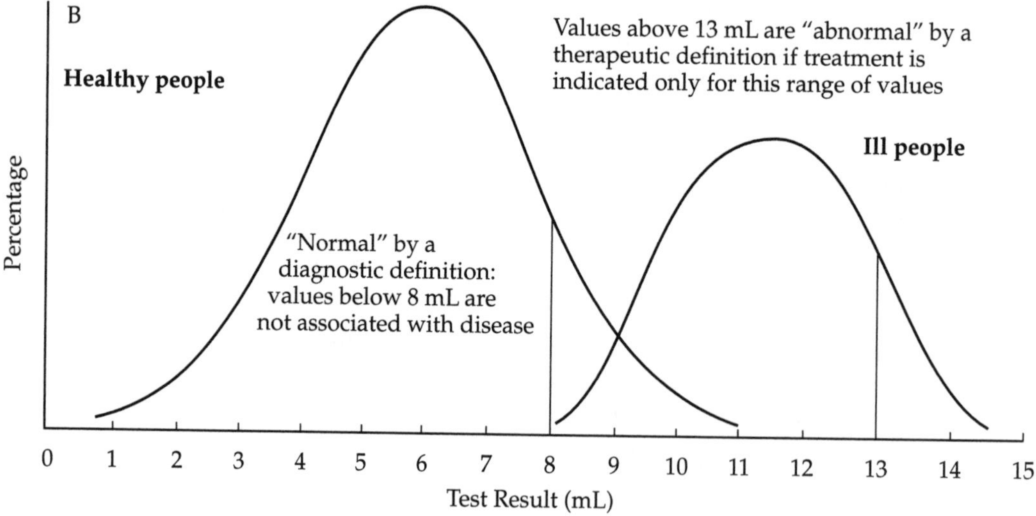

FIGURE 10.1 Illustrations of several definitions of normal. **(A)** Statistical definitions. The **Gaussian definition** is based on a normal distribution and identifies as "normal" the range of values between, usually, two standard deviations above and below the mean (the middle 95% of the values in the distribution). Here, the range between 3 mL and 9 mL would be considered "normal," whereas values beyond the range at either end (2.5% of the values at either end) would be considered "abnormal." A **percentile definition** identifies the lower (or upper) 95% of the range of values as normal; in this case, the range from 0 to 8.6. In this definition, only the upper (or lower) 5% of values would be considered to be "abnormal." **(B)** Clinical definitions. A **diagnostic definition** indicates the probability of disease for a given test result; here, a score below 8 mL indicates that disease is absent. A **therapeutic definition** indicates the usefulness of therapy for a given test result. For example, medical evidence may indicate that medications are appropriate only for patients with values of, say, 13 mL or higher. In other words, for a therapeutic definition, a positive result will change the way a patient is managed.

bution or the bell-shaped curve). Unfortunately, test results are seldom normally distributed (2). Sometimes, however, test scores can be mathematically "transformed" to create a more normal distribution so that the "normal" range can be determined *(see Guidelines 2.14 and 2.15)*. The values of the "normal" range are then transformed back into the original units for clinical applications. This process does not address the underlying problem, however; uncommon scores do not necessarily indicate illness, and normal scores do not necessarily indicate the absence of illness.

- A **percentile definition** of normal expresses the normal range arbitrarily as the lower (or upper) percentage of the total range. For example, any value in the lower 95% of all test results may be defined as normal, and only the upper 5% may be defined as abnormal. Again, there may be no clinical meaning to the definition, only a statistical one.
- A **social definition** of normal is based on popular beliefs about what is and is not normal. Desirable weight, for example, or developmental milestones, such as when a baby's teeth should appear, often have social definitions of "normal" associated with them, which may or may not have valid medical implications.

CHARACTERISTICS OF THE TEST

10.4 Describe the biological principle on which the test is based.

Knowing how the test works will help readers evaluate the validity of the test. The level of detail should be appropriate for the purpose of the study and the needs of the audience.

10.5 Report the validity of the index test that is under study and the reference test to which it was validated.

Validity is the ability of the index test under study to provide accurate measurements, as determined by how closely the results match those of a reference test. The reference test may be another test in common use; ideally, it will be the **criterion standard** (or "gold standard"), which is the test accepted as the definitive measurement of the condition. For example, the results of exercise stress testing can be compared to those of coronary angiography, a reference test that is also the criterion standard for the diagnosis of coronary heart disease.

It is sometimes useful to report the proportion of diseased and disease-free patients identified by the reference test and by the index test.

The accuracy of the reference test should be addressed (5). If the reference test is inaccurate, the estimates of the index test's characteristics will be biased. Reference tests may be markedly inaccurate, even though they are widely used clinically. In addition, many criterion standards may not be clinically available in a study because they can be performed only at autopsy.

The index test result (positive or negative) must be independent of the verification of disease (present or absent) (2,4,5,10–15). Independence is best established with the masked ("blinded") assessment of the test against a criterion standard.

The independence of the index test and the verification against a criterion standard can be affected by at least three biases (5):

- *Work-up* (or *verification) bias* can occur when the result of an earlier diagnostic test affects who will be considered to receive the index test. An earlier negative test result may reduce the likelihood that some patients will receive the index test, whereas an earlier positive test result may increase the likelihood that other patients will receive the index test.
- *Diagnostic review bias* can occur if the results of previous tests are known by those interpreting the index test. For example, if a pulmonary nodule is apparent on a CT scan, an otherwise undetected lesion on a chest roentgenogram may become more obvious (12). Masking can reduce this form of bias during the evaluation phase of test development. But because clinicians are not masked to other tests in the day-to-day course of providing care, masked studies may be unrealistic (7).
- *Incorporation bias* can occur when the diagnosis is established with the results of the index test rather than with the criterion standard. Incorporating the test results into the diagnosis violates the independence of the test and the criterion standard.

10.6 Report the reliability of the test.

Reliability is the ability of the test to produce consistent results. Several factors can affect reliability:

- *Differences in how the test was administered (2).* The results of echocardiography, for example, may vary depending on the skill with which the probe is positioned.
- *Differences in how the test sample was processed.* Different laboratories may

use different procedures, calibrate their equipment differently, use different reagents, and so on.

- *Differences in the conditions under which the patient is tested.* For instance, the results of a blood test may be different at different times during the day, at different stages of a disease, or in different patient populations, such as in women who are or are not pregnant (8,16).
- *Interobserver reliability,* or the degree to which two or more judges differ in their interpretation of the same results, as often occurs in the interpretation of imaging tests, such as roentgenograms, CT scans, or ultrasound charts.
- *Intraobserver reliability,* or the degree to which a single judge varies in interpreting the same result at different times.

EXAMPLES:

- Reliability was 100% for participants with systolic pressures greater than 180 mm Hg and 85% for those with systolic pressures less than 100 mm Hg.
- Interobserver agreement was high (kappa = 0.8).
- Correlation between observations from a single rater on the same images was low (intraclass correlation coefficient = 0.3).

10.7 Explain the meaning of equivocal results and how such results were incorporated into the calculation of the test's characteristics.

Not all tests give clear-cut positive or negative results. Perhaps not all of the barium dye was consumed; perhaps bowel gas interfered with the ultrasound imaging of abdominal structures; perhaps the bronchoscopic biopsy neither ruled out nor confirmed the diagnosis; perhaps observers could not agree on the interpretation of clinical signs. The number and proportion of nonpositive and non-negative results are important because such results affect the clinical usefulness of the test and the need for retesting or additional tests.

Simel and colleagues (17) identify three types of equivocal results:

- **Intermediate results** are those that fall between a negative result and a positive result. In a tissue test based on the presence of cells that stain blue, "bluish" cells that are neither unstained nor the required shade of blue might be considered intermediate results.

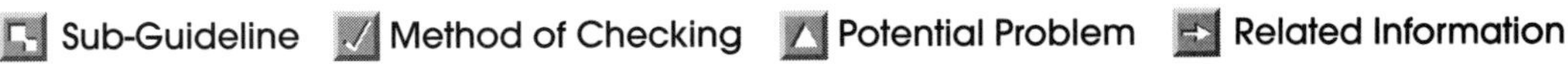

- **Indeterminate results** are results that indicate neither a positive nor a negative finding. A pattern of responses on a psychological inventory may provide no insight into whether the respondent is or is not alcohol-dependent.
- **Uninterpretable results** are produced when a test is not conducted according to specified performance standards. Rectal temperatures obtained from patients not able to remain in a metabolic chamber at 50 °F for the required length of time may be uninterpretable.

How such results were counted when calculating sensitivity and specificity should be reported. These characteristics will vary depending on whether the results are counted as positive or negative or were not counted at all (*see also Guideline 10.8 and Table 10.1*).

TABLE 10.1 Summary of the Characteristics of Diagnostic Tests.*

Test Result	Actual Condition of Population: Patients with Disease	Actual Condition of Population: Patients without Disease	Totals
Positive	a (true-positives) Sensitivity	b (false-positives)	a + b
Negative	c (false-negatives)	d (true-negatives) Specificity	c + d
Totals	a + c	b + d	a + b + c + d

* The formulas assume that the true prevalence of the disease is represented in the sample used to create the table.

Sensitivity = proportion of true positives = a/(a + c). A sensitive test is a good screening test because it identifies most of the people who have the disease, and perhaps a few who do not.

Specificity = proportion of true negatives = d/(b + d). A specific test is a good diagnostic test because it identifies most of the people who do *not* have the disease, and maybe a few who do.

False-positive rate = proportion of false positives = b/(b + d) = 1 – specificity.

False-negative rate = proportion of false negatives = c/(a + c) = 1 – sensitivity.

Prevalence = proportion of population affected with the disease = (a + c)/(a + b + c + d).

Positive predictive value* = the number of diseased patients with positive tests divided by the number of patients with positive tests: (prevalence)(sensitivity)/[(prevalence)(sensitivity) + (1 – prevalence) (1 – specificity)]. If the table reflects the prevalence, then PPV = a/(a + b).

Negative predictive value* = the number of nondiseased patients with negative tests divided by the number of patients with negative tests: (1 – prevalence)(specificity)/[1 – prevalence)(specificity) + (prevalence)(1 – sensitivity)]. If the table reflects the prevalence, then NPV = d/(c + d).

Diagnostic accuracy (efficiency) = proportion of correct results = (a + d)/(a + b + c + d) or: (prevalence)(sensitivity) + (1 – prevalence)(specificity).

Likelihood ratio for a positive test = [a/(a + c)]/[b/(b + d)] = sensitivity/(1 – specificity).

Likelihood ratio for a negative test = [c/(a + c)]/[d/(b + d)] = (1 – sensitivity)/specificity.

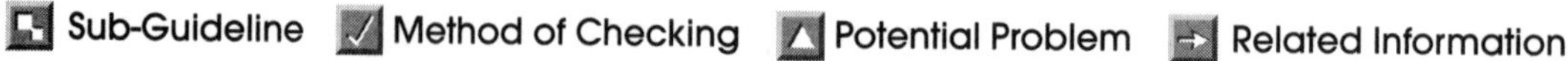

10.8 Report the diagnostic sensitivity and specificity of the test, including the associated (95%) confidence intervals.

The ideal diagnostic test would return a positive result for all patients who have the disorder and a negative result for all patients who do not have the disorder. Few tests are perfect, however; most have some measure of error associated with them (their validity and reliability are less than 100%) and so will return some false-positive and some false-negative results.

In addition, the test results of normal and ill participants often overlap (**Figure 10.2**). When the high values of one distribution overlap the low values of the other, the values in the overlapping region do not discriminate between healthy and ill subjects. Even an accurate test result, then, can lead to a diagnostic error if it occurs in this overlapping region.

The qualities of a test that indicate its diagnostic accuracy are **sensitivity** and **specificity. Table 10.1** shows how these measures are calculated (16,17).

- **Sensitivity** answers the question "If the patient has the disease, how likely is she to have a positive test?" (4). A sensitivity of 90% means that of 100 people with a *verified diagnosis,* the test is likely to detect 90 of them (a true-positive rate of 90%). The remaining 10 negative results are said to be "false-negative" results.
- **Specificity** answers the question: "If the patient does not have the disease, how likely is she to have a negative test?"(4). A specificity of 75% means that of 100 people *proven not to have a disease,* the test is likely to be negative for 75 of them (a true-negative rate of 75%). The remaining 25 positive results are said to be "false-positive" results.

Guideline 10.7: Explain the meaning of equivocal results

Give the rationale for selecting a given cutpoint. There is a trade-off between sensitivity and specificity (**Figure 10.2**). Because the normal and abnormal ranges of values often overlap, a cutpoint in the overlapping range is used to define a "decision threshold" that can be varied to alter the test's sensitivity and specificity.

A sensitive test is a good *screening* test because it identifies most of the people who have the disease, and perhaps a few who do not.

A specific test is a good *diagnostic* test because it identifies most of the people who do *not* have the disease, and perhaps a few who do.

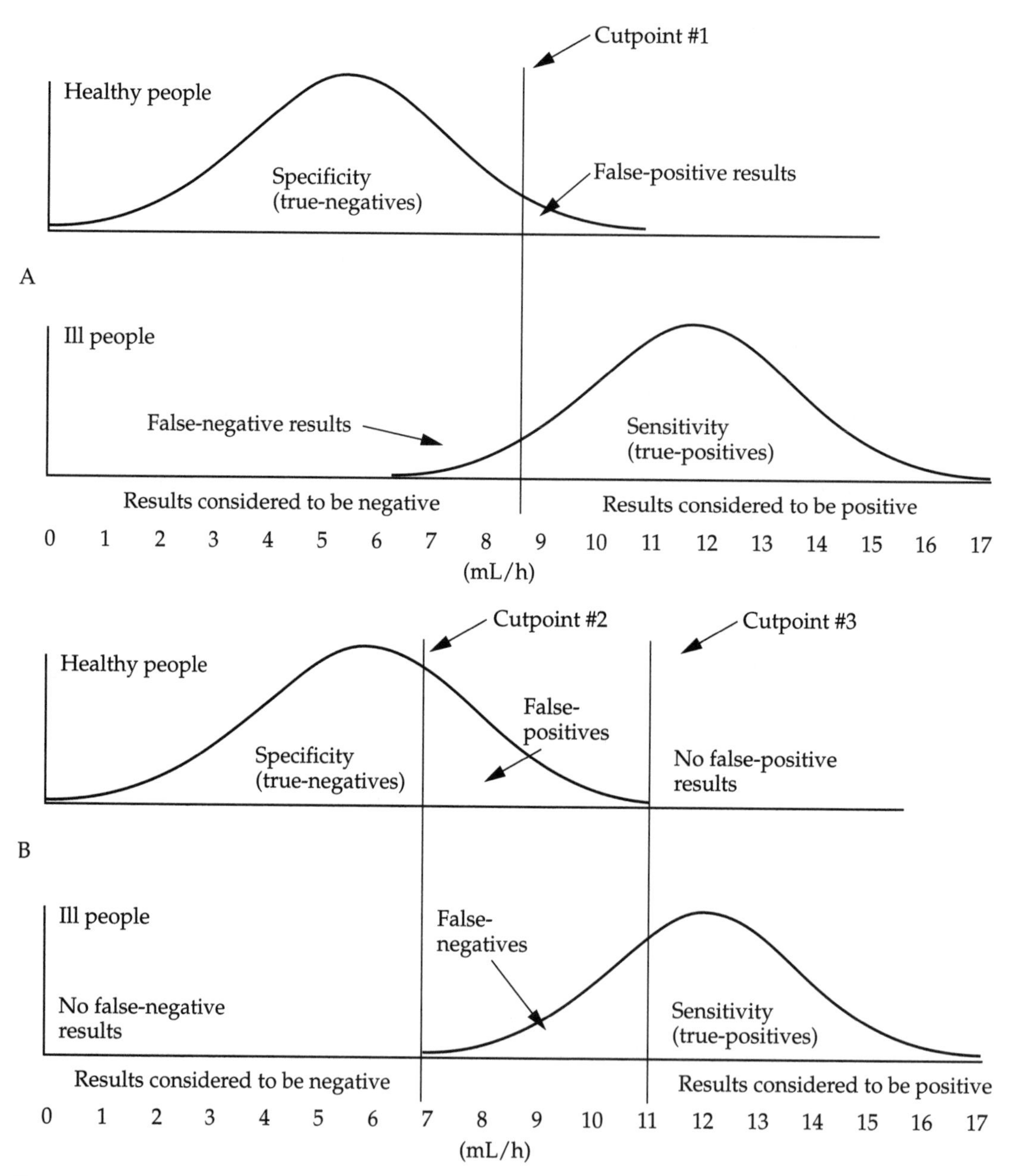

FIGURE 10.2 When, as is often the case, the distributions of values for healthy and diseased patients overlap, the sensitivity and specificity of a test can be varied by moving the decision threshold or "cutpoint" to a new value. Here, the distributions overlap in the range from 7 to 11 mL/h. **(A)** A cut point (#1) in the middle of this range balances the number of false-positive and false-negative results. **(B)** Moving the cutpoint to 7 mL/h (#2) eliminates false-negative results but increases the proportion of false-positive results. Likewise, moving the cutpoint to 11 mL/h (#3) eliminates false-positive results but increases the proportion of false-negative results.

Another characteristic that is sometimes reported with sensitivity and specificity is **diagnostic accuracy** or **diagnostic efficiency (Table 10.1)**. Diagnostic accuracy is the percentage of all correct decisions (the number of true positives and true negatives, divided by the number of all decisions). The accuracy of a test depends on the prevalence of the disease, however. A better but more sophisticated indication of accuracy is provided by the ROC curve (*see Guideline 10.10*), in which the area under the curve indicates the accuracy of the test with different cutpoints (which also change the sensitivity and specificity); that is, the ROC curve is independent of the prevalence of the disease.

10.9 Report the positive and negative likelihood ratios of the test.

Likelihood ratios are another measure of the diagnostic accuracy of a test, and they are becoming increasingly popular for reporting the characteristics of diagnostic tests. The likelihood ratio simply combines in one number the sensitivity and specificity of the test. Thus, the **likelihood ratio for a positive test** is the sensitivity (the proportion of true-positive results) divided by 1 minus the specificity (the proportion of false-positive results; see **Table 10.1**). In other words, the likelihood ratio for a positive test is

$$\frac{\text{the likelihood of a positive result in patients } \textit{with} \text{ disease}}{\text{the likelihood of a positive result in patients } \textit{without} \text{ disease}}$$

For example, if the likelihood ratio of a positive test is 6.2, a positive test result is 6.2 times more likely to occur in a patient with disease than in a patient without disease. The likelihood ratio for a negative test gives the chances that a negative result will be expected in a patient who actually has the disease, as opposed to one who does not.

10.10 When a diagnostic test is an essential part of the research, and when its interpretation depends on a cutpoint on a continuum, illustrate its characteristics with a receiver operating characteristics (ROC) curve.

A useful way to present the characteristics of a diagnostic test is the receiver operating characteristics (ROC) curve **(Figure 10.3).** The ROC curve is a graph in which the Y axis represents sensitivity (the proportion of true-positive results) and the X axis represents 1 minus specificity (or the proportion of false-positive results). As the decision threshold of the test is varied (that is, as the cutpoint that separates healthy patients from ill ones is changed (*see also Guideline 10.8*), the sensitivity and specificity of the test also change. These values are plotted and joined to produce the ROC curve.

An ROC curve that operates no better than chance for detecting disease will lie along the 45-degree line that runs from the intersection of the X and Y axes to the upper right corner of the graph (**Figure 10.3**). Points on this line indicate that the test provides an equal number of true- and false-positives; that is, it does not discriminate between healthy and ill participants. The most accurate ROC curve is one that arches up to the upper left-hand corner of the graph before moving to the upper right corner of the graph (**Figure 10.3**). The best cutpoint for balancing the sensitivity and

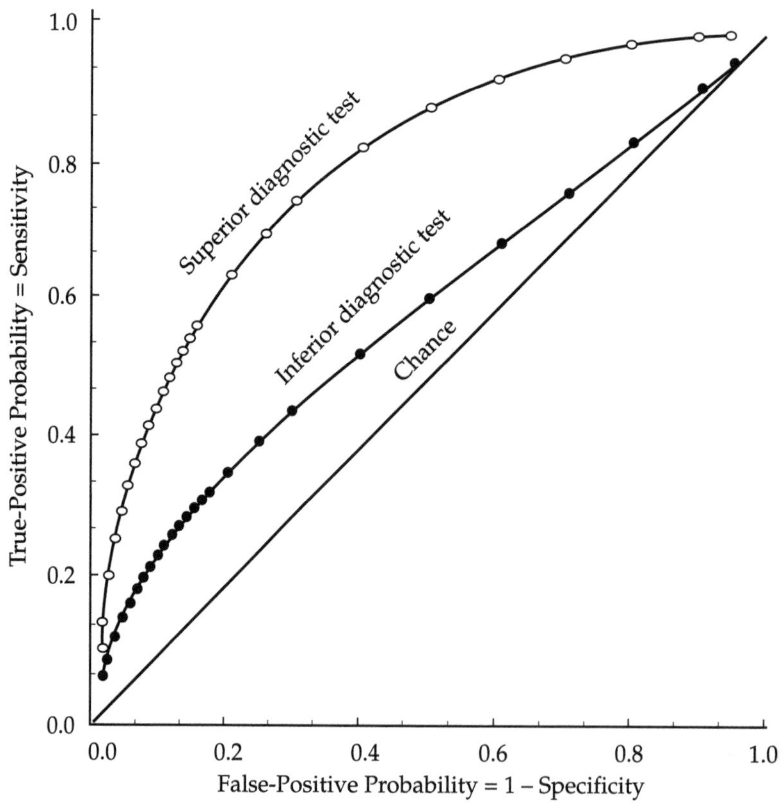

FIGURE 10.3 For tests whose results are expressed as a continuous variable, the receiver operating characteristics (ROC) curve plots the true-positive rate (sensitivity) against the false-positive rate (1 – specificity) over a range of cutpoints. Points along the diagonal indicate results no better than chance. Points closest to the upper left corner indicate the cutpoints that maximize the number of true-positive results and minimize the number of false-positive results. When comparing tests, the test with the largest "area under the ROC curve" is preferred, assuming that the goal is to balance sensitivity and specificity.

specificity of the test is the one represented by the point on the curve closest to the upper left-hand corner.

Both the likelihood ratio (***see Guideline 10.9***) and the ROC curve are derived from the test's sensitivity and specificity ***(see Guideline 10.8).***

✓ **When comparing diagnostic tests in which sensitivity and specificity are considered to be equally important, the test with the largest "area under the ROC curve" is considered to be the more accurate test (see Figure 10.3).**

10.11 When a test is an essential part of the research, report the number and proportion of patients with and without the disease who were tested to determine the specificity and sensitivity.

By convention, the numbers of healthy and ill study participants chosen to establish the sensitivity and specificity of the test are generally equal, which ensures the greatest power of the test (10). Because these proportions are seldom encountered outside of study populations, additional measures—the positive and negative predictive values—are necessary to help interpret the results when the test is applied in clinical practice. Whereas sensitivity and specificity are characteristics of the test itself (when calculated under the conditions described) and do not vary with disease prevalence, the positive and negative predictive values of a test *do* depend on the prevalence of the condition in the population, as well as on its sensitivity and specificity.

→ **Guideline 10.8: Sensitivity and specificity**

CLINICAL APPLICATION OF THE TEST

10.12 Describe how the test is to be administered.

If the test is to be adopted, its administration in clinical practice should be described. Describe, if applicable, the following:

- The protocol for administering the test.
- How the results are to be interpreted.
- How patients are to be prepared for the test (for example, special diets, activity restrictions, medications, fluid requirements).
- What patients may experience during and after the test.

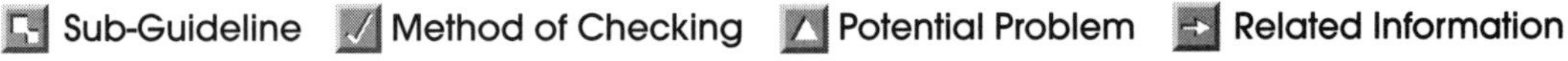
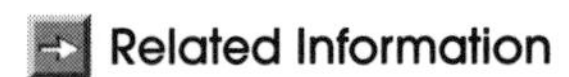

- What precautions need to be taken before, during, and after the test.
- How specimens should be taken, stored, transported, or analyzed.
- What uncertainties remain before, during, and after the test (2).

10.13 Report the positive and negative predictive values of the test, as well as the prevalence of the disease associated with these values.

When determined correctly, sensitivity and specificity *(see Guideline 10.8)* are characteristics of the diagnostic test itself and are independent of the prevalence of the disease. The usefulness of a test result for an individual patient, however, depends on the prevalence of the disease in the population being tested. That is, a positive test result is more likely to be true if the disease is widespread than if the disease is rare: "If you hear hoofbeats, don't expect to see zebras." In other words, although zebras have hooves, the sound of hoofbeats has to be interpreted in light of the fact that horses are more common than zebras. The probability that the hoofbeats belong to horses is therefore far higher than the probability that they belong to zebras. Disease prevalence can be combined with sensitivity and specificity to create two other useful measures of diagnostic accuracy: the positive and negative predictive values (**Tables 10.1** and **10.2**).

TABLE 10.2 **Positive and Negative Predictive Values for a Diagnostic Test with a Sensitivity of 80% and a Specificity of 90% for Various Prevalence Rates (the "Pre-test Probability" That a Given Patient Will Have the Disease).**

	Pre-test Probability of Disease (Prevalence)			
Characteristic	**1%**	**10%**	**50%**	**90%**
Positive Predictive Value (%)*	7.5	47.1	88.9	98.6
Negative Predictive Value (%)†	99.8	97.6	81.8	33.3
Diagnostic Accuracy (%)	89.9	89.0	85.0	81.0

* When disease prevalence is 1%, only 7 or 8 of 100 (7.5%) patients with a positive test result will likely have the disease; the rest will have false-positive results. When disease prevalence is 90%, 98 or 99 of 100 (98.6%) patients will likely have the disease.

† When disease prevalence is 1%, it is likely that all 100 (99.8%) patients with a negative test result will likely be disease-free; there will be few if any false-negatives. When disease prevalence is 90%, however, only 34 of 100 (33.3%) patients with negative results will likely be disease-free, and the rest will have false-negative results.

- The **positive predictive value** (or accuracy for positive prediction) answers the question "If the patient has a positive test, how likely is he or she to have the disease?" A high positive predictive value is desirable for detecting the presence of disease. A positive predictive value of 83% means that 83 of 100 patients who test positive will likely have the disease.
- The **negative predictive value** (or accuracy for negative prediction) answers the question "If the patient has a negative test, how likely is he or she *not* to have the disease?" A high negative predictive value is desirable for ruling out the presence of disease. A negative predictive value of 94% means that 94 of 100 women testing negative will likely not have the disease.

A useful way to report the predictive values of the test is shown in **Figure 10.4** (18). In this figure, predictive value is plotted against the prevalence of the disease, and the sensitivity and specificity are reflected in the shape of the two curves for the positive and negative predictive values. Clinicians can then estimate the predictive values using the prevalence figure for their patients.

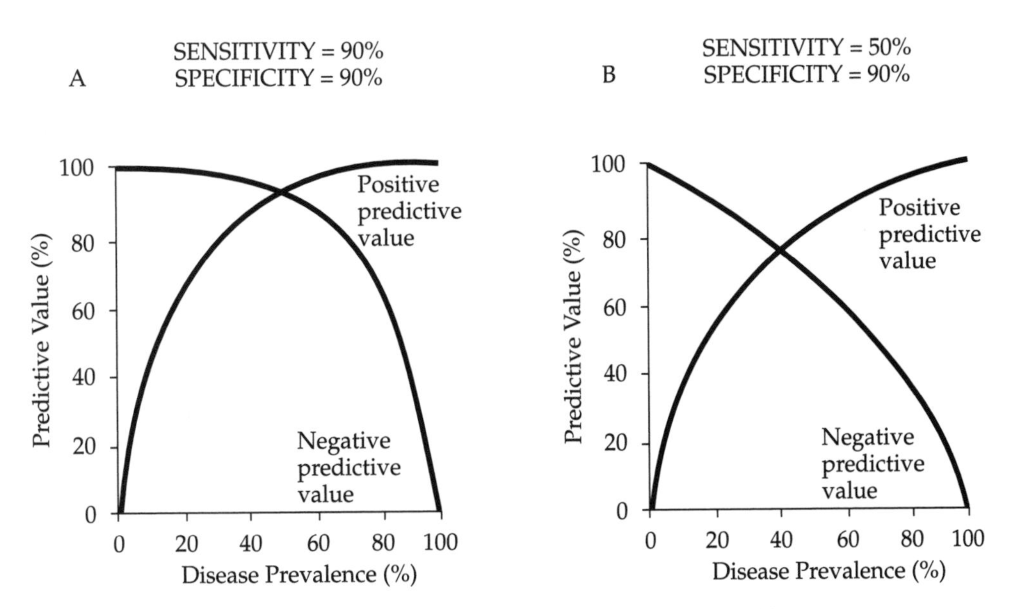

FIGURE 10.4 A graph for reporting the characteristics of diagnostic tests. In clinical practice, the predictive values of a test may be more useful than its sensitivity and specificity. (**A**) A test with a sensitivity of 90% and a specificity of 90%. (**B**) A test with a sensitivity of 50% and a specificity of 90%. (Reprinted with permission from Eisenberg MJ. Accuracy and predictive values in clinical decision-making. Cleve Clin J Med. 1995; 62[5]:311-6.)

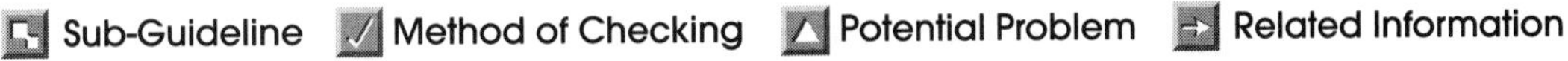

Predictive values are often computed with the use of **Bayes' theorem**. This theorem is an equation giving the relationships between a "prior (or pre-test) probability," a "conditional probability," and a "posterior (or post-test) probability." In simple terms, Bayes' theorem uses new information (the conditional probability) to update old information (the prior probability). The updated result is called the posterior probability, or, in this case, the predictive values (***see also Chapter 14***).

- The **prior** (or **pre-test**) **probability of the disease** may be simply the prevalence of the disease; in other words, the probability that a patient selected at random will have the disease. However, it may also include other information that has raised the "index of suspicion" about a particular diagnosis.
- The **conditional probability** is the probability that, in this case, a diagnostic test will return a certain result under specified conditions. Two such "specified conditions," or conditional probabilities, are expressed in the likelihood ratio ***(see Guideline 10.9)***. In the likelihood ratio of a positive test, the conditional probability expressed in the numerator is the likelihood of a *positive* test in patients *with* the disease; in other words, the sensitivity of the test. The conditional probability expressed in the denominator is the likelihood of a *positive* result among patients *without* the disease, which is equal to 1 minus the specificity of the test (**Table 10.1**).
- The **posterior** (or **post-test**) **probability of the disease** is the probability that a patient will have the disease if the prevalence and the results of the diagnostic test are known: the positive or negative predictive values of the test.

> **EXAMPLE:** If the pretest probability of disease (say, the prevalence of the disease in a population routinely screened for the disease) is 0.1 (10%), and the likelihood ratio of a positive test is 20 (meaning that a positive test is 20 times more likely to occur in a patient with the disease than in one without), then the post-test probability of disease for a positive test result will be about 0.7 (70%). So, in this case, in the population screened, a patient with a positive test result will have a 70% chance of having the disease. This result can easily be determined with a nomogram (**Figure 10.5**) (1,20).

A useful diagnostic test has a high conditional probability (a high likelihood ratio) and thus markedly alters the "post-test probability" of having the disease.

FIGURE 10.5 A nomogram allows the positive and negative predictive values (the post-test probabilities of disease) to be determined from the likelihood ratios of the test and the prevalence of the disease in the population (the pre-test probability of disease). (Reprinted with permission from Fagan TJ. Nomogram for Bayes' theorem [letter]. N Engl J Med. 1975; 293:257. Copyright 1975, Massachusetts Medical Society.)

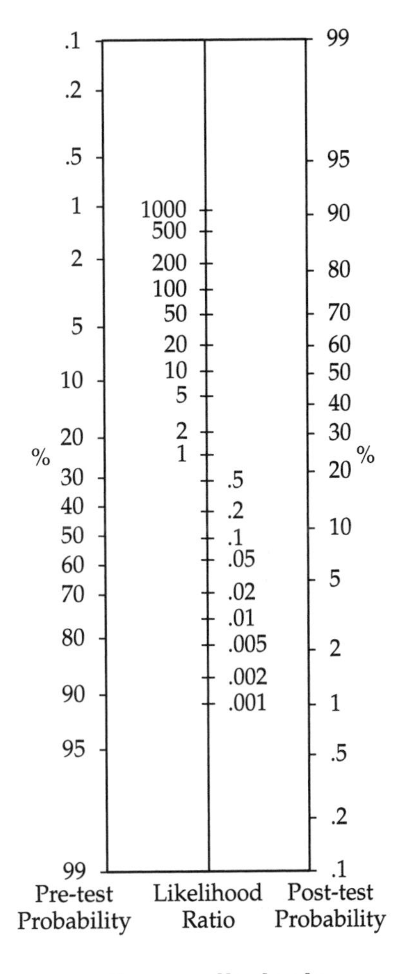

10.14 When reporting the use of two or more diagnostic tests in combination, indicate the order in which the tests were given, the characteristics of each, and the contribution of each test to the final result.

Tests with different degrees of sensitivity and specificity can be used simultaneously or sequentially to enhance their diagnostic utility, to save money, or both. In fact, tests are more often used in sequence than in isolation (5). In such cases, a diagram showing the relationships and characteristics of the tests is desirable (**Figure 10.6**).

Chapter 13. Reporting Decision Analyses and Clinical Practice Guidelines

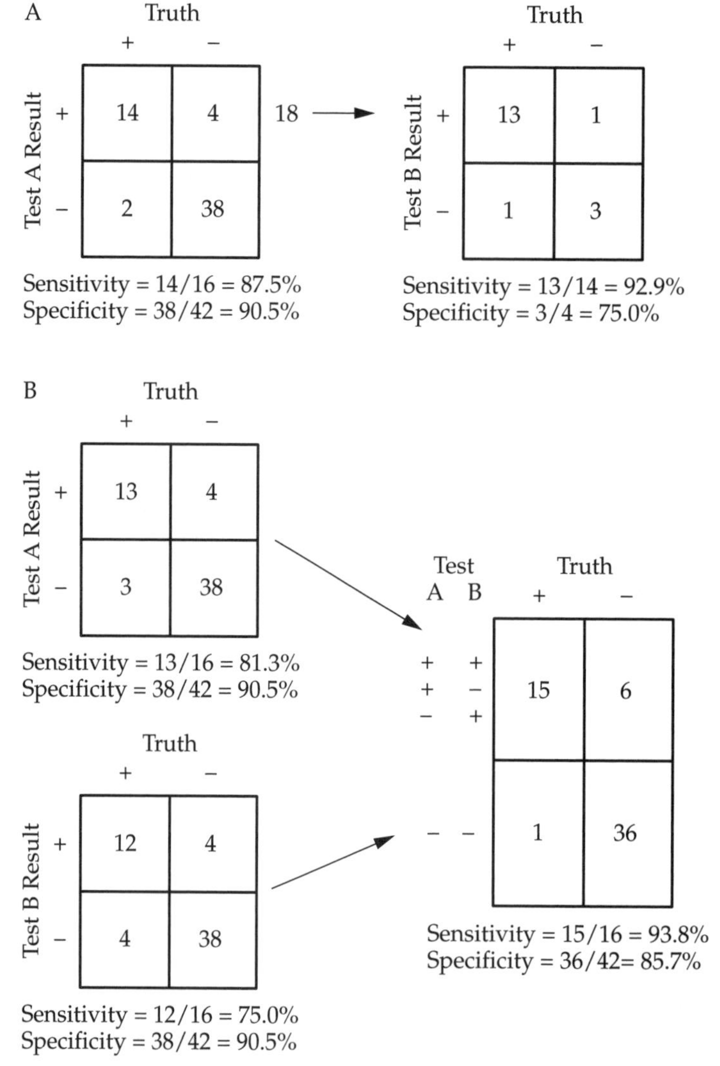

FIGURE 10.6 Diagnostic tests can be run sequentially (**A**) or simultaneously (**B**) to increase the utility of the test, reduce the costs of testing, or both. The contribution of each test to the final determination should be specified. Here, the sample reflects a 30% prevalence of disease. In **A**, the 18 patients who tested positive with Test A are tested again with Test B, which increases the sensitivity from about 88% to about 93%. In **B**, two tests are run concurrently, and all patients with a positive result on either test are considered to be positive, thus increasing the sensitivity compared with either of the two component tests alone.

CONSIDERATIONS IN ADOPTING THE TEST

If the focus of the article is to promote the adoption of a test, the guidelines below should be addressed (*see also Chapter 12*).

10.15 Present other pertinent information about the test.

A great many diagnostic tests are adopted prematurely because they have not been adequately evaluated. Tests that have proven valuable in each of the five phases described below are more likely to be clinically valuable than those that have not (20):

Phase 1: The test accurately and reliably identifies cases of obvious pathology under closely controlled conditions.

Phase 2: The test accurately and reliably differentiates between healthy controls and patients with a narrow, well-defined spectrum of disease.

Phase 3: The test accurately and reliably differentiates between healthy controls and patients with a broader spectrum of disease, including less typical and less severe presentations.

Phase 4: The test accurately and reliably differentiates between more heterogeneous groups of controls and patients. In particular, patients with comorbidities should be included in each group. These comorbidities should include diseases or conditions most likely to be confused with the diagnosis of interest and those that may interfere with the test or whose treatment may interfere with the test.

Phase 5: The test accurately and reliably differentiates the disease among patients who would be encountered in a typical clinical setting. In such a study, the sample would include consecutive patients with the full spectrum of disease, without the disease, with and without comorbidities, and for whom the test would most likely be ordered.

It is also useful to know the impact of the test on patient management and on the course of the disease (5,21).

The effectiveness of the test may change over time with technological improvements or with increased experience of operators (5).

10.16 Describe the human, financial, and physical resources necessary to offer the test in a given setting.

The increasing sophistication of medical technology means that the ability to offer a test may require more resources than is immediately apparent.

- Required **human resources** may include skilled operators, qualified maintenance and repair technicians, and trained clinical support personnel.
- Required **financial resources** may include those needed to cover: acquisition costs, maintenance costs, overhead costs, materials costs, operating costs, training costs, insurance costs, and replacement costs.

- Required **physical resources** may include laboratory space, computing and data management capacity, and environmentally controlled space.

10.17 Describe the medical costs and benefits of adopting the test.

The medical implications of a test may include its

- Diagnostic validity
- Invasiveness
- Potential for causing or preventing adverse reactions
- Potential for requiring or preventing hospitalization
- Potential for delaying care until the results are known
- Effect on health care delivery if conditions are diagnosed at increasing rates
- Impact on patients misdiagnosed or misclassified as a result of the test

10.18 Describe the financial costs and benefits of adopting the test.

Although tests that provide earlier, more accurate diagnoses improve the ability to provide better care, they can also alter the financial implications of care. Financial implications may include the following:

- Per-patient and total costs of administering the test
- Changes in who pays for the test
- Cost of procedures necessitated or avoided by implementing the test
- Money saved in replacing a more expensive test
- Elimination of intermediate tests with their associated costs
- Impact of test failures

10.19 Describe how the test compares with similar tests.

The comparative advantages of the new test over alternative tests should be discussed. The important question is "What makes the test better than the criterion standard?" (2). Tests can be compared based on their

- Accuracy (compare the ROC curves if possible [5])
- Reliability
- Ease of administration
- Cost of administration
- Impact on patients (invasiveness, discomfort, convenience)

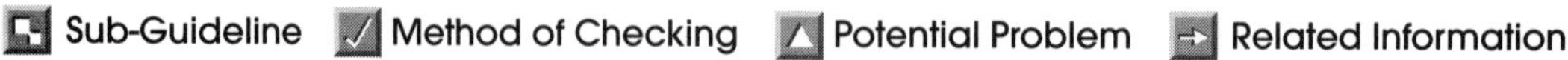

REFERENCES

1. **Jaeschke R, Guyatt GH, Sackett DL.** Users' guides to the medical literature. III. How to use an article about a diagnostic test. B. What are the results and will they help me in caring for my patients? The Evidence-Based Medicine Working Group. JAMA. 1994;271(9):703-7.
2. **Haynes RB.** How to read clinical journals: II. To learn about a diagnostic test. Can Med Assoc J. 1981;124(6):703-10.
3. **Wald N, Cuckle H.** Reporting the assessment of screening and diagnostic tests. Br J Obstet Gynaecol. 1989;96(4):389-96.
4. **Ransohoff DF, Feinstein AR.** Problems of spectrum and bias in evaluating the efficacy of diagnostic tests. N Engl J Med. 1978;299 (17):926-30.
5. **Begg CB.** Biases in the assessment of diagnostic tests. Stat Med. 1987;6(4):411-23.
6. **Begg CB, Pocock SJ, Freedman L, Zelen M.** State of the art in comparative cancer clinical trials. Cancer. 1987;60(11):2811-5.
7. **Reid MC, Lachs MS, Feinstein AR.** Use of methodologic standards in diagnostic test research. JAMA. 1995;274(8):645-51.
8. **Griner PF, Mayewski RJ, Mushlin AI, Greenland P.** Selection and interpretation of diagnostic tests and procedures. Principles and applications. Ann Intern Med. 1981;94 (4 part 2):557-92.
9. **Diamond GA, Forrester JS.** Clinical trials and statistical verdicts: probable grounds for appeal. Ann Intern Med. 1983;98(3): 385-94.
10. **Metz CE.** Basic principles of ROC analysis. Semin Nucl Med. 1978;8(4):283-98.
11. **Cooper LS, Chalmers TC, McAlly M, Berrier J, Sacks HS.** The poor quality of early evaluations of magnetic resonance imaging. JAMA. 1988;259:3277-80.
12. **Jaeschke R, Guyatt GH, Sackett DL.** Users' guides to the medical literature. III. How to use an article about a diagnostic test. The Evidence-Based Medicine Working Group. A. Are the results of the study valid? JAMA. 1994;271(4):389-91.
13. **Sox HC Jr.** Probability theory in the use of diagnostic tests. An introduction to critical study of the literature. Ann Intern Med. 1986;104(1):60-6.
14. **Sheps SB, Schechter MT.** The assessment of diagnostic tests. A survey of current medical research. JAMA. 1984;252(17):2418-22.
15. **Arroll B, Schecter MT, Sheps SB.** The assessment of diagnostic tests: a comparison of medical literature in 1982 and 1985. J Gen Intern Med. 1988;3:443-7.
16. **Riegelman RK, Hirsch RP.** Studying a Study and Testing a Test. 2nd ed. Boston: Little, Brown and Company; 1989.
17. **Simel DL, Feussner JR, Delong ER, Matchar DB.** Intermediate, indeterminate, and uninterpretable diagnostic test results. Med Decis Making. 1987;7(2):107-14.
18. **Eisenberg MJ.** Accuracy and predictive values in clinical decisison-making. Cleve Clin J Med. 1995;62(5):311-6.
19. **Sackett DL.** Interpretation of diagnostic data: 5. How to do it with simple math. Can Med Assoc J. 1983;129(9):947-54.
20. **Nierenberg AA, Feinstein AR.** How to evaluate a diagnostic marker test. JAMA. 1988; 259(11):1699-1702.
21. **Guyatt GH, Tugwell PX, Feeny DH, Haynes RB, Drummond M.** A framework for clinical evaluation of diagnostic technologies. Can Med Assoc J. 1986;134:587-94.

Chapter 11

Combining the Results of Several Studies

Reporting the Results of Meta-Analyses

Meta-analysis provides a logical framework to a research review: similar measures from comparable studies are listed systematically and the available effect measures are combined where possible.

K. Dickersin and J.A. Berline (1)

"Meta-analyses are studies of studies . . ."(2). Sometimes called "statistical overviews" or "systematic reviews," meta-analyses resemble traditional narrative review articles in that they are based on thorough reviews of the literature about a single topic. Meta-analyses differ from review articles in that they statistically combine the results of several studies into a single outcome measure. By combining the samples of the individual studies, a meta-analysis greatly increases the overall sample size, which increases the statistical power of the analysis as well as the precision of the estimate of the treatment effects. Because the "data" for meta-analyses usually come from articles published in scientific journals, the quality of meta-analyses depends heavily on the quality of these studies, how well their findings are reported, and how they come to the attention of the meta-analyst.

Meta-analysis is not without controversy. The issues include the wisdom of combining studies that differ in important respects, such as study populations, experimental designs, and quality controls; the existence of "publication bias," or the fact that studies with positive treatment effects are more likely to be published than those finding no treatment effect; and the fact that, in some cases, the results of meta-analyses and large, randomized controlled trials—the so-called "mega-trials"—on the same topic have been contradictory (3). (For a discussion of the controversy, see the entire issue of the *Journal of Clinical Epidemiology*, 1995;48[1]).

The guidelines below are listed more or less in the order in which they might appear under each heading of a scientific article that reports the results of a meta-analysis.

GUIDELINES ADDRESSED IN THE INTRODUCTION

11.1 State the purpose of the study. Identify the relationship that was studied and the reasons for studying it.

As in all scientific research, the purpose of the study should be clearly defined. In addition to the usual requirements that the study be concerned with a topic of clinical importance and be biologically plausible, meta-analyses may have several purposes:

- To summarize a large and complex body of literature on a topic
- To resolve conflicting reports in the literature
- To clarify or quantify the strengths and weaknesses of studies on a topic
- To document the need for a major clinical trial
- To avoid the time and expense of conducting a clinical trial
- To increase statistical power by combining many smaller studies
- To improve the precision of an estimated treatment effect
- To detect smaller treatment effects than have been reported
- To investigate variations in treatment effects through subgroup (or stratified) analysis
- To improve the generalizability of known treatment effects

11.2 Describe the population(s) studied and to which the results are to be generalized.

Because meta-analyses combine the results of many different studies, the populations involved may be many and diverse. Populations may be identified primarily by diagnosis (for example, patients with symptomatic coronary heart disease), by demographic variables (working class men older than 50 years of age), or by treatment (patients undergoing coronary angioplasty). However, there is often a trade-off between combining heterogeneous populations to improve the generalizability of the results (at the expense of variability) and combining more homogeneous populations to reduce the variability in the results (at the expense of generalizability).

GUIDELINES ADDRESSED IN THE METHODS

11.3 State whether the research was guided by a written protocol.

A written protocol helps reduce bias in the many judgments that must be made when conducting a meta-analysis. The protocol should address all the issues raised in this section, but especially those for the following:

- Searching for the studies to be considered in the analysis
- Including or excluding studies from the analysis
- Extracting data from the studies
- Analyzing the data statistically

It is also appropriate to include a statement in the Results section confirming that the protocol was followed closely during the study.

11.4 Provide operational definitions for the explanatory and response variables (the outcomes or endpoints).

Operational definitions describe variables in observable, measurable terms. Such definitions are even more important in meta-analyses because different definitions of the same variable may not be suitable for combining. For example, one study on lowering serum cholesterol may define its outcome measure as total serum cholesterol, whereas another may use the ratio of high-density lipoprotein to low-density lipoprotein. It may be unwise to combine studies with different operational definitions of the same variables.

11.5 Report the minimum difference in the response variable that is considered to be clinically important.

Specifying the nature of a clinically important finding before the study begins helps to avoid bias in interpreting the results and keeps the research focused on clinical importance, as opposed to statistical significance.

11.6 Report the period of time covered by the literature search.

Reporting the time period during which the desired studies are to have taken place puts the meta-analysis in perspective with developments in medicine that may precede, coincide with, or follow the meta-analysis. Reporting the time period is also necessary to allow other investigators to replicate the meta-analysis.

11.7 Describe in detail the information sources and search strategies used to find the studies to be analyzed.

The "subjects" or "units of observation" studied in a meta-analysis consist of accounts of research studies on identical or similar topics. It is essential to identify as many of these accounts as possible so that the "sample" used in the meta-analysis will be as large and as representative of the total "population" of these studies as possible. An incomplete search can introduce "selection bias" into the meta-analysis by failing to identify important studies.

The key to avoiding selection bias in meta-analysis is to search thoroughly and systematically. Several search strategies are better than one. Typical search strategies include the following:

- Key-word searches of computerized databases, such as MEDLINE; *these index terms should be reported in the published meta-analysis* (4). Indicate the databases searched, the dates covered by the search, and whether the search was conducted by a professional medical librarian.
- Cross-checking citations to appropriate studies, either through reviewing the bibliographies of published articles already identified or through indexing and citation services, such as the Science Citation Index.
- Surveying investigators, government funding agencies, and pharmaceutical companies for information on studies, published or unpublished.
- Searching registries of pertinent studies, such as the Oxford Database of Perinatal Trials.

Typical issues raised in the search are:

- Should reports in languages other than English be included?(5)
- Should unpublished data that have not undergone peer review, including dissertations and conference presentations, be included in the analysis? (2,6–8)
- Should proprietary studies, such as those conducted by pharmaceutical companies, be solicited?

Computer literature searches should not be the only strategy used to identify studies (1,5). Even trained medical librarians have failed to identify a large percentage of published studies on a topic, suggesting the existence of important indexing errors or indexing variability (7). For example, a MEDLINE search by a trained librarian identified only 29% of trials on neonatal hyperbilirubinemia and only 56% of the trials on intraventricular hemorrhage listed in the Oxford Database of Perinatal Trials.

Another study found that consistency between indexers was only 45% to 50% (1,7). Yet another study identified more than *30 000* published controlled trials that had not been appropriately indexed in MEDLINE. (These trials have since been indexed appropriately [9].)

Many trials produce multiple publications. Different publications from large trials are often written by a different set of authors and may not reference the source study, which can result in the same trial being represented in the meta-analysis more than once (7).

Abstracts do not usually contain enough information to be useful in meta-analysis. Abstracts may confirm the existence of published or unpublished studies, however (7).

11.8 State the measures taken to reduce and identify publication bias.

Publication bias refers to the fact that studies with statistically significant results are more likely to be published than those without statistically significant results (10). Because meta-analyses are usually based on published reports, the potential under-representation of negative studies in the literature is a major concern (8). The wisdom of including unpublished data, however, is contested (1,2). Unpublished studies have not undergone formal peer review, and the fact that the study was not submitted for publication raises questions about the quality of the work.

One common way to adjust for publication bias is to compute the number of negative trials that would be needed to invalidate the results of the meta-analysis—the "fail-safe N" method proposed by Rosenthal (1,5,7,8,11,12). If the number is larger than the probable number of unidentified negative trials, the results can be accepted with more confidence. For example, in a study of 345 published trials, Rosenthal calculated that 65123 unpublished studies with negative results would be required to negate the combined statistical significance of the 345 published studies (11).

A useful technique for identifying possible publication bias in larger meta-analyses is the funnel plot (**Figure 11.1**) (1,5,7). Assuming that the results of individual published trials will cluster around the "true" result, a scatter plot of the effect size versus the sample size of the individual studies should be symmetrical about the "true" result, with smaller studies showing more variation than larger ones. If studies showing negative results are missing from the plot, the scatter will be asymmetrical, indicating the possibility of publication bias.

Still another way to adjust for publication bias is to analyze large stud-

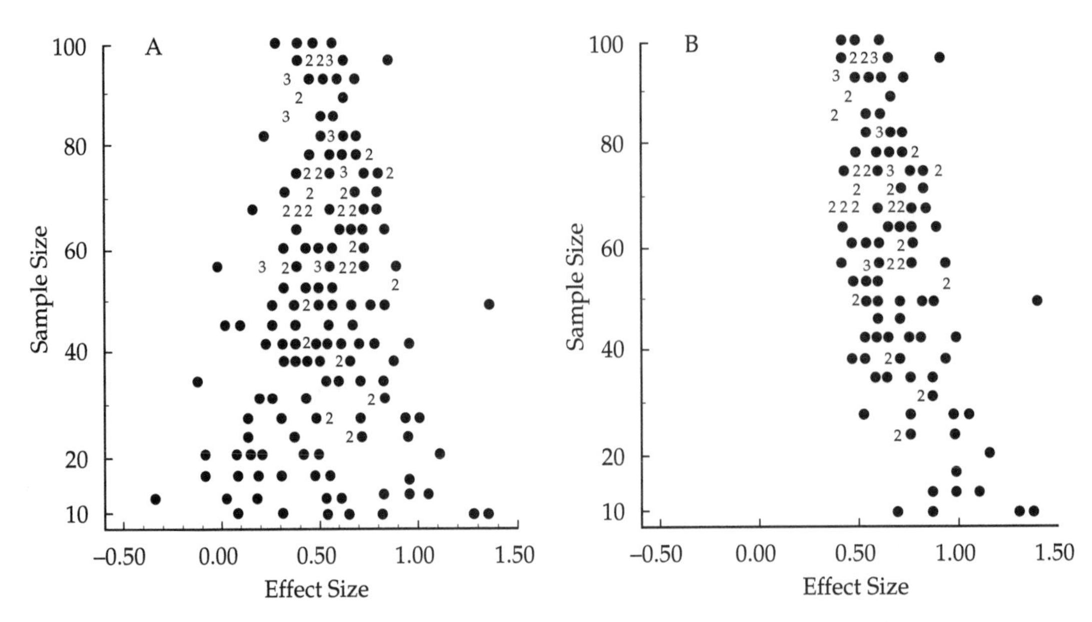

FIGURE 11.1 A funnel plot used to assess publication bias. **A,** All studies. **B,** Published studies. The lack of published studies reporting nonsignificant findings in small studies may indicate such a bias. (Reprinted with permission from Light RJ, Pillemer DB. Summing Up: The Science of Reviewing Research. Cambridge, MA: Harvard University Press; 1984:888. Copyright © 1984 by the President and Fellows of Harvard College. [Adapted from Klitgaard, Dadabhoy, and Litkouhi; "Cognitive equality and educational policies: an example from Pakistan," Pakistan Developmental Review; 18:79-88, 1979].)

ies separately from smaller ones, in the belief that large studies are less likely to be affected by publication bias than small studies; that is, larger studies are more likely to be reported whether or not they have positive results (5,7).

Publication bias may work both ways. Reports of adverse drug reactions or of environmental toxins (such as asbestos), for example, may be more likely to be published if the results are *not* statistically significant (5,7). Similarly, articles that challenge long-standing beliefs or that are otherwise newsworthy may also be published primarily for these reasons. Also, ". . . publication bias may be a function not just of statistical significance but of the ebb and flow of editorial and consensus opinion" (7).

11.9 Report the criteria used for including or excluding studies from the meta-analysis.

The issue here is whether the studies chosen are suitable for combining in a meta-analysis (1,2,11,13). Although meta-analysis has been criticized for comparing "apples and oranges and the occasional lemon" (14) the differences among studies are also what make the findings of meta-analysis more robust: if similar results are obtained under many different conditions, they are more likely to reflect real biological relationships and not artifacts or chance.

Inclusion and exclusion criteria should be as specific as possible so that only compatible, relevant studies of suitable quality are compared. The studies compared must be similar in several important respects (2):

- The studies should test the same hypothesis (6) and should therefore have the same outcome or endpoint (8).
- The studies should compare similar patients (for example, similar in age, sex, diagnosis, state of disease, or comorbidities) or similar interventions (5,6). A study that tests a drug against a placebo should not be compared with one that tests it against a competing drug, for example.
- The trials should meet a minimum standard of scientific quality. Such standards may include the following: an adequate sample size, random assignment between treatment and control groups, masking of patients and caregivers (that is, a "double-blind" trial), quality controls on data collection and management, and formal statistical analyses.

Selection bias is the main reason for discrepant results among meta-analyses (7). Reporting specific inclusion and exclusion criteria will aid researchers in comparing the results of meta-analyses.

A meta-analysis may legitimately address issues other than the primary comparisons in the individual studies (5). For example, the primary comparison of a single study might be to test the efficacy of a drug, whereas the purpose of the meta-analysis is to test for the likelihood of adverse reactions in a particular subgroup of patients.

Occasionally, a source study will describe several comparisons in the Methods section but report only those that were statistically significant. Such studies may need to be excluded from a meta-analysis (7).

11.10 Describe the criteria used in extracting the data from the studies. Include a measure of inter-extracter reliability to establish the consistency of extraction.

Describe the "who, what, and how" of the extraction process. Ideally, the extraction criteria will have been specified in advance on a "data extraction sheet." The accuracy of extraction is then often measured by

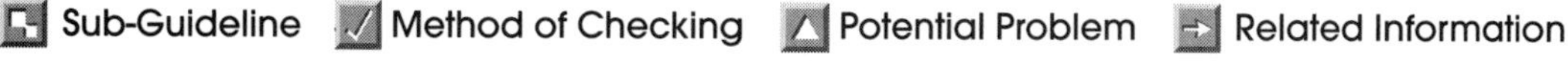

having two or more reviewers extract data from the same articles and comparing the results for agreement. Extracting data may also involve calculating new measures from the data reported (7).

Data extraction is often a subjective and tedious process. Extraction criteria that are too general allow data extractors more freedom of interpretation, which may introduce bias into the process.

11.11 Describe the statistical analyses used to analyze the data.

In meta-analysis, each study's results are combined statistically with those of other studies, a feature that makes meta-analysis different from narrative review articles. Because differences in statistical methods can result in different results, the method must be reported.

The specific statistical method used depends on several factors, such as the hypothesis being studied and the nature of the response variable. Most methods, however, estimate an "effect size," which combines the differences and standard deviations of the response variable into standardized units across studies. Often, an odds ratio is used for each study. These estimates, and sometimes the study results on which they are based, are then combined in some way to yield an overall result.

The statistical methods may also involve one of two types of models, which should also be reported. A **fixed-effects model** makes more assumptions about the variability in the analysis and may be a better summary of the effects reported in the individual studies of the meta-analysis. A **random-effects model** makes fewer assumptions about the variability in the analysis and so is more conservative. This type of model, however, is sometimes better suited for generalizing the results to other settings.

Beware of the "head counting" or "vote counting" approach in which the highest number of "positive" or "negative" studies determines the results of the analysis (11,13–15). In the most simplistic terms, all studies have one of three outcomes: significant positive effects, significant negative effects, or nonsignificant effects. Simply tallying the number of studies in each category to determine the "winner" is easy but potentially misleading. Such an approach ignores the effects of sample size, research design, alpha level, and effect size on the final conclusion, and it does not adequately account for the existence of trials with conflicting results.

Beware of the process of simply combining significance tests (11). A second quick way to summarize the results in a meta-analysis is to mathematically combine only the P values of each of the studies into a single P

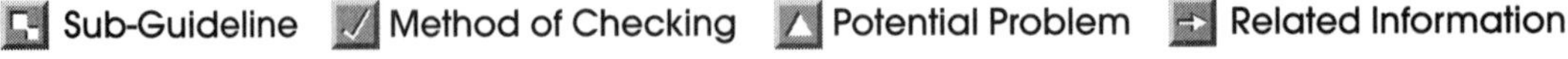

value for the meta-analysis. Such an approach does not consider the distribution of outcomes across all studies, so one study may have a disproportionate effect on the final calculation. Also, this method is based entirely on *P* values, and nonsignificant studies (studies with *P* values greater than, say, 0.05) are published less often, making this method prone to publication bias.

GUIDELINES ADDRESSED IN THE RESULTS

11.12 Provide a summary measure, with a confidence interval, of the estimated size and direction of the effect of the treatment.

The most common measure used to report the results of meta-analyses is the odds ratio (16). In meta-analyses, the odds ratio refers to the likelihood (actually, the odds) of an outcome occurring in the treatment group divided by the likelihood (actually, the odds) that the outcome will occur in the control group (***see also Guideline** 7.25*). Thus, an odds ratio greater than 1 indicates increased risk in the treatment group; less than 1, a decreased risk in the treatment group. A ratio of 1 indicates no difference in risk; that is, that the treatment is neither harmful nor protective; it is just as likely to occur in the treatment group as it is in the control group.

Another common measure used to report the results of meta-analyses is the "pooled estimate of the risk difference," or the percent reduction in risk (5).

11.13 Summarize the results of the individual studies and of the meta-analysis in a graph or a table.

The typical graph of a meta-analysis is a plot of the odds ratio and its 95% confidence interval of each study included in the analysis (**Figure 11.2**). The studies may be arranged in several ways to reveal certain features of the findings:

- By publication date
- By sample size
- By the quality of the study
- By the duration of treatment
- By the size of the dose
- By study design (randomized trials versus nonrandomized, observational studies)

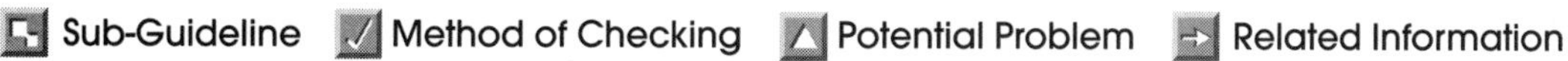

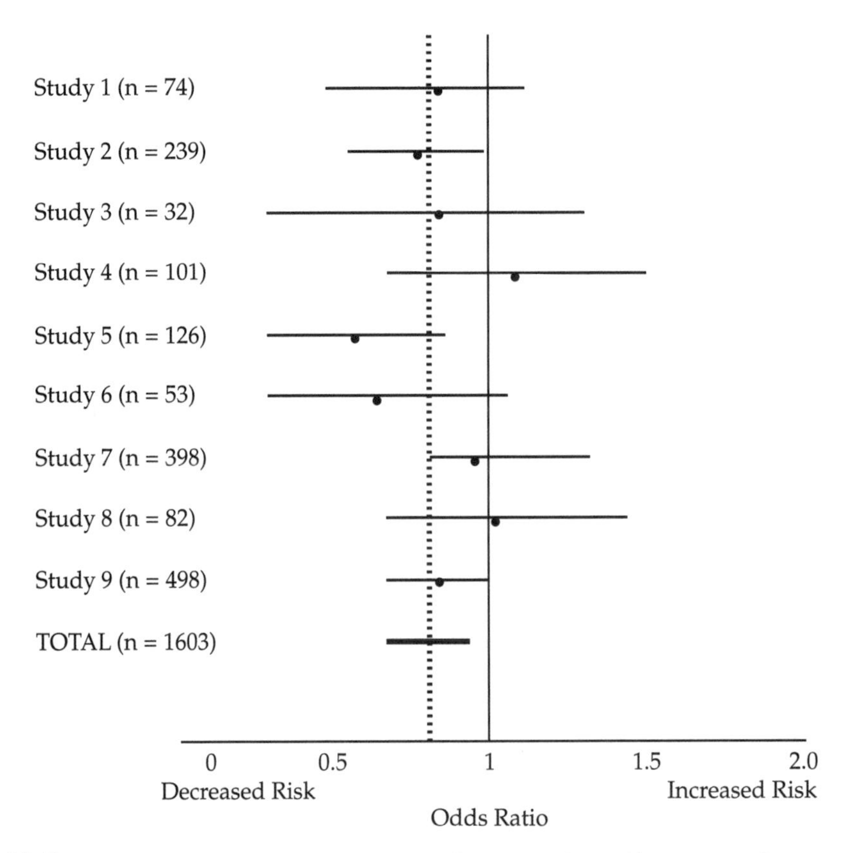

FIGURE 11.2 A chart for presenting the results of meta-analysis. The estimated mean odds ratio and 95% confidence limits are shown for each study, and the overall estimated odds ratio is indicated by the dotted line. An odds ratio of 1 means that the treatment neither increases nor decreases the risk of the outcome of interest.

11.14 State the statistical power of the analysis.

The effect of statistically pooling the results is to increase the sample size and, hence, the statistical power of the meta-analysis over that of the individual studies it summarizes. Meta-analysis is thus useful for analyzing multiple studies of low power and with studies showing small effects for which a more precise estimate is required (for example, complication rates of rare problems.) A power of 0.8 or 0.9 (which may be expressed as a beta of 0.2 or 0.1, respectively) to detect a specified difference, if such a difference exists, is desirable. A power statement answers the question: "Given the sample size and other factors, what is the probability of finding a difference of a specified size if it truly exists?"

Guideline 4.4: Report the details of an a priori power calculation

11.15 Provide an assessment of the quality of each study included in the analysis.

Characterizing the quality of the studies allows researchers to use more specific inclusion or exclusion criteria and sometimes to assign weights to studies of different quality when combining them in the analysis.

Commonly, two or more reviewers will individually assess the quality of each study—masked as to the authors and the results of the study—and then meet to resolve any differences. In such cases, it is helpful to include a measure of inter-rater reliability to establish the consistency of the quality assessment (5,7).

11.16 List the studies excluded from the meta-analysis and the reason for their exclusion.

Because selection bias is the single most common reason for differing results in meta-analyses, knowing which studies were excluded, and sometimes why they were excluded, will enable other meta-analysts to draw their own conclusions about the selection process.

11.17 Test important choices and assumptions with sensitivity analysis to determine whether their impact on the result is warranted.

In sensitivity analysis, some studies are excluded to determine how their exclusion affects the results. If the effect is great, the studies may have an undue impact on the results. If the effect is small, the results may be more representative of all the studies. Studies that may produce greater effects are likely to be larger, of higher quality, more recently conducted, or to use random assignment and masking.

GUIDELINES ADDRESSED IN THE DISCUSSION

11.18 Discuss the variability (or "heterogeneity") of the results of the individual trials.

Because meta-analysis combines the results of several studies, the degree of agreement among the results of these studies—the "homogeneity" or "heterogeneity" of the results—can affect the interpretation of the meta-analysis and so must be addressed. Homogeneous results are more easily interpreted because they are similar; heterogeneous results are more difficult to interpret because wide variation in the results may need to be explained.

In particular, differences in the *direction* of the results can be troublesome. If the results of some studies favored the treatment group whereas the results of others favored the control group, the combined results are said to be heterogeneous because they do not support the same conclusion.

Similarly, differences in the *magnitude* of the results can also be important. If some studies conclude that the drug was highly effective whereas others concluded that it was only marginally effective, the results can again be described as heterogeneous.

One indication of heterogeneity is whether the differences among the results of the individual studies are statistically significant. The differences can be compared with a hypothesis test (such as a chi-square test or an F test), and if P is less than, say, 0.1, then factors other than chance may be involved: perhaps the studies were too dissimilar to compare in the first place or perhaps differences in eligibility requirements, patient populations, measurement technique, or treatments account for the differences (1).

A useful way to report the heterogeneity of the results is with the L'Abbé plot (**Figure 11.3**), which plots the response rate of the control group against the response rate of the treatment group for each study (5). Thus, points spread over the graph indicate heterogeneous results, whereas points in a tighter cluster represent more homogeneous results.

11.19 Discuss the populations represented in the meta-analysis and the generalizability of the results of the meta-analysis to other populations.

The variability in the populations included in the meta-analysis may make interpreting the results difficult. How well do hospital-based studies reflect what can be expected in outpatient-based programs, for example? Still, for the meta-analysis to be useful, the patient populations to whom the results might apply must be identified.

11.20 Discuss the implications of the results.

In meta-analysis, as in all research, the implications of the results to scientific understanding or to the delivery of health care should be addressed. The discussion should integrate the strength of the evidence, the threshold at which the benefits exceed the risks of the treatment, and the size of and precision of the estimated effect (17).

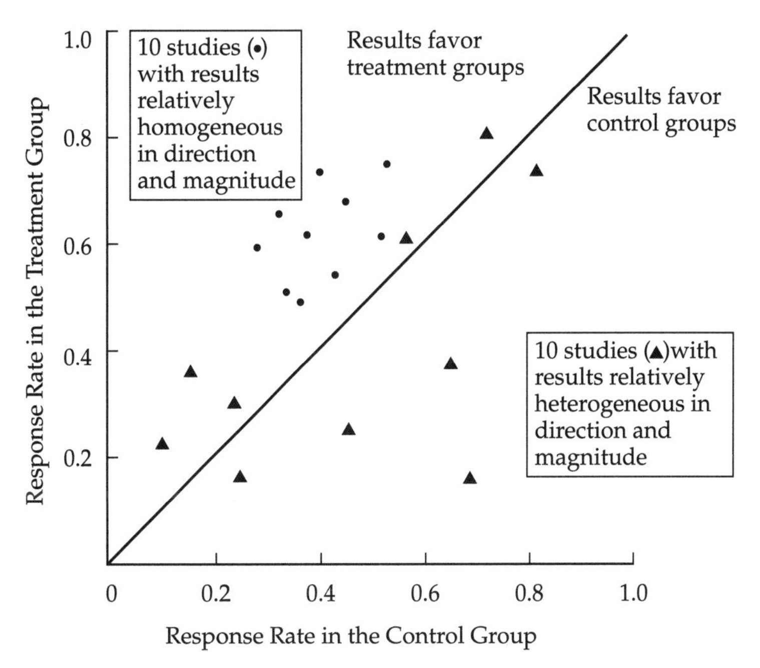

FIGURE 11.3 The L'Abbé plot indicates the heterogeneity of the results of the individual studies by plotting the response rate of the control group against the response rate of the treatment group for each study. Points scattered over the graph indicate heterogeneous results; points clustered in a tighter area indicate more homogeneous results. In addition, points along the 45-degree diagonal line indicate similar results in both treatment and control groups, and points farther away from zero indicate larger response rates.

A NOTE ABOUT CUMULATIVE META-ANALYSIS

Cumulative meta-analysis is the practice of conducting a meta-analysis over time, adding additional studies to the meta-analysis as they become available and recomputing the results after each study is added. Such a practice may allow the results of a treatment to be confirmed as early as possible, perhaps settling the question and reducing the number of additional studies and the number of additional patients that may be put at risk.

For example, Lau and colleagues (18) conducted a cumulative meta-analysis on the effectiveness of streptokinase in treating acute myocardial infarction. They analyzed 33 randomized controlled trials of streptokinase conducted over 29 years and involving a total of 36 974 patients. Their results, shown in **Figure 11.4**, indicate that the effectiveness of streptokinase was established statistically with the publication of the seventh study. However, 25 more studies involving 34 542 additional patients were

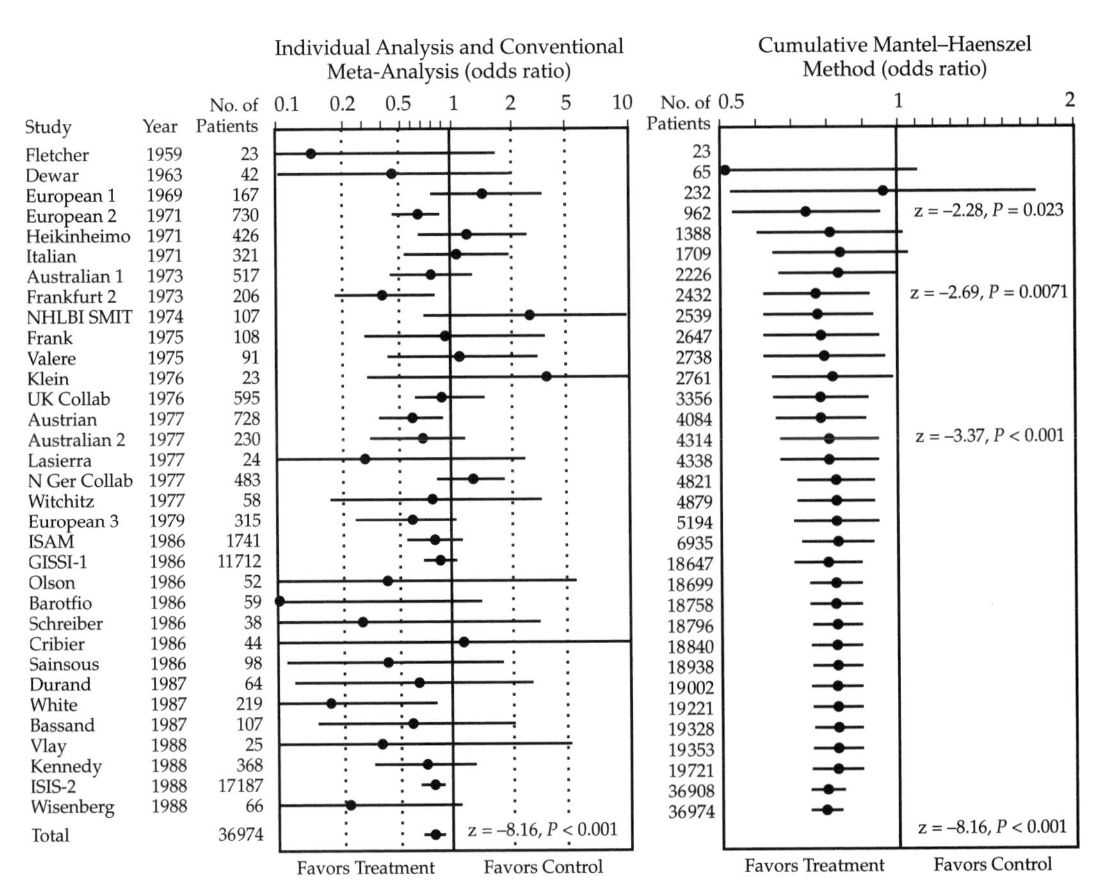

FIGURE 11.4 A chart for presenting the results of a cumulative meta-analysis. As each study is added to the computations, the effective sample size increases, and the precision of the estimated result improves, as indicated by the shortening of the horizontal line that represents the 95% confidence interval. This chart shows that the results were statistically significant after the seventh study. The estimated value of the result also stabilizes as the sample size increases. (Reprinted with permission from Lau J, Antman EM, Jimenez-Silva J, Kupelnick B, Mosteller F, Chalmers TC. Cumulative meta-analysis of therapeutic trials for myocardial infarction. N Engl J Med. 1992;327 [4]:250. Copyright 1992, Massachusetts Medical Society.)

conducted over the next 15 years before streptokinase was generally accepted as an effective treatment.

The guidelines for reporting meta-analyses are also suitable for reporting cumulative meta-analyses, with the addition of a figure similar to that shown in **Figure 11.4** to illustrate the cumulative effect of each additional study. Also, because cumulative meta-analysis involves data as they accumulate, any adjustments for multiple analyses should be reported.

Chapter 5. The Multiple Testing Problem

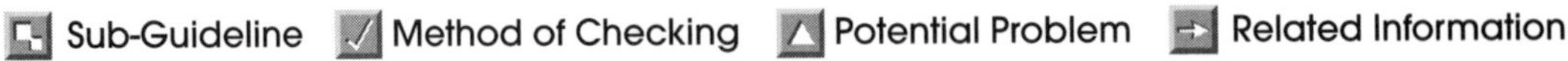

REFERENCES

1. **Dickersin K, Berlin JA.** Meta-analysis: state-of-the-science. Epidemiol Rev. 1992;14: 154-76.
2. **Kassirer JP.** Clinical trials and meta-analysis. What do they do for us? [Editorial]. N Engl J Med. 1992;327(4):273-4.
3. **Borzak S, Ridker PM.** Discordance between meta-analyses and large-scale randomized, controlled trials. Examples from the management of acute myocardial infarction. Ann Intern Med. 1995;123:873-7.
4. **Journal of the American Medical Association.** Instructions for preparing structured abstracts. JAMA. 1993;271(2):162-4.
5. **Wilson A, Henry DA.** Meta-analysis. Part 2: Assessing the quality of published meta-analyses. Med J Aust. 1992;156:173-87.
6. **West RR.** A look at the statistical overview (or meta-analysis). J R Coll Physicians Lond.1993; 27(2):111-5.
7. **Felson DT.** Bias in meta-analytic research. J Clin Epidemiol. 1992;45(8):885-92.
8. **Simes J.** Meta-analysis: its importance in cost-effectiveness studies. Med J Aust. 1990; 153(Suppl):S13-6.
9. **Bero L, Rennie D.** The Cochrane Collaboration. Preparing, maintaining, and disseminating systematic reviews of the effects of health care. JAMA. 1995;274 (24):1935-8.
10. **Dickersin K.** The existence of publication bias and risk factors for its occurrence. JAMA. 1990;263:1385-9.
11. **Light RJ, Pillemer DB.** Summing Up: The Science of Reviewing Research. Cambridge, MA: Harvard University Press; 1984.
12. **Andersen JW, Harrington D.** Meta-analyses need new publication standards [Editorial]. J Clin Oncol. 1992;10(6):878-80.
13. **Henry DA, Wilson A.** Meta-analysis. Part 1: An assessment of its aims, validity and reliability. Med J Aust. 1992;156:173-87.
14. **Jones DR.** Meta-analysis of observational epidemiological studies: a review. J R Soc Med. 1992;85(3):165-8.
15. **Walter SD.** Methods of reporting statistical results from medical research studies. Am J Epidemiol. 1995;141(10):896-906.
16. **Laupacis A, Sackett DL, Roberts RS.** An assessment of clinically useful measures of the consequences of treatment. N Engl J Med. 1988;318;1728-33.
17. **Guyatt GH, Sackett DL, Sinclair JC, Hayward R, Cook DJ, Cook RJ.** Users' guides to the medical literature. IX. A method for grading health care recommendations. The Evidence-Based Medicine Group. JAMA. 1995; 274(22):1800-4.
18. **Lau J, Antman EM, Jimenez-Silva J, Kupelnick B, Mosteller F, Chalmers TC.** Cumulative meta-analysis of therapeutic trials for myocardial infarction. N Engl J Med. 1992;327:248-54.

Chapter 12

WEIGHING THE COSTS AND CONSEQUENCES OF TREATMENT

Reporting the Results of Economic Evaluations

The principal value of formal cost-effectiveness analysis in health care is that it forces one to be explicit about beliefs and values that underlie allocation decisions.

M.C. WEINSTEIN AND W.B. STASON (1)

The components of the health care system are increasingly under pressure to control their costs, to improve the quality of patient outcomes, to provide more consistent care, and to be accountable for their decisions. As a result, several related topics have become popular: technology assessment, outcomes research, pharmacoeconomics, decision analysis, practice guidelines, evidence-based medicine, and a broad area called **economic evaluation,** a branch of medical economics concerned with evaluating the costs, outcomes, and trade-offs between alternative medical therapies.

An important impetus for economic evaluations has been the introduction of **pharmacoeconomics,** or the study of the economic implications of medication use. Such studies may now be required as part of the drug-approval process, and they are often used in sales and advertising campaigns. Proponents of pharmacoeconomics talk of the need to make sound, cost-effective prescribing decisions based on hard data; opponents see pharmacoeconomics as a new marketing ploy by pharmaceutical companies and as a field of study plagued with considerable bias.

Consequently, many of the guidelines for reporting economic evaluations are directed to preventing overt bias in pharmacoeconomic studies. However, the methodology can be used to guide the applications of other therapies, as well as drug therapies: health care policies, clinical procedures, diagnostic tests, or patient education programs. Economic evaluations provide insight, not necessarily answers, and are most often used by administrators and policymakers, not individual physicians.

Included here are descriptions of cost-identification, cost-minimization, and cost-of-illness studies. Most of the guidelines, however, apply to cost-benefit, cost-effectiveness, and cost-utility analysis, in which two or more therapies are compared. Any type of economic evaluation should be described accurately, clearly, and completely, and replication must be possible.

GUIDELINES ADDRESSED IN THE INTRODUCTION

12.1 State the purpose of the study. Identify the treatments that were studied and the reasons for studying them.

As in all scientific research, the research question should be an answerable question stated in unambiguous terms. Primary goals should be distinct from secondary ones. The purpose statement should specify the following:

- The therapies to be evaluated or compared
- The diagnoses or indications for use and the associated patient populations to which the therapies are targeted
- The settings in which the therapies are usually applied
- The providers who usually make the therapies available
- The type of economic evaluation undertaken (***see Guideline 12.2***)
- Why these therapies are being compared, and why now

In general, an economic evaluation is appropriate to evaluate high-cost therapies, therapies that have wide application and therefore high total costs, or therapies that may provide greater benefits even though they may have greater costs than alternative therapies.

It may also be appropriate to indicate why the therapies are being evaluated at this time. One issue in economic evaluations is the timing of the evaluation with respect to the development of the intervention. Because technology tends to improve over time, evaluations too early in the development of an intervention may not adequately reflect its eventual value.

EXAMPLES:

- Is it cost effective to vaccinate healthy people older than 65 years of age against Hong Kong flu?

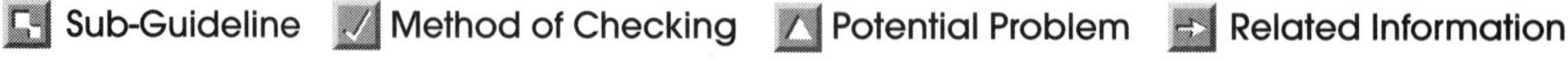

- What schedule of colonoscopic cancer screening examinations will provide the optimum cost-benefit for patients with chronic ulcerative colitis?
- Would it be cost-effective to routinely substitute t-PA for streptokinase in patients requiring thrombolytic therapy for acute myocardial infarction?

12.2 State the type of economic evaluation undertaken.

The terms for different economic evaluations are often confused. The most common types of economic evaluation are identified below.

- **Cost-identification analysis** seeks to identify the costs of providing the treatment. This type of analysis is the first step in all of the other types of analyses, but it is often the only economic evaluation undertaken or reported in a study.
- **Cost-minimization analysis** seeks to identify the least expensive alternative intervention. This type of analysis assumes that differences in outcome are nonexistent or unimportant, so only the monetary costs of the therapies are compared. For example, a hospital might undertake such a study to determine whether to replace or to repair an x-ray machine.
- **Cost-of-illness analysis** estimates the total cost of a disease or disability to a society by studying the total value of medical diagnosis and treatment and lost productivity. Such analysis results in a single dollar amount that provides a general sense of the impact of the illness on an entire economy. For example, the statement that heart disease costs the United States $128 billion each year is the result of a cost-of-illness study.
- **Cost-benefit analysis** assesses one or more therapies on the basis of monetary costs and monetary benefits. In cost-benefit analysis, all outcomes are expressed in dollars, including lives or years of life. Thus, the cost-benefits of glaucoma prevention programs can be compared with those of heart transplantation, and both can be compared with the cost-benefits of other programs, such as highway development or job training.
- **Cost-effectiveness analysis** compares two or more therapies on the basis of monetary costs and clinical effectiveness. Results are usually reported in units of "dollars per clinical outcome," such as dollars per life saved, dollars per additional years of life, or dollars per number of new cases diagnosed. The outcomes of therapies to be compared with cost-effectiveness analysis must be expressed in the same units.

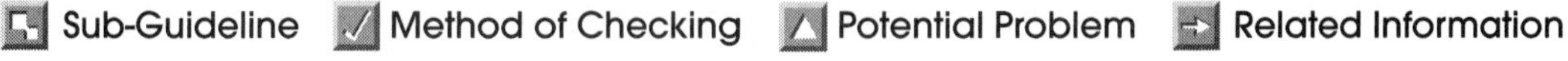

- **Cost-utility analysis** assesses two or more therapies on the basis of monetary costs and a measure of "utility," which is the product of a clinical outcome, such as years of life, and a subjective weighting of the quality of life to be had during those years. This measure is usually taken from any of several *health status indexes.* Utility is expressed, then, in units such as quality-adjusted life years (QALYs) or sometimes as the number of "well-years."

Cost-identification, cost-minimization, and cost-of-illness analyses are usually descriptive, and many of the Guidelines here can be applied to reporting the results of such analyses. Cost-benefit, cost-effectiveness, and cost-utility analyses are usually comparative, and all the Guidelines in this section may be applicable.

12.3 State the perspective of the designers of the evaluation.

Economic evaluations must be interpreted in view of the needs, interests, and values of its designers. For example, total costs might be of concern to a health maintenance organization, whereas only nonreimbursable costs might concern a community hospital. Designers may represent any of several perspectives:

- Society at large
- A pharmaceutical company
- A third-party payer (for example, an insurance company)
- A managed care group
- A community hospital
- A patient population or diagnostic group

On occasion, some perspectives may conflict with others. For example, insurance carriers have traditionally reimbursed patients for hospitalization costs but not for home health care costs. This reimbursement policy has led many physicians to keep less affluent patients in the hospital longer (a rational choice from the physician's perspective of providing individual patients with comprehensive care), to reduce the patients' out-of-pocket costs (desirable from the patient's perspective), but at the expense of higher insurance costs (undesirable from a payer's perspective) and overall medical costs (undesirable from a societal perspective).

Although the societal perspective is the broadest and is often considered to be the most desirable for an economic evaluation, most allocation decisions are made by parties with other perspectives (2).

Highlight any part of the evaluation that deviates from the stated perspective (3). It is not always possible to obtain data consistent with the desired perspective. A drug study conducted from a societal perspective could be expected to use wholesale costs, but retail prices or bills may have to be used instead. Such a departure from the stated perspective should be noted.

12.4 Identify who funded the study and describe the relationship between the researchers and the funding agent.

The results of economic evaluations often heavily influence the adoption of one intervention over another and thus can have enormous financial impact. Because pharmaceutical companies fund many economic evaluations (the field of pharmacoeconomics) and may use the results to help market their products, the need to establish the independence and the objectivity of the investigator has become important.

All economic evaluations involve uncertainties that can be resolved (biased) for or against the intervention under study. The need for straightforward, unbiased reporting is thus critical in economic evaluations. So strong is the notion that financial arrangements can create an incentive for bias, that some journals will not publish economic evaluations by authors who have a financial conflict of interest with the sponsoring agency (4).

At the same time, researchers who are stock owners, paid consultants, or employees of companies with financial interests in the treatments under study are not necessarily biased or unethical, but they do need to report their relationship with the organization who funded the study. Further, if the funding organization placed any constraints on the investigation, these should be disclosed in the published article (5).

GUIDELINES ADDRESSED IN THE METHODS

12.5 Describe the treatments being compared and give the reasons for comparing them.

Economic evaluations are concerned with assessing one or more *specific* therapies for a *specific* set of indications (6). For each intervention, identify the following:

- Who provides it
- Who receives it (which patient population or diagnosis)
- Who pays for it
- Its intensity of use (how often it is given per patient or how many patients receive it in a given time)
- Its expected outcomes
- Its effect on groups other than patients, payers, and providers

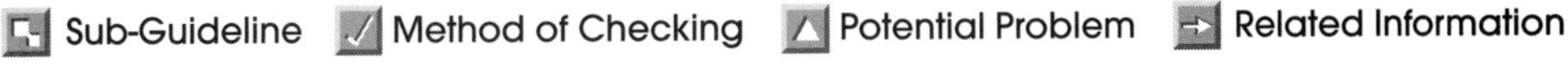
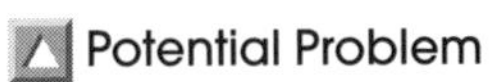
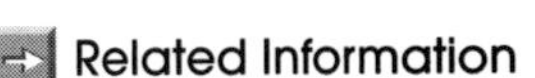

Does the comparison include the leading alternative treatments? (7–9) The choice of alternative treatments should be based on clinical relevance, not on the potential desirability of the results (5). Comparing a new treatment with an obviously inferior treatment can be a marketing ploy; the new treatment will predictably compare favorably. Thus, all reasonable alternative treatments should be considered, but especially the following:

- The least expensive alternative
- The most common alternative (the "usual standard of care" in the community)
- The most effective alternative
- The "do nothing" alternative (when appropriate)
- Nonpharmacologic alternatives (when appropriate)

Therapies from different countries should be compared with caution (10). The costs and availability of competing interventions and other medical infrastructure characteristics differ from country to country and can affect the costs, use, and outcomes of a treatment. Differences in exchange rates must also be considered when evaluating costs in different countries.

12.6 Verify the clinical effectiveness of each treatment being evaluated.

Given the time and effort needed to conduct an economic evaluation, the effectiveness of each treatment should be established before the study begins. In particular, each treatment should be accompanied by a documented description of its

- *Safety.* Does the treatment do more good than harm when applied properly?
- *Efficacy.* Does the treatment do what it is supposed to do under controlled circumstances, such as in clinical trials?
- *Effectiveness.* Does the treatment do what it is supposed to do under real-world conditions? (Do availability, patient adherence, or cost adversely affect its correct use?)
- *Distribution.* Is the treatment geographically available on a scale that makes it a reasonable alternative for comparison?
- *Availability.* Is the treatment financially and otherwise accessible on a scale that makes it a reasonable alternative for comparison?

Economic evaluations assume a treatment's effectiveness—they do not establish it (9).

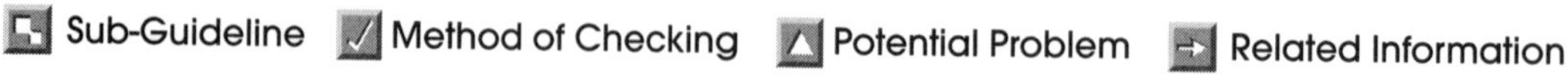

The discovery that there is no good evidence of benefit for a treatment is an important result of an economic analysis (6).

12.7 Describe any pilot studies undertaken in preparation for the primary study.

Pilot studies are often conducted before a full economic evaluation to identify the costs and outcomes to be considered, to determine any potential problems in methodology and data collection, to obtain preliminary estimates for planning the full analysis, to determine the probable scope of the full analysis, and so on. However, pilot studies can also be a potential source of bias by creating expectations among researchers. Also, sponsors have been known to fund economic evaluations in stages and to abandon the research if the results appear to be unfavorable at any stage.

12.8 State whether the study was conducted according to a written protocol.

Following a written protocol established in advance of data collection helps avoid bias during the conduct of the study.

Economic evaluations are sometimes conducted as part of a clinical research study to test the efficacy of an intervention (11–13). The advantage of this concurrent approach is that more specific data can be collected from individual patients randomly assigned to the treatment and control groups. The disadvantages are that an economic evaluation adds to the burden of an already-complex clinical study; the results may not generalize well to other, less-controlled settings; and if the clinical trial indicates that the intervention is not effective, the economic evaluation may have little value. Alternatively, separate economic evaluations of some therapies may not be ethically sound because an inferior therapy should not be compared to a superior one, especially if the study is primarily for marketing purposes.

Deviations from or modifications to the protocol made during the study should be reported (5).

12.9 Identify the "time horizon" over which the costs and benefits of the treatments are expected to accrue.

The time horizon should be relevant to the diagnoses and therapies under study. For example, the effects of stopping a child from smoking at age 11 years can accrue over an entire lifetime in the form of fewer respiratory ailments, improved physical capacity, and reduced risk of cancer and heart disease. The time horizon of an anesthetic that reduces postoperative hypotension is very short in comparison.

The duration of the time horizon is also important in determining how costs and outcomes will be discounted so that future costs and savings are expressed in current dollars (*see also Guideline 12.19*).

The duration of the time horizon may also present an important ethical consideration, in that evaluations using years-of-life saved or well-years as outcome measures inherently favor therapies delivered to younger populations (14).

12.10 Identify the key assumptions and value judgments used in the evaluation.

All economic evaluations require several assumptions and value judgments that can affect the results. For example, the quality of life may be seen as more important than the length of life in some conditions but not others; short-term spending may be preferable to long-term savings for some organizations but not for others. Given the potential and incentive for bias in economic evaluations, it is important to identify these choices and the rationale for choosing among the alternatives. Conservative assumptions (those biased against the therapy) are preferred (3,5).

When appropriate and possible, the effect of key assumptions and value judgments should be assessed with sensitivity analysis to determine their effect on the overall results (*see Guideline 12.20*).

12.11 Identify the types of costs included in the evaluation (and important costs that were not included) and state how these costs were determined.

Costs are the economic consequences of choosing an intervention (15). They generally include the short-term, long-term, direct, and indirect costs, as well as savings, that result from the treatment **(Table 12.1).** Patients, providers, and payers may all have costs and "averted costs," or savings. In addition, some treatments may have "induced costs," which are new costs created by offering the treatment, such as the cost of treating adverse side effects.

However, there are as yet no widely accepted standards or components for cost evaluations (16). (Costs listed in **Table 12.1** are illustrative, not comprehensive.) Further, there are many controversies about which types of costs to include and how to evaluate them. For example, should institutional overhead costs be included? Are future medical costs—those incurred because a patient lives longer—to be assessed?

TABLE 12.1 Types of Costs Typically Included in Economic Evaluations. Costs May be Incurred in the Short Term or the Long Term.

Medical

Fixed direct costs (equipment purchases)
Variable direct costs (consumable supplies; procedure fees; length of hospital stay)
Fixed indirect costs (provider salaries; facilities overhead; administration)
Variable indirect costs (training and education; fluctuating staff levels)
Induced cost created by the intervention (increased adverse event rates; future medical costs incurred by prolonged survival)
Averted cost, or savings created by the intervention (fewer diagnostic tests; reduced rehabilitation needs)

Financial (related to the larger economy)

Transfer payments (changes in social security payments resulting from changes in life span)
Inflation
Discounting (the opportunity cost of spending money now rather than investing it elsewhere)

Nonmedical

Access costs (transportation costs; communication costs)
Coping costs (child care; household services; rehabilitation equipment)
Lost work productivity

Intangible

Pain and suffering
Opportunity cost of patients' time

Costs are not the same as charges. A **cost** is the amount that a provider must pay for goods or services, whereas a **charge** is the amount that the provider bills the payer. Thus, a syringe may cost a hospital $0.50, but the hospital may charge the patient $1.50. Often, charges are used instead of costs in economic evaluations because they are more readily available. Both costs and charges can vary widely by institution and geographical area, which compounds the problem of comparison. **Payments,** the amount the payer actually returns to the provider, are sometimes used in lieu of costs or charges but are associated with even greater uncertainty.

Beware of "gaming:" cost-shifting and cross-subsidization of services that can affect cost evaluations. For example, in many institutions, nursing services are considered to be overhead costs, whereas respiratory care

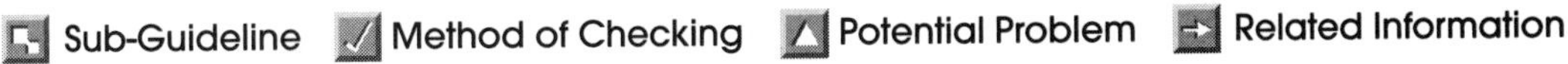

services are considered to be direct costs, which are reimbursable. Thus, the hospital will charge a patient if a ventilator is set up by a respiratory therapist but not if it is set up by a nurse. The hospital may increase the number of respiratory therapists as a means of generating additional income.

Costs can be divided into two general categories: **monetary costs** that are typically already expressed in dollars, and **nonmonetary costs,** such as lost productivity or grief, that must be converted to dollars (cost-benefit analysis) or to a measure of utility (cost-utility analysis). The three most common methods of **economic conversion** are the human capital approach, the willingness-to-pay approach, and the indirect approach.

In the **human capital approach** (or the "lost earnings" approach), the earning potential of the patient is projected for the duration of the disability. If a technician makes $15/hour and loses 2 weeks (80 hours) of work, the value of the lost productivity is $1200. However, this approach is biased toward patients in traditional occupations and becomes more speculative as the duration of the disability is extended to, say, 30 or 40 years and includes occupations without fixed renumeration, such as people who are self-employed, salespeople who work on commission, or those in the unpaid domestic workforce.

In the **willingness-to-pay approach,** a community is surveyed to determine how much people would be willing to pay to avoid having a particular symptom or disability. For example, people may be asked how much money they would be willing to spend each week to avoid having the symptoms of arthritis. If the answer is $30, then the "cost" for 1 year of arthritis would be valued at $1560 (52 weeks × $30 per week), and for 25 years, $39 000. Willingness to pay, however, may vary considerably among ethnic and economic communities.

In the **indirect approach,** data from various sources are examined to derive a monetary value for a given symptom or condition. So, for example, if the average insurance settlement to a 30-year-old head-of-household for a lost limb is $200 000, the loss of a limb early in life from say, diabetes, could be valued at $200 000 with some justification.

12.12 Identify the outcomes (benefits) of the treatments being compared and how these outcomes were determined.

As with cost evaluations, outcomes include the short-term, long-term, direct, indirect, and intangible consequences of the treatment for patients, providers, and payers.

Therapies usually have multiple outcomes, all of which should be addressed, if not included, in the analysis. Many therapies considered in economic evaluations affect the length and the quality of life. Thus, most therapies have at least four direct outcomes: success, mortality, morbidity, and post-treatment quality of life (6).

Some evaluations may use **surrogate endpoints** rather than direct health benefits. For example, patients with amyotrophic lateral sclerosis usually die when their respiratory muscles no longer function. Some patients elect to be maintained on ventilators, however, so going on a ventilator is sometimes used as a surrogate endpoint for death. How closely the date of going on the ventilator approximates the date of "death," however, is difficult to determine.

Economic evaluations that assess outcomes express them differently:

- In **cost-benefit analysis,** outcomes are expressed in dollars. Thus, lives saved or lost must be given a dollar figure. Any of the three methods of economic conversion described above (the human capital approach, the willingness-to-pay approach, and the indirect approach) can be used to assign dollar amounts to intangible outcomes.
- In **cost-effectiveness analysis,** outcomes are expressed in clinical terms or as "functional status," such as new cases diagnosed, lives saved, or injuries avoided. A common unit is the "year of life saved," or "life-years." One awkward issue here is whether providing 1 person with 40 more years of life is equivalent to providing 40 people with 1 additional year—both equal 40 life-years.
- In **cost-utility analysis,** outcomes are usually reported with the aid of a "health status index," which allows the computation of "utilities," such as the number of "well-years" or "quality-adjusted life years" (QALYs). A QALY is the product of the number of years of life times the quality of those years, as measured from 0 (indifference between life and death) to 1 (full health) on a quality-of-life questionnaire. Thus, an operation that provides an average of 12 more years of life with a quality rating or utility of 0.4 is said to provide 4.8 QALYs (12 years × 0.4 = 4.8 QALYs).

Report the method used to evaluate quality of life. Quality of life can be assessed in several ways. (For an excellent review of these methods, see Ref. 17.) The most common methods of measuring utility are described below (18–20). Because improved quality of life may differentiate one therapy from another or justify adopting a therapy with a higher cost, the method of determining quality of life should be reported.

- **Rating scales,** such as visual analog scales, use a line with clearly defined endpoints, such as death at one end and robust health at the other. Patients with the condition under study indicate their quality of life by marking a point along the line. In a related procedure called **category scaling,** patients choose from several ranked categories.

- The **standard gamble** presents respondents with two alternatives. One alternative has two possible outcomes: a return to normal health for a given length of time or a death. The other alternative is the certainty of living at a specified quality of life for the remainder of one's life. Respondents must choose one of the two alternatives. The probabilities of the two possible outcomes for alternative one are varied during testing until the respondents are as likely to choose the health state as they are to "gamble" on the chance of health at the risk of death.
- The **magnitude estimation technique** asks respondents to assign a ratio of undesirability for a pair of health states. For example, one state may be seen as twice as bad as another or three times as bad as a third. By asking a series of questions, the states can be ranked on a scale of "disutility" or undesirability.
- The **time-trade-off technique** presents respondents with two alternatives: living X years with a given quality of life, or death. The length of life, X, is then varied until respondents are indifferent to the choice.
- The **person trade-off technique** asks respondents which of two groups needs the most help: a group of X people with condition A or a second group of Y people with condition B. The numbers in each group (X and Y) and the quality of life for each group (A and B) are varied in a series of questions until respondents are as likely to choose one group as the other. The conditions or utilities can then be ranked on a scale of undesirability.

Different forms of assessment yield different utilities (10,18,21). Two basic issues in the measurement of utility or quality of life are 1) Who provides the assessment? The patient, who is experiencing what is being measured; the caregiver, who has observed a wider range of patients in the same condition; or the public, who may be unfamiliar with the condition? and 2) Is the measure a single question, such as "What is your quality of life?," or a composite score that combines answers on several dimensions, such as physical, psychological, functional, social, and spiritual?

12.13 Report any mathematical model used to compare costs and outcomes.

The costs and outcomes included in economic evaluations can sometimes be expressed in an equation, which may be useful in reporting the study. For example, a model used to evaluate the cost-utility of treating mild-to-moderate hypertension is shown below (22):

$$\frac{C}{B} = \frac{(\Delta C_{RX} + \Delta C_{SE} - \Delta C_{morb})}{(\Delta Y_{LE} - \Delta Y_{SE} + \Delta Y_{morb})}$$

where C is *net health care costs* of antihypertensive therapy per patient and B is the *net health care benefits* (presented here as a utility) of antihypertensive therapy per patient, expressed in quality-adjusted life-years, and

ΔC_{RX} = change in direct medical costs of treating hypertension

ΔC_{SE} = change in medical costs of treating the side effects of antihypertensive medication

ΔC_{morb} = change in savings in health care costs from prevention of morbid events

ΔY_{LE} = change in life expectancy from life-long antihypertensive treatment, expressed in life-years

ΔY_{SE} = change in quality of life as a result of the side effects of antihypertensive medication, expressed in quality-adjusted life-years

ΔY_{morb} = change in quality of life as a result of averted morbid events, such as stroke, expressed in quality-adjusted life-years

Other statistical methods may be used in economic evaluations, including Cox regression models, receiver operating characteristics curves (ROC curves), and Markov models and decision trees.

12.14 Describe the sources of data and the methods of data collection.

Most economic evaluations require a variety of cost and outcome data: adverse event rates, disease prevalence rates, operative success rates, measures of patient satisfaction, the preferred intensity of medical follow-up, changes in salaries and wages, and so on. Further, these data may be obtained from any of several sources: published meta-analyses, clinical trials run concurrently with the economic evaluation, local or national data bases, production records, expert opinion, marketing studies, patient surveys, and so on. In any event, the sources of data should be identified, the criteria for selecting them should be given, and their strengths, weaknesses, and potential biases should be discussed.

GUIDELINES ADDRESSED IN THE RESULTS

12.15 Report the individual and aggregate *costs* for each treatment. Establish that the costs were identified fully, measured well, and valued appropriately.

Report the results of the cost evaluation. The specific goods and services evaluated and the dollar value that was calculated for each, as well as the total aggregate costs, can be given in a table (**Table 12.2**).

12.16 Report the individual and aggregate *outcomes* for each treatment. Establish that the outcomes were identified fully, measured well, and valued appropriately.

Report the results of the outcome evaluation. The outcomes may be the likelihoods of morbidities or mortality, quality-of-life measures, number of cases prevented, increases in life expectancy, and so on. Outcomes generally are best give in a table (**Table 12.3**).

12.17 Report both average and incremental cost-outcome ratios for each treatment.

Average cost-outcome ratios are computed by dividing total costs by total outcomes (**Table 12.4**). The unit of outcome (a measure of benefit, effectiveness, or utility) differs according to the type of economic evaluation performed.

✓ **When comparing treatments, the lower the average cost-outcome ratio, the better.** In **Figure 12.1,** treatments are compared on the basis of total costs and outcomes and average and incremental cost-outcome ratios; although treatment B has the lowest total cost and treatment C has the highest outcome, the preferred treatment is E, which has the lowest average cost-outcome ratio, 1 life-year for $3750.

Incremental or **marginal cost-outcome ratios** indicate the cost of providing one additional unit of outcome. Incremental ratios are important because average cost-outcome ratios can be misleading if they are the only criteria used to choose among therapies. The marginal cost-outcome ratio is:

$$\frac{\text{cost of new} - \text{cost of old}}{\text{outcome of new} - \text{outcome of old}}$$

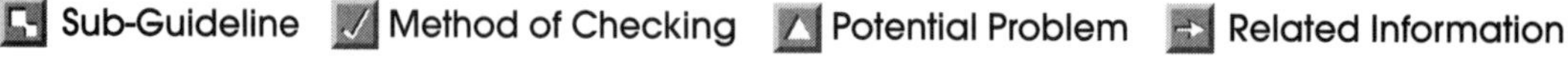

TABLE 12.2 Illustration of a Table Reporting the Actual Costs Used in an Economic Evaluation.*

Cost	Hospital Cost ($)	Physician Fees ($)
Initial Hospitalization†		
ICU stay, 1 day, no complications	1400	126
ICU stay, 1 day, mild complications	2070	187
ICU stay, 1 day, severe complications	2760	250
Nursing unit stay	475	54
Diagnostic cardiac catheterization	1670	400
Coronary angioplasty	6200	1356
Coronary bypass surgery	8800	2564
Emergency room visit	300	125
Rehospitalization†		
Coronary bypass surgery	19 000	2823
Fatal myocardial infarction	4745	. . .
Heart failure and shock	3440	. . .
Initial hospital day	. . .	111
Subsequent hospital day	. . .	55
Initial clinic visit	. . .	98
Subsequent clinic visit	. . .	45

* Data are illustrative only.
† Indicate the source of the data in a footnote.

TABLE 12.3 Illustration of a Table Reporting the Actual Outcomes Used in an Economic Evaluation.*

Outcome	Without Vaccination (n)	With Vaccination (n)	Cases Prevented (n)
Chickenpox cases	149 050	9375	139 675
Morbidities			
Pneumonia	1500	15	1485
Encephalitis	775	9	766
Long-term disability from encephalitis	10	2	8
Mortality	7	0	7

* In a cost-benefit analysis, each outcome would be converted into a dollar amount. In a cost-effectiveness analysis, each outcome would be expressed as a clinical measure, such as cost per infection prevented. In a cost-utility analysis, outcomes would be assigned a utility and expressed in terms such as well-years gained per vaccination. (Data are illustrative only.)

TABLE 12.4 Cost-Outcome Ratios for Three Hypothetical Interventions Assessed with Cost-Benefit, Cost-Effectiveness, and Cost-Utility Analyses.

Cost of Outcome	Intervention 1	Intervention 2	Intervention 3
Treatment cost ($) (known from the study)	17 000	30 000	98 000
Treatment benefits ($) (known from the study)	22 000	30 000	42 000
Effectiveness (life-years) (known from the study)	0.5	3	5
Quality of life weighting (0 to 1.0) (known from the study)	0.9	0.6	0.5
Utility (quality-adjusted life-years) (Effectiveness × QOL)	0.45	1.8	2.5
Average cost-benefit ratio (cost/benefits)	0.77	1.0	2.33
Average cost-effectiveness ratio ($/life-years) (cost/effectiveness)	34 000	10 000	19 600
Average cost-utility ratio ($/QALY) (cost/utility)	37 777	16 666	39 200

For example, the guaiac test for occult blood in the stool is a screening test for colon cancer. In one study, the average cost-effectiveness ratio was $1175; the "marginal" cost for each case of cancer detected after screening with a single test was thus also $1175. But the test is imperfect, so retesting may identify additional cases. The *average cost* to perform the sixth test was $2541, but the *marginal cost* for the sixth test—the cost of each additional case of cancer detected by the sixth test—exceeded $47 million! (23). In other words, among a large number of tests, only a few cases of cancer were found.

When one treatment is compared with or "challenges" another, the incremental cost-outcome ratio of the two treatments illustrates the trade-offs of changing from one to the other. In **Figure 12.1**, treatment A is assumed to be the current standard of care. Comparing each of the alternatives to A, it can be seen that

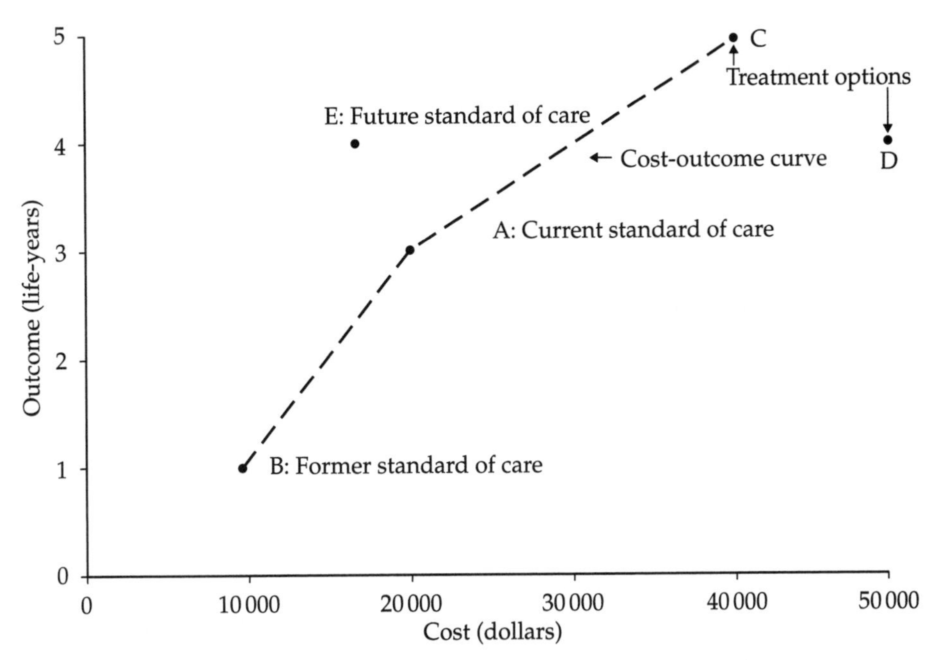

FIGURE 12.1 Average cost-outcome ratios for five hypothetical therapies. Dotted lines represent the "envelope" of the *cost-outcome curve.* Providers can choose to "operate" at any point along the curve. Incremental cost ratios can be indicated by the slope of the line drawn between two points; the steeper the slope, the lower (and more desirable) the incremental ratio. Negative slopes (from E to A) are rare but represent the ideal medical advance of providing increased total outcomes at reduced total costs.

- Compared with the former standard of care, B, A has a lower average cost-outcome ratio ($20 000/3 life-years = $6667/life-year) and a favorable (low but not the lowest) incremental cost-outcome ratio ($5000/life-year); moving from B to A was wise.
- Moving from A to C would incur an incremental cost of $10 000/life-year [($40 000 – $20 000)/(5 life-years – 3 life-years)], which is higher than the current average cost of $6667 ($20 000/3 life-years) and therefore is not wise.
- Moving from A to D would incur an incremental cost of $30 000/life-year [($50 000 – $20 000)/(4 life-years – 3 life-years)], a relatively expensive option.
- Moving from A to E would save $5000/life-year [($15 000 – $20 000)/(4 life-years – 3 life-years)]; in other words, not only does E cost less than A, but it produces 1 additional life-year for this reduced cost. In this case, E is said to "dominate" A. From an economic standpoint, treatment E should become the future standard of care.

Several incremental cost-ratios may be of interest, depending on the unit under study (***see also Guideline 12.18***). Consider the options in a pharmacoeconomic study: cost per pill, cost per dose, cost per day, cost per treatment, cost per patient, and cost per outcome.

12.18 Provide a measure of "therapeutic effort to clinical yield" (an effort-to-yield ratio) for each treatment.

Another useful cost-outcome ratio is the therapeutic effort-to-yield ratio. The most common is the number of patients who need to be treated to prevent one adverse outcome; or the number of tests necessary to detect one additional positive case: the **number needed to treat.**

> **EXAMPLE:** The usefulness of the effort-to-yield ratio is illustrated below. Each expression is statistically correct and scientifically appropriate, but each leaves the reader with a different impression of the effectiveness of the drug (24,25):
>
> - *Results expressed in absolute terms (the* **absolute** *or* **attributable risk reduction** [**ARR**]): In the Helsinki study of hypercholesterolemic men (26), after 5 years, 84 of 2030 patients on placebo (4.1%) had heart attacks, whereas only 56 of 2051 men treated with gemfibrozil (2.7%) had heart attacks ($P < 0.02$), for an absolute risk reduction of 1.4% (4.1% – 2.7% = 1.4%).
> - *Results expressed in relative terms (the* **relative risk reduction** [**RRR**]): In the Helsinki study of hypercholesterolemic men (26), after 5 years, 4.1% of the men treated with placebo had heart attacks, whereas only 2.7% of the men treated with gemfibrozil had heart attacks. The difference, 1.4%, represents a 34% relative risk reduction in the incidence of heart attack in the gemfibrozil-treated group (1.4%/4.1% = 34%).
> - *Results expressed in an effort-to-yield measure:* In the Helsinki study of 4081 hypercholesterolemic men (26), after 5 years, the results indicate that about 200 000 doses of gemfibrozil were ingested for each heart attack prevented.
> - *Results expressed in another effort-to-yield measure (the* **number needed to treat** [**NNT**]): The results of the Helsinki study of 4081 hypercholesterolemic men (26) indicate that 71 men need to be treated for 5 years to prevent a single heart attack.

Compute the absolute and relative risk reductions and the number needed to treat to help determine the therapeutic effectiveness of the treatment.

- **Absolute risk reduction (ARR)** = Pc – Pt, where Pc is the event rate of the control group and Pt is the event rate in the treatment group. In the example above, the absolute risk reduction is 4.1% – 2.7% = 1.4%.
- **Relative risk reduction (RRR)** = (Pc – Pt)/Pc, where Pc is the event rate of the control group and Pt is the event rate in the treatment group. In the example above, the relative risk reduction is 1.4%/4.1% = 34%.
- **Number needed to treat (NNT)** = 1/absolute risk reduction. In the example above, the number needed to treat is 1/0.014 = 71 men.

12.19 State the method of discounting used to adjust for costs and benefits that accrue during different time periods.

The costs and outcomes of an intervention typically are realized at different times and often over a long "time horizon." To adjust for these differences, a process called **discounting** or **present value analysis** must be done to weigh future dollars by a **discount factor** to make them comparable to present dollars.

Although inflation is a factor that makes future dollars worth less than current dollars, the primary reason for discounting is the "opportunity cost" of not investing the money elsewhere. For example, a hospital can spend $10 000 now on new equipment or invest it. After, say, 5 years at 5% interest, the $10 000 will be worth $12 763. By the same token, a projected savings of $10 000 5 years from now would have a current discounted value of $7835.

A 5% discount rate is standard. Costs and outcomes may not need to be discounted for therapies whose results are realized in the short term.

Assuming a discount rate of 5%, $X spent in n years has a present value of $X/(1.05)^n$ (1).

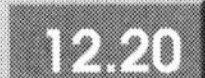

12.20 Test important choices and assumptions with sensitivity analysis to determine their impacts on the result.

Sensitivity analysis provides a measure of how "sensitive" the results of the analysis are to changes in assumptions. The most important assumptions in the analysis are usually varied one at a time over the range of possible values. If the basic conclusions do not change when an assumption is varied, the conclusions can be accepted with more confidence. For example, the results may vary depending on whether treatment costs are expected to increase by 5%, 7%, or 10% over 3, 5, or 7 years.

Typical assumptions tested for sensitivity are the following:

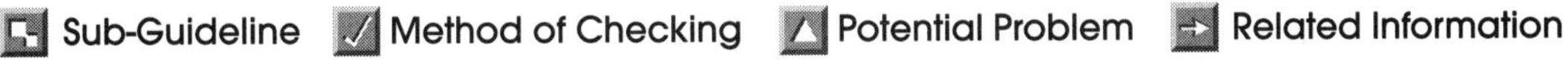
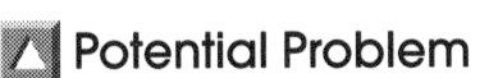

- Estimates of the degree of clinical effectiveness of the treatments
- Weightings of the quality-of-life measures
- Discount rates of costs and outcomes, including a rate of 0%
- Adverse event rates
- Prevalence rates
- Survival rates

One-way sensitivity analysis varies one assumption at a time. Two- and three-way analyses may also be performed (**Figures 12.2** and **12.3**).

Three special cases may be of interest:

- The best case, in which the most optimistic assumptions are used.
- The worst case, in which the most conservative assumptions are used.
- The break-even case, which is the combination of values at which the costs equal the benefits. For example, if to achieve the break-even

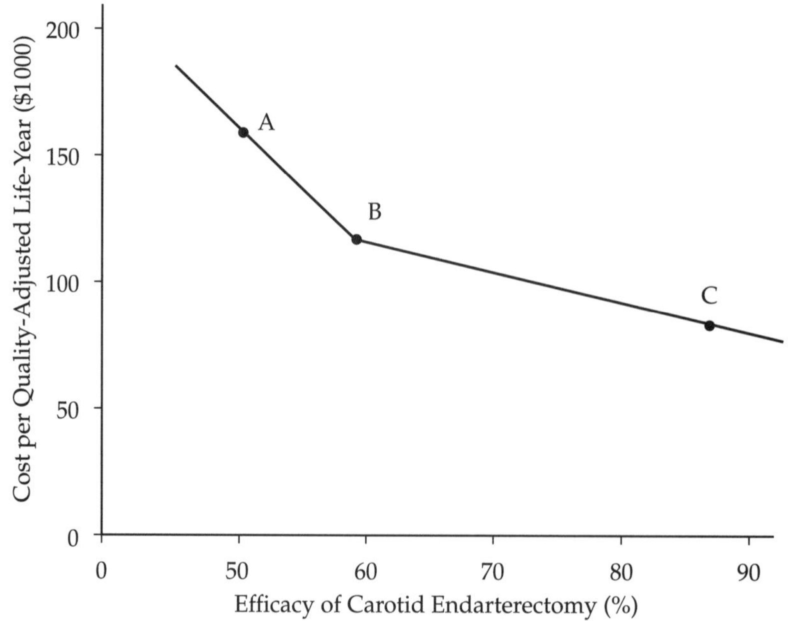

FIGURE 12.2 In one-way sensitivity analysis, the range of a variable is graphed on the X axis and the corresponding outcome is read on the Y axis. Here, the cost per quality-adjusted life-year (QALY) will vary between about $150 000 (point A) and $90 000 (point C), depending on whether the efficacy of carotid endarterectomy is assumed to be 50% or 87%, respectively. The efficacy of carotid endarterectomy is more of a factor in the 50% to 70% range (specifically at point B) than it is in the 70% to 90% range, because the cost per QALY varies more at the lower range than at the higher range. If other data support a higher efficacy for carotid endarterectomy, say, 80%, the model will be more stable. If the data support only a 55% efficacy, the model will have more variability.

point, the accuracy of a common diagnostic test must be dropped to as low as 20% from reported values of 80% to 90%, the results are not particularly sensitive to the accuracy of the test. Because the break-even point is well beyond the expected variation of at least this aspect of the evaluation, the results can be accepted with more confidence.

GUIDELINES ADDRESSED IN THE DISCUSSION

12.21 Discuss the generalizability of the results.

Even if an economic evaluation takes a societal perspective, local and regional differences in prices, competing health interventions, differences in the health care infrastructure, and population characteristics often limit

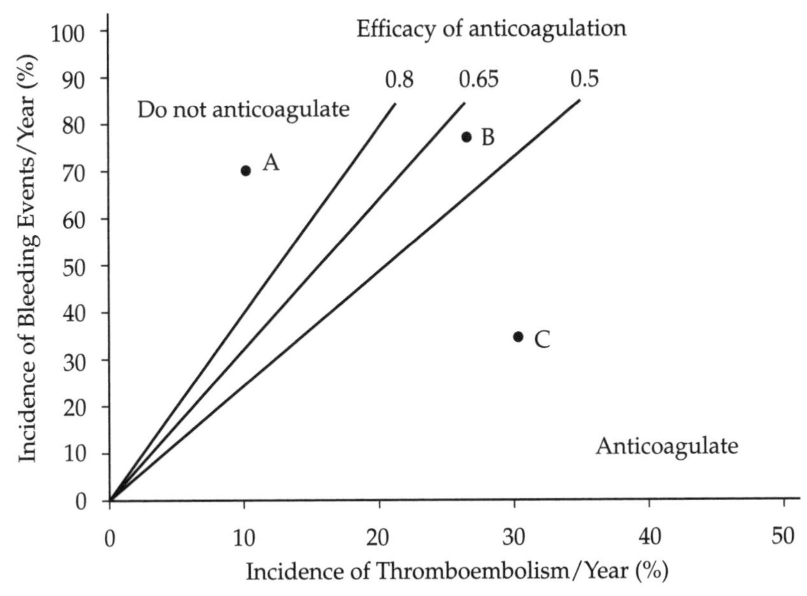

FIGURE 12.3 In three-way sensitivity analysis, three variables are shown over the ranges of interest. Here, the annual incidence of bleeding events varies from 0% to 100% on the Y axis; the annual incidence of thromboembolism varies from 0% to 50%; and the efficacy of anticoagulation is modeled at 50%, 65%, and 80%. The diagonal lines indicating the efficacy of anticoagulation are called "thresholds of equivalence," at which point there is no advantage of one treatment over the other. Points falling to the left of these lines (whichever efficacy value is chosen as the more appropriate) indicate that patients should not be anticoagulated, whereas points to the right indicate that patients should be anticoagulated. Thus, patients meeting the assumptions of point A (a 10% risk of thromboembolism and a 70% chance of bleeding) probably should not be anticoagulated, but patients meeting the assumptions of point C probably should be. The best course of action for patients at point B depends on the assumed efficacy of anticoagulation: if the assumption is 65%, anticoagulation is indicated. If the assumption is 50%, anticoagulation is not indicated.

its applicability to other circumstances. Nevertheless, it is worthwhile to project the results to other patients, settings, and times.

12.22 Describe the distributional effects of the alternative treatments, including the types and number of people who stand to benefit and to lose.

Any intervention affects at least three groups of people: patients, providers, and payers. When comparing two or more treatments for setting health care priorities, the overall implications of choosing one over the other for these three groups need to be addressed. For instance, access to lung transplantation benefits an older, wealthier, smaller population; increases the demand for pulmonary physicians and surgeons and intensive care rooms; and likely increases insurance costs to cover more high-cost treatments, whereas school programs to prevent sexually transmitted diseases benefit a larger, younger, more diverse population; increases the demand for health educators and instructional materials; and may reduce insurance rates if the incidence of these diseases drops.

The total costs of the treatment must also be considered. The number of patients receiving long-term hemodialysis each year is much less than the number being treated for myocardial infarction. So, although the costs per QALY may be similar, the total cost of treating patients for myocardial infarction will be substantially greater (11).

Most economic evaluations assume that freed resources will not be wasted (9). It may be unwise to assume that money saved on one intervention will be spent on another.

12.23 Discuss the feasibility of implementing the treatment.

In addition to medical and financial considerations, political, historical, psychological, and ethical issues may affect the likelihood of implementing a new treatment program, for example,

- People identify with a 38-year-old housewife who has terminal breast cancer but not with an anonymous woman who never got cervical cancer because she was treated early after seeking a routine screening test (6).
- Older patients are seen as less worthy of additional care than younger patients (14,27).
- Many people are more excited about high-technology interventions, such as magnetic resonance imaging, than they are about low-technology interventions, such as more frequent physical examinations (6).

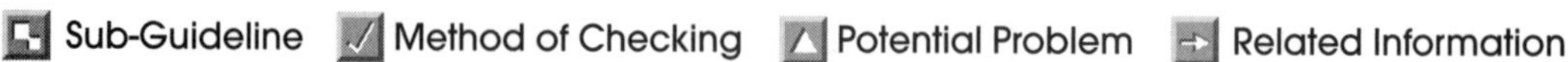

Cost-outcome ratios should not be the only criteria for choosing among alternative therapies (10).

12.24 Discuss the limitations of the study.

Few research studies go as planned; most encounter difficulties in data collection, management, or interpretation. The complexities and uncertainties associated with economic evaluations are particularly likely to create difficulties that limit their quality or validity. These limitations should be reported to help put the study in perspective and to inform other researchers of potential problems with similar investigations.

REFERENCES

1. **Weinstein MC, Stason WB.** Foundations of cost-effectiveness analysis for health and medical practices. N Engl J Med. 1977;296 (13):716-21.
2. **Weinstein MC.** Principles of cost-effective resource allocation in health care organizations. Int J Technol Assess Health Care. 1990;6(1):93-103.
3. **Hillman AL.** Economic analysis of health care technology. A report on principles. The Task Force on Principles for Economic Analysis of Health Care Technology. Ann Intern Med. 1995;123:61-70.
4. **Kassirer JP, Angell M.** The Journal's policy on cost-effectiveness analysis. N Engl J Med. 1994;331(10):669-70.
5. **Hillman AL, Eisenberg JM, Pauly MV, Bloom BS, Glick H, Kinosian B, Schwartz JS.** Avoiding bias in the conduct and reporting of cost-effectiveness research sponsored by pharmaceutical companies. N Engl J Med. 1991;324(19):1362-5.
6. **Eddy DM.** Clinical decision-making: from theory to practice. Cost-effectiveness analysis: Is it up to the task? JAMA. 1992;267 (24):3342-8.
7. **Ganiats TG, Wong AF.** Evaluation of cost-effectiveness research: a survey of recent publications. Fam Med. 1991;23(6):457-62.
8. **Lee JT, Sanchez LA.** Interpretation of "cost-effective" and soundness of economic evaluations in the pharmacy literature. Am J Hosp Pharm. 1991;48(12):2622-7.
9. **Stoddart GL.** How to read journals: VII. To understand an economic evaluation (Part B). Can Med Assoc J. 1984;130(12):1428-34.
10. **Mason J, Drummone M, Torrance G.** Some guidelines on the use of cost effectiveness league tables. BMJ. 1993;306(6877):570-2.
11. **Kupersmith J, Holmes-Rovner M, Hogan A, Rovner D, Gardiner J.** Cost-effectiveness analysis in heart disease, part I: general principles. Prog Cardiovasc Dis. 1994;37(3):161-84.
12. **Adams ME, McCall NT, Gray DT, Orza MJ, Chalmers TC.** Economic analysis in randomized control trials. Med Care. 1992:30 (3): 231-43.
13. **Guyatt GH, Tugwell PX, Feeny DH, Haynes RB, Drummond M.** A framework for clinical evaluation of diagnostic technologies. Can Med Assoc J. 1986;134(6):587-94.
14. **Welch GH.** Comparing apples and oranges: Does cost-effectiveness analysis deal fairly with the old and young? Gerontologist.1991; 31(3):322-36.
15. **The Zitter Group.** Outcomes Backgrounder: An Overview of Outcomes and Pharmacoeconomics. San Francisco: The Zitter Group; 1994:1-56.
16. **Warner KE.** Issues in cost effectiveness in health care. J Public Health Dent. 1989;49 (5 Spec No):272-8.

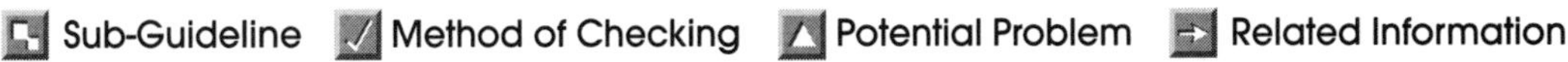
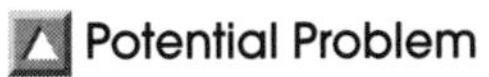
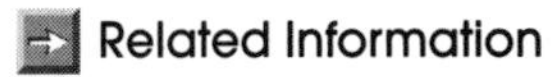

17. **Kaplan RM, Feeny D, Revicki DA.** Methods for assessing relative importance in preference based outcome measures. Qual Life Res. 1993;2:467-75.
18. **Laupacis A, Feeny D, Detsky AS, Tugwell PX.** How attractive does a new technology have to be to warrant adoption and utilization? Tentative guidelines for using clinical and economic evaluations. Can Med Assoc J. 1992;146(4):473-81.
19. **Nord E.** Methods for quality adjustment of life years. Soc Sci Med. 1992;34(5)559-69.
20. **Testa MA, Simonson DC.** Assessment of quality-of-life outcomes. N Engl J Med. 1996; 334(13):835-40.
21. **Guyatt GH, Sackett DL, Sinclair JC, Hayward R, Cook DJ, Cook RJ.** Users' guides to the medical literature. IX. A method for grading health care recommendations. Evidence-Based Medicine Group. JAMA. 1995; 274(22):1800-4.
22. **Kawachi I, Malcom LA.** The cost-effectiveness of treating mild-to-moderate hypertension: a reappraisal. J Hypertens. 1991;9:199-208.
23. **Maynard A.** The design of future cost-benefit studies. Am Heart J. 1990;119(3 Part 2): 761-5.
24. **Brett AS.** Treating hypercholesterolemia: How should practicing physicians interpret the published data for patients? N Engl J Med. 1989;321(10):676-80.
25. **LeBlond RF.** Improving structured abstracts [Letter]. Ann Intern Med. 1989;111(9):764.
26. **Frick MH, Elo O, Haapa K, et al.** Helsinki heart study: primary prevention trial with gemfibrozil in middle-age men with dyslipidemia: safety of treatment, changes in risk factors, and incidence of coronary heart disease. N Engl J Med. 1997;317:1237-45.
27. **Detsky AS, Naglie IG.** A clinician's guide to cost-effectiveness analysis. Ann Intern Med. 1990;113:147-54.

Chapter 13

CONSIDERING MEDICAL RISKS AND PATIENT PREFERENCES

Reporting Decision Analyses and Clinical Practice Guidelines

Decision analysis is the application of explicit, quantitative methods to analyze decisions under conditions of uncertainty.

W.S. RICHARDSON AND A.S. DETSKY (1)

The practice of medicine involves making decisions about how best to diagnose and treat patients. Good medical care requires that these decisions be made appropriately and efficiently from the patients', providers', and payers' points of view. However, medical advances have increased the number of diagnostic and treatment options, which has in turn increased the number and complexity of potential care decisions that need to be made. In addition, the need to be cost-conscious and to consider patients' preferences for care further increases the number of factors in each decision.

Not surprisingly, research into the delivery of health care has indicated several problems with the collective decision-making of health care providers:

- Many medical therapies have not been tested with, or are not supported by, scientific research (2). The Congressional Office of Technology Assessment estimated that randomized controlled trials support the efficacy of less than 20% of all medical procedures available in the United States (3).
- Much medical care appears to be unnecessary (4,5). In fact, "Every study that has looked for the overuse of medical services has found it" (6).
- The rate with which a given therapy is administered, even in adjacent geographical areas, is often widely variable (6,7). This variability appears to be the result of a lack of consensus as to what constitutes

appropriate care, not as a result of different patient populations or the availability of the therapies.

In response to these issues, many clinicians are attempting to "... move away from unexamined reliance of professional judgment toward more structured support for, and accountability of, such judgment" (6). This movement toward "evidence-based medicine" (8) has stimulated the development of several methods for weighing health effects, economic effects, and patient preferences in making medical decisions (9). Such methods attempt to improve decision-making by detailing appropriate indications for specific medical interventions and may allow clinicians to improve the quality of care and to reduce the cost of care at the same time (6). The potential benefits and concerns about the use of these methods are summarized in **Table 13.1.**

Among these methods are **decision analysis** and the writing of **clinical practice guidelines.** *Decision analysis* is the "systematic approach to decision making under conditions of uncertainty" (10), whereas clinical *prac-*

TABLE 13.1 Potential Benefits and Concerns of Adopting the Use of Decision Analyses and Clinical Practice Guidelines.

Benefits	Concerns
Promotes the application of medical research to patient care	May lead to "cookbook" medicine and to disinterest in practicing medicine
May improve a clinician's effectiveness	May lead to nonphysician (governmental) control of medicine
May reduce the amount of inappropriate care	May stifle innovations in care
Makes trade-offs explicit and identifies the probabilities of each choice	Trade-offs may not be evaluated appropriately; data may be inadequate
May improve the cost-effectiveness of medical decisions	Savings may not offset the cost of developing and updating guidelines
Accommodates the complexity of new technologies	Technology may change more quickly than the guidelines can be developed
May serve as an "affirmative defense" in malpractice cases	May serve as culpable evidence in malpractice cases
Explicitly incorporates patients' values and desires	May reduce all decisions to mathematical probabilities

(Adapted from Walker RD, Howard MO, Lambert MD, Suchinsky R. Medical practice guidelines. West J Med. 1994;161[1]:39-44.)

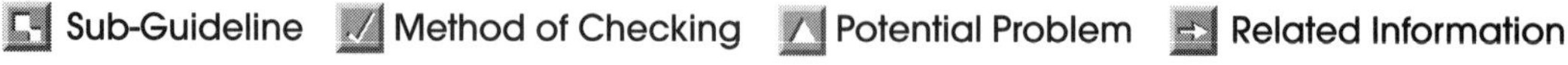

tice guidelines, critical pathways, prediction rules, or the *AMA's Practice Parameters* (11) are "systematically developed statements to assist practitioner and patient decisions about appropriate health care for specific circumstances" (6,8,12–15). Decision analysis differs from practice guidelines in that a decision analysis is usually more quantitative and a practice guideline is usually more "narrative" and specific to a particular practice setting. A decision analysis attempts to provide insight into the *process* of clinical decision making, whereas a clinical practice guideline is more prescriptive about clinical decisions (16). Indeed, a practice guideline may be based on a decision analysis. However, the two methods are similar and complementary, so we present guidelines for reporting the development and characteristics of both. For the sake of consistency, we use the terms for decision analysis and refer to clinical practice guidelines only when presenting information that is not part of a decision analysis.

Decision analysis begins with the question of how best to treat a specific medical condition. It then defines the treatment options and the potential complications of each option, identifies the eventual clinical endpoints of each option, and incorporates a measure of patient preference for the desirability of each endpoint. By making the treatment decisions explicit and by estimating the likelihood and desirability of each option and endpoint, these methods allow patients and providers to make better informed decisions.

SAMPLE PRESENTATION

Our goal was to determine whether women with a dominant breast mass detected on physical examination should routinely undergo needle biopsy to detect malignancy without first undergoing mammography or whether the combination of mammography and biopsy would be a more efficient approach to detecting breast cancer.

The decision tree is shown in **Figure 13.1.** Data from a national study conducted by Smith and colleagues indicate that of every 1000 women with a breast mass, about 14% will have positive mammograms, about 10% will have inconclusive mammograms, and about 76% will have negative mammograms.

The likelihood that cancer will be confirmed in a woman with a positive mammogram is based on data from a randomized controlled trial by

Continued

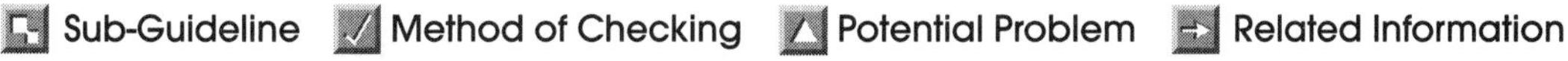
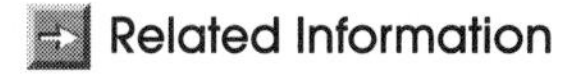

SAMPLE PRESENTATION – *Cont'd.*

Jones and colleagues. The sensitivity of mammography for breast cancer was thus determined to be 53% and the specificity, 96%. The United Health Congress Consensus Conference reported that cancer was eventually detected in women with inconclusive mammograms at a rate of 34%, and in women with negative mammograms at a rate of 4%.

Using the biopsy threshold of 10% reported by Brown for a large randomly selected sample of women in Chicago, we conclude that only women with dominant breast masses and positive or inconclusive mammograms should be referred for needle biopsy. The risk of cancer in these two groups is 53% and 34%, respectively, well above the 10% risk at which women in the Chicago sample would elect to have the biopsy. Women with a negative mammogram have only a 4% risk of cancer, which is below the 10% threshold.

Adopting the above policy means that biopsy would be indicated in 240 of every 1000 women with a dominant breast mass; that is, in all women with positive or inconclusive mammographic findings.

Because current practice is to perform a biopsy on each woman in whom a mass is detected, our results indicate that if 1000 such women first had mammography, 760 biopsies could be avoided. In addition, 30 cases of malignancy would be missed, an error rate of 0.03. (This example is modified by one presented in Eddy [17].)

Here,

- The decision to be made is stated (should needle biopsy be routine?), as is the patient population (women with a dominant mass in the breast found during a physical examination) and the outcome of interest (diagnosing malignant breast tumors).
- A decision tree (**Figure 13.1**) presents the possibilities to be considered and the probabilities associated with each possibility. The sources for the data used to construct the tree are also given.
- The biopsy threshold is the level of risk below which women do not wish to undergo biopsy and above which they do choose biopsy. In this case, "Brown" (a fictitious name for this example) has reported that women prefer that a biopsy be performed only if the chance of having cancer is greater than 1 in 10. Such patient preferences are an important feature in decision analyses and clinical practice guidelines.
- The implications of a change in policy are given; namely, that for every 1000 women considered, 760 biopsies could be avoided at the cost of missing malignancy in 30 cases and the cost of 1000 mammograms.

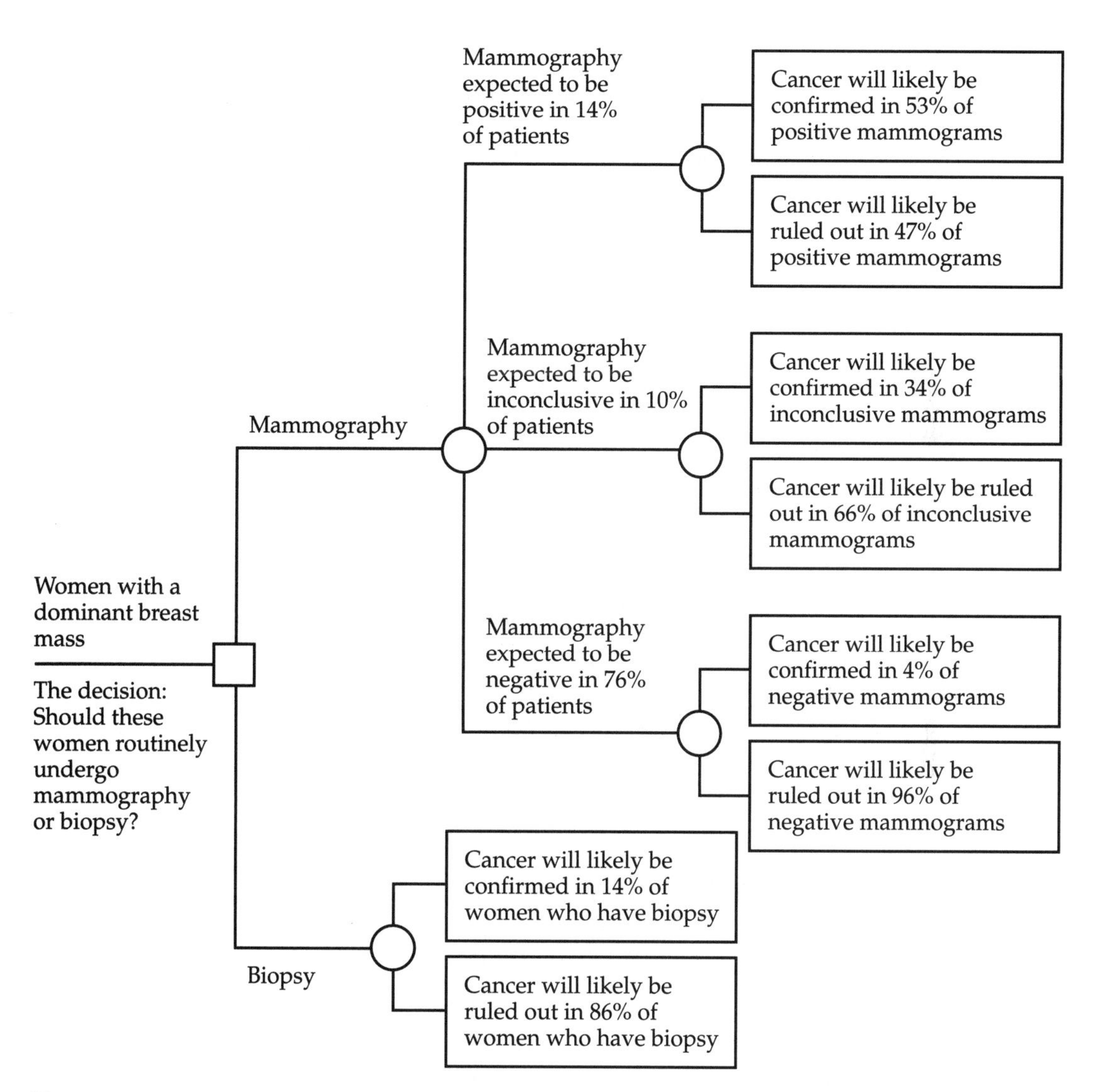

FIGURE 13.1 A decision tree comparing the options and probable consequences of routinely performing needle biopsies or mammography on all women in whom a dominant breast mass is discovered during a physical examination. The probabilities of each branch are shown. Square nodes are called "decision nodes" because the branches represent options that can be chosen. Circular nodes are called "chance nodes" because the branches represent biologically determined responses. The sum of the probabilities for each level of the decision tree is 1.0.

GUIDELINES ADDRESSED IN THE INTRODUCTION

13.1 State the question under study. Specify the diagnosis and the patient population of interest and, if appropriate, the providers and the setting involved and the time horizon over which the analysis is to be applied.

Both decision analyses and clinical practice guidelines should begin with a clear problem statement. The targeted patient population, the targeted diagnosis, and the targeted treatments should be thoroughly described. For example, the purpose of the analysis may be to prevent, screen, diagnose, treat, or palliate.

The time horizon is the time period over which the events and decisions in the analysis are expected to occur. The time horizon for patients with silent gallstones may extend for 30 years, whereas the time horizon for the decision to perform a diagnostic test may be negligible.

EXAMPLES:

- To identify the optimal cost-effective screening strategy for breast cancer in asymptomatic women, we compared the results of breast physical examination with those of radiographic examination of both breasts. These screening tests were compared for various age groups of women, for various frequencies of testing, and for asymptomatic women with and without specified risk factors.
- Should patients older than 65 years of age with systolic hypertension be treated with antihypertensive medication? (2)

13.2 Indicate why the analysis was undertaken.

Decision analyses or practice guidelines may be developed for several reasons (12):

- To promote more effective and efficient physician practices
- To evaluate physician practices (for utilization review and quality assurance studies)
- To promote more consistent physician practices
- To clarify or resolve clinical controversies
- To set limits on physician choices (for recertification and cost-containment programs)
- To communicate important new findings from clinical studies

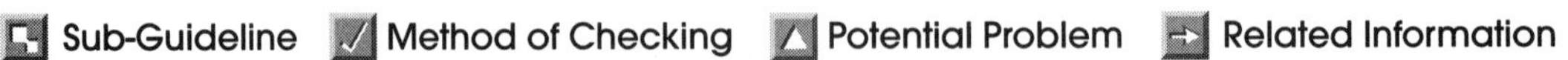

Decision analyses and practice guidelines may also be developed for use with individual patients, for general use with a class of patients, or to develop health policies (18).

Given the time and resources necessary to develop clinical practice guidelines, the objective should have important clinical or financial implications.

13.3 State the perspective from which the analysis was conducted.

A decision analysis or practice guideline used to treat a single patient may incorporate different preferences than one used to guide policy, in which the goal may be to provide the greatest good for the greatest number of patients (19). Also, because the assumptions required in a decision analysis or a practice guideline are easily influenced by the perspective of the developers, this perspective should be identified.

The importance of declaring the identity (*see **Guideline 13.4***) and the perspective of the developer is illustrated by Trobe (4), who cites the findings of three different groups who evaluated the ability of the contrast sensitivity test to determine whether a patient would benefit from cataract surgery:

- The American College of Eye Surgeons (characterized as "high-volume cataract surgeons") was much in favor of the test.
- The American Academy of Ophthalmology (characterized as "ophthalmologists with many different subspecialty interests") acknowledged the occasional value of the test.
- The Agency for Health Care Policy and Research (characterized as "ophthalmologists, nonophthalmologic physicians, optometrists, nurses, social workers, and patients") reported that the evidence for the efficacy of the test was not convincing.

13.4 Identify the persons, groups, or both, who developed, funded, or have endorsed the practice guideline.

Listing the people and organizations associated with the practice guideline may aid readers in evaluating the guideline. The American Medical Association also recommends that relevant physician organizations be given the opportunity to review and comment on practice guidelines during their development (11).

Several professional societies and government agencies are involved with developing clinical practice guidelines, such as the American Medical Association, the American College of Physicians, the Canadian

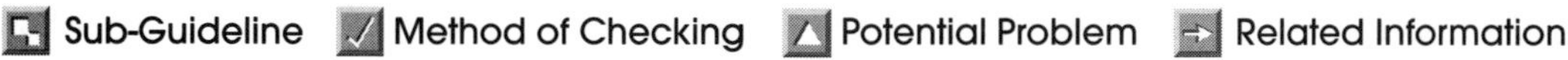

Task Force on the Periodic Health Examination, the US Preventive Health Task Force, and the National Institutes of Health Consensus Development Program (4,13).

GUIDELINES ADDRESSED IN THE METHODS

13.5 Identify the decisions and implications under study: the starting point, branching points, and outcomes that were considered in the analysis.

Decision analysis involves studying choices and their consequences, so those included in the analysis must be identified. All therapies have "benefits, harms, and costs" that should be considered (2). In addition, the context and boundaries of the decision need to be known so that the analysis can be put into perspective (10). Most common in decision analysis is the decision tree, described below.

The *starting point* is the question posed.

The *branching points* are points at which alternatives become possible. There are two types: decision nodes and chance nodes. **Decision nodes** are branching points at which alternative choices are indicated, such as the choice between medical or surgical therapy or between one drug and another. Sometimes, patient preferences for each alternative are given, as in the opening example, where women choose not to undergo biopsy until the risk of cancer is more than 10%. **Chance nodes** indicate the probable biological consequences of a decision or condition: adverse event rates, survival rates, failure rates, and so on.

Outcomes are the clinical states at which the decision analysis concludes. Each outcome is often assigned a weight or utility (a qualitative measure of desirability) so that it may be compared with alternative outcomes. Report the outcomes (the benefits, harms, and costs) in clinically relevant terms, such as the number-needed-to-treat (or another effort-to-yield ratio), or likelihood ratios (2,14) (***see Guidelines 10.9 and 12.18***).

Economic outcomes are as difficult to evaluate as therapeutic outcomes and are often not included in clinical practice guidelines.

As in economic evaluations, when structuring the problem to evaluate competing treatments, the comparison may need to include the following:

- The most common therapy
- The most effective therapy
- The least expensive therapy
- The do-nothing option

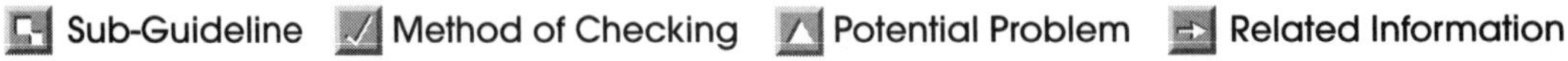

In decision analyses, the structure of the problem may be a "decision tree" or a "decision table." In clinical practice guidelines, the structure may be referred to as a "care path" or as a "treatment algorithm." Sometimes the problem can be structured with a receiver operating characteristics (ROC) curve or as a cost-outcome curve (***see Guidelines 10.10 and 12.17, respectively***).

13.6 Describe the criteria used to include, exclude, combine, or otherwise evaluate the data used in the analysis.

Because the quality of a decision analysis or a clinical practice guideline depends on the quality of the data on which it is based, how the data were selected is an important part of the development process. Literature reviews may be restricted to randomized controlled trials, for example, or to studies with a minimum sample size.

Guideline 11.7: Describe the information sources and search strategies used to find the studies to be analyzed

The quality of the data may also be indicated to aid in analysis (8). One common illustration of the strength of scientific evidence is shown below in ascending order, from weakest to strongest.

1. Anecdotal case reports of single patients
2. Case series without controls
3. Case series with controls from the literature
4. Analyses of clinical databases or registries
5. Case–control observational studies
6. Case series based on historical control groups
7. Single randomized controlled trials
8. Confirmed randomized controlled trials
9. Meta-analyses (controversial; ***see Chapter 11***)
10. Cumulative meta-analyses (controversial; ***see Chapter 11***)

Determinants of poor study quality include, among many other factors: inadequate sample size, recruitment bias, losses to follow-up, unmasked outcome assessment, atypical patient groups, unreproducible interventions, and impractical clinical settings (20).

Because appropriate, well-conducted scientific studies may not be available for many topics, expert opinion is often required to resolve questions of medical practice. In such cases, "consensus conferences" or expert panels may be convened, or a consensus-building technique such as the Delphi process may be used. In the **Delphi process,** a summary statement

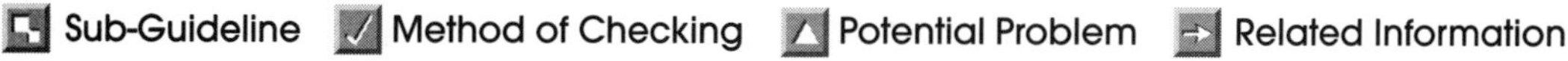

of the topic is circulated to a group of experts, who comment on it. Their comments are synthesized into a revised summary statement, and the new statement is circulated again to the same experts. Comments are again added and synthesized. The process continues until consensus is reached or until the discrepancies are defined.

However, "There is no consensus on how consensus is achieved . . . " (13) and "The nature of appropriate use of expertise is one of the most hotly debated areas in guideline development (8)." For these reasons, the process by which consensus was reached (or not) should be described in detail.

In **Monte Carlo simulations,** a large, hypothetical cohort of patients is put through the decision analysis to generate a distribution of expected probabilities for each outcome. The means and standard deviations of these distributions can then be used to estimate the probabilities in the formal decision model. Monte Carlo simulations can also be used to estimate the utilities of outcomes and to evaluate the results of a Markov process (*see also Guideline 13.9*).

13.7 Describe the methods used to identify and collect the data on which the analysis is based.

Data for clinical practice guidelines should be collected systematically and with great thoroughness. Data may come from several sources:

- Literature reviews, especially of meta-analyses and economic evaluations
- Fee schedules
- Clinical registries and health care databases
- Expert opinion
- Consensus panels
- Input from patients
- Input from providers

Different sources of data may emphasize different aspects of treatment (12). For example, the results of literature reviews, expert opinion, and local experience may differ.

In **consensus conferences**, experts discuss the current state of the knowledge about a practice, but the evidence and rationale for the recommendations are often obscure (9). Randomized controlled trials may not be representative of actual medical practices (19). At issue is whether a tightly controlled trial that establishes the efficacy of a treatment can be used to infer the effectiveness of the treatment under real-world conditions where patient adherence is not as good, procedures may not be applied as rigorously, and so on.

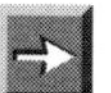 **Guideline 1.1: State the purpose of the study**

13.8 State how utilities (patient values or preferences) for different choices or outcomes were determined.

A utility is a measure of desirability and is usually expressed on a scale from 0 (most undesirable) to 1 (most desirable). The value of decision analyses and practice guidelines is that they explicitly accommodate preferences, usually those of patients but sometimes of providers and payers. Thus, it is important to specify the people (for example, generalists, specialists, patients, payers) and the methods used to assign values.

"Linking treatment options to outcomes is largely a question of fact and a matter of science. In contrast, assigning preferences to outcomes is largely a question of opinion and a matter of value" (8).

It may be useful to state the ethical principles on which these preferences were determined (8):

- *Patient autonomy,* which emphasizes personal freedom of choice
- *Nonmalfeasance,* which emphasizes the desire not to cause harm
- *Distributive justice,* which emphasizes fairness within a defined group

"It is crucial for practitioners to describe the outcomes to their patients and to elicit their preferences" (21). Patient preferences may be established for different alternatives (for example, medical versus surgical treatment), for decision thresholds (for example, the degree of acceptable risk), or for outcomes (for example, quality-of-life measures). Among the techniques used to assign preferences are the standard gamble (or lottery technique), magnitude estimation, and the time-trade-off techniques (22,23) (*see* ***Guideline 12.12***).

The degree of consensus (or ambivalence) among those involved should be indicated, and relevant dissenting opinions may also need to be reported (8). Also, utilities may not be constant over time (19).

13.9 Identify the statistical techniques and the associated statistical package or program used in the analysis.

Each alternative in the structure of a decision tree is associated with a probability that it will occur or that it will result in a particular outcome. Several statistical techniques can be applied to calculate these probabilities. The most common are described below.

The **Markov** or **state-transition process** is used in complex decision trees, in which the number of branches and alternatives is large, the associated probabilities may change over time, and events may occur more than once. In this process, a set of "health states" is defined, as are the criteria for moving from one health state to another. The likelihood that a patient will move from one health state to another in any given period is called the "transition probability" (23). In addition, each health state is weighted by a measure of utility, such as a quality-of-life adjustment, which indicates on a scale of 0 (indifferent to life and death) to 1 (health) how desirable the health state is rated to be ***(see also Guideline 12.12).*** The Markov process may also use "subtrees" to represent repetitive segments of the decision tree.

In **Bayes' theorem,** three probabilities are involved:

- The "prior probability" of the condition or event that is known in advance of the study (for example, the prevalence of patients having a given allergy).
- The "conditional probability," typically the success rate of the treatment or the sensitivity of the test (here, the probability that the patch test will result in true-positive findings).
- The "posterior probability," or the probability determined from the first two probabilities using Bayes' theorem (here, the probability of actually truly being allergic to the allergen, given a positive patch test) (***see also Chapter 14***).

Numerical models encompass a range of general linear models (for example, linear regression or analysis of variance) and structural equation models.

Receiver operating characteristics (ROC) curves are useful in indicating the trade-offs between false-positive and false-negative results from diagnostic tests, including those applied simultaneously or sequentially to improve diagnostic accuracy.

Cost-outcome curves indicate the trade-offs between monetary costs and monetary benefits (cost-benefit curves), therapeutic measures (cost-effectiveness curves), or health states (cost-utility curves). Once the curves are constructed, patients and providers can "operate" at any point along the curve to identify the combination of inputs to outcomes that best meets their needs.

Computer programs developed to perform decision analyses include the following:

- DATA (Decision Analysis by TreeAge Software, Inc), which does decision trees and Markov models
- LISREL (Linear Structural Relationships), which does structural equation modeling
- Decision Tree Software
- Decision Maker

- SML TREE
- SPlus

13.10 Identify the major assumptions and areas of potency, variability, and uncertainty in the analysis.

"A fundamental tenet of decision analysis is that even though available information is incomplete, a decision must be made. Thus analyses often contain assumptions about or estimates of missing data" (19). Variables subject to uncertainty and variation may include infection rates, relapse rates, mortality and morbidity rates, false-positive and false-negative rates, patient preferences, surgical success rates, and so on. The value of these variables in the model may need to be assumed if the analysis is to proceed, and the impact of the assumptions should be tested with sensitivity analysis.

Guideline 13.15: Report any sensitivity analyses used to test the assumptions

Decision analyses and practice guidelines require considerable time and resources to develop. They must be developed carefully because of their *potency*—if implemented, they will likely affect the care of large numbers of people. A flaw in an analysis could adversely affect thousands of patients (13,21). In addition, the more complex the clinical problem and the greater the number of possible treatment options, the more *uncertainty* there is likely to be throughout the analysis, and uncertainty is the main cause of mistakes (21). Finally, the larger the population treated according to the analysis, the more *variability* there is likely to be at every point (24). It is important, therefore, to indicate the areas of potency, uncertainty, and variability in the development process.

GUIDELINES ADDRESSED IN THE RESULTS

13.11 Report the estimated probability for each alternative of each chance node, as well as the misclassification rate at each alternative.

The probability for each alternative in a chance node should be specified. Probabilities may include those associated with the natural history of the condition (such as the rate of calcium loss) or the effects of the therapy under study (such as the infection rate) (19).

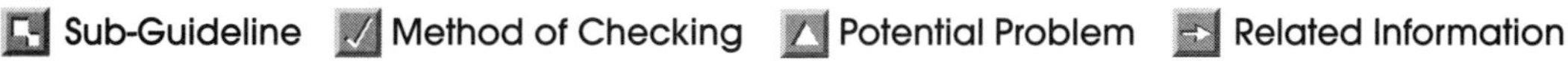

The fact that two or more therapeutic alternatives do not result in markedly different outcomes (the "toss-up result") is also valuable (18).

The sum of the probabilities from the alternatives at each branching point should be 1.

13.12 Report the estimated probability of each alternative of each decision node.

In a decision analysis or economic evaluation, the probabilities of each alternative in a decision node may need to be specified so that the probability of each outcome or the number of patients achieving each outcome can be predicted. In a clinical practice guideline, the probabilities may not be necessary because the purpose of the guideline is to guide care, not to quantify the relationships between options and outcomes.

13.13 Report the utility measure for each outcome and for each decision node, if applicable.

One of the purposes of decision analysis is to incorporate patient preferences into the decision-making process. This purpose is achieved by quantifying the risk and benefits of the various choices, including the desirability of the final outcome.

13.14 When possible and appropriate, illustrate the analysis with a decision tree.

A decision tree is a diagram that depicts the chance nodes, decision nodes, and outcomes of the decision analysis (**Figure 13.1**). We use the term *decision tree* here in a general sense; other terms are common, although some have slightly different meanings. In particular, *algorithms* usually consist of several yes-no branching points without probabilities or utilities. Algorithms are often perceived as being too simplistic for clinical use.

Clinical care paths, flow diagrams, and *classification and regression trees (CART)* are other common terms for these diagrams. These diagrams indicate courses of action and the conditions under which each is preferred (**Figure 13.2**).

13.15 Report any sensitivity analyses used to test the assumptions.

Sensitivity analysis is a procedure in which important variables are varied over their range of values to determine their impact on the outcome.

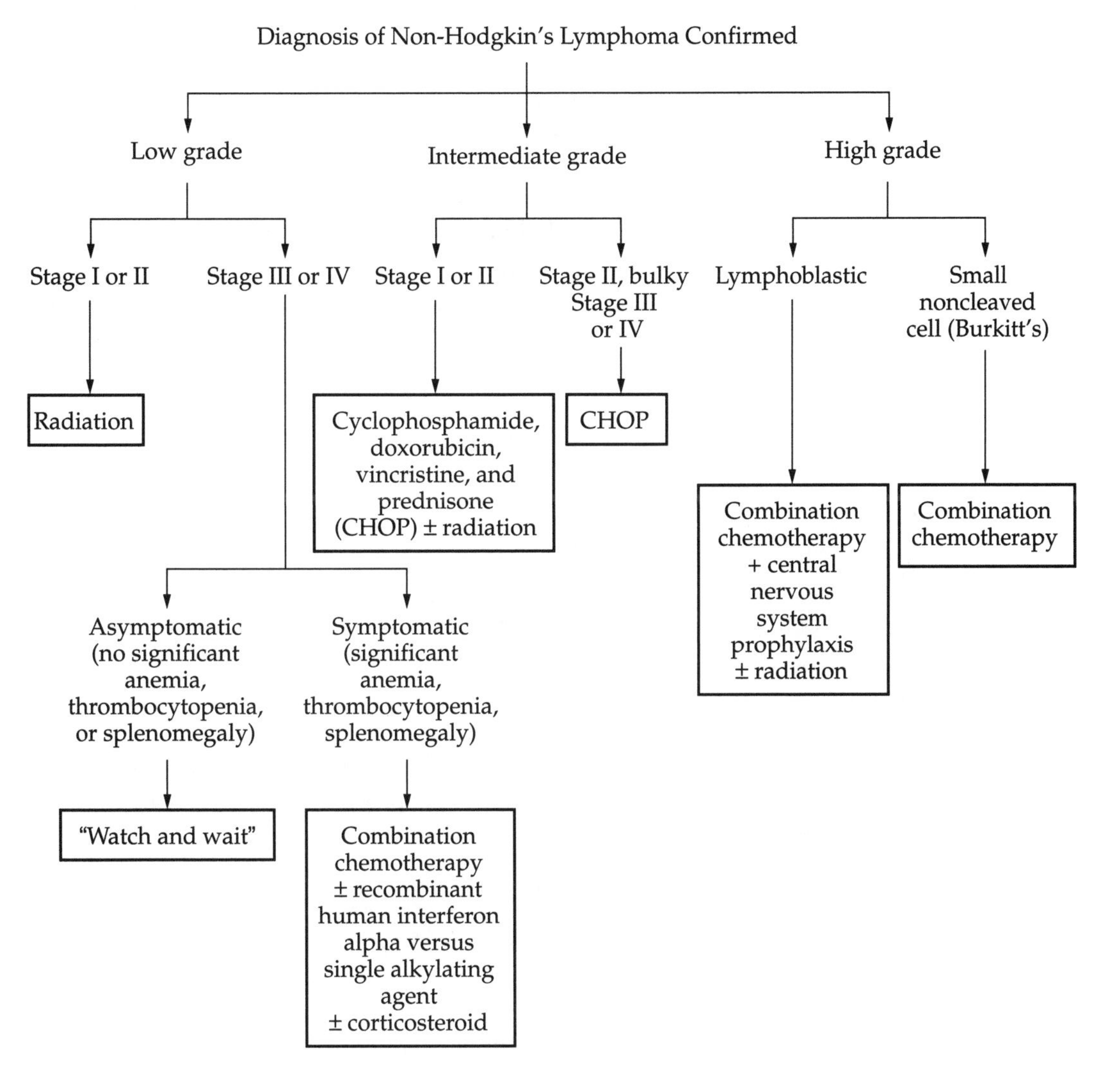

FIGURE 13.2 A clinical practice guideline indicates the preferred course of action in different conditions. Probabilities or utilities may not be assigned to alternatives and endpoints, as in decision analysis, but the guideline may otherwise be developed through a process similar to that of decision analysis. (Reprinted with permission from Fisher RI, Oken MM. Clinical practice guidelines: non-Hodgkin's lymphomas. Cleve Clin J Med. 1995; 62(suppl I):516-42.)

For example, the incidence of an adverse reaction to a treatment may be known only within wide limits. In the decision analysis, the incidence can be changed from the minimum incidence to the maximum incidence. If the outcome changes little, the incidence rate adds little to the uncertainty of the outcome and the model can be applied with more confidence. If the outcome changes greatly, it may be wise to define the incidence rate more closely before applying the model.

In **threshold analysis,** the probabilities and utilities are varied to determine the "break-even" point of each variable in the model; that is, the points at which outcomes are equivalent in the strategies being compared (19).

One-way, two-way, and **three-way sensitivity analyses** may also be performed, in which one, two, and three variables, respectively, are varied together to determine changes in outcome (**Figures 12.2 and 12.3**). These figures may contain "strategy lines." The point at which strategy lines intersect is called a "decision threshold," meaning that the optimal treatment differs on either side of the threshold.

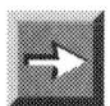
Figures 12.2 and 12.3 in Economic Evaluations

GUIDELINES ADDRESSED IN THE DISCUSSION

13.16 State the recommendations and the conditions under which alternatives at each decision node are and are not appropriate.

For clinical practice guidelines, give the indications, contraindications, and differential risks for each treatment (2). The recommendations should be both practical and clinically important (8,20).

13.17 Indicate the strength of the recommendations and the flexibility with which the decision analysis or practice guideline can be applied.

In any decision analysis, there must be a good "fit" among the question being asked, the structure of the mathematical model, and the data available. Sometimes the analyst finds a good match between only two of these three factors (18). The better the "fit," the stronger the recommendations.

Eddy (21) has proposed that practice guidelines be identified as being from one of three categories that indicate the flexibility with which the guideline can be applied. Classification into these categories depends on 1) the degree of certainty associated with the outcome, 2) the degree to which the preferences of patients are known, and 3) the range of preferences among patients (9,21).

- A **standard** is a practice guideline that should be applied in virtually all cases. Exceptions will be rare and difficult to justify, and violation of the standard may be considered to be malpractice. The evidence for the predictability of the therapeutic and economic outcomes must be compelling. There must be unanimity among patients about the overall desirability (or undesirability) of the outcomes.

- A **guideline** is a practice guideline that should be followed in most cases. It can and should be modified for individual circumstances, but deviations are expected and do not in themselves constitute malpractice. The predictability of at least some of the outcomes should be known within reasonable limits. An appreciable majority of patients must desire (or not desire) the outcomes.
- An **option** is a practice guideline that neither recommends nor warns against a particular clinical practice. Here, the outcomes may not be known, patient preferences may not be known or they may be divided among equivalent options, or patients may be indifferent to the outcomes.

Other terms that may be used to describe the recommended treatment include a **pathway**, which identifies a preferred course of action (12), a **boundary,** which indicates the limits within which appropriate practice takes place, and a **provisional practice guideline,** which identifies the guideline as tentative, pending additional evidence (12).

13.18 Identify any dissenting opinions or disagreements among the guideline developers.

Because the options, probabilities, and utilities used in a decision analysis may be greatly influenced by judgment, it is important to report any major differences in opinion that become apparent during the analysis.

13.19 Describe any evaluation or validation process to which the decision analysis or practice guideline was subjected.

Ideally, the validity of the decision analysis or practice guideline will be assessed before implementation. Common validation procedures include the following:

- Peer review by other professional groups
- Comparison with related guidelines developed by other groups
- Field testing
- Subjecting the guideline to the rigors of a randomized controlled trial

"Custom-tailored clothes and over-fit decision rules often don't look good when worn by someone else" (24).

13.20 Indicate the similarities and differences of the decision analysis or practice guideline to other analyses or guidelines covering similar content areas.

Comparison with similar guidelines may help validate the recommendations **(Guideline 13.19)** and may highlight practices that clinicians will have to change if they adopt the recommendations.

13.21 Describe the expected benefits, problems, and costs that may affect patients if the recommendations are implemented.

To help clinicians adopt the recommendations, provide some indication of what they may expect on adoption. Include:

- Expected changes in the rates at which procedures are required
- The possible consequences of mislabeling patients at any point in the analysis

13.22 Give the dates of the most recent evidence considered in the analysis.

Decision analyses and practice guidelines should be based on the most recent data. However, the time between starting and publishing an analysis can be long enough that important new data can be missed. Placing the analysis in time by indicating when the data were current helps readers evaluate the recommendations.

13.23 Identify in-progress or recent developments that may be relevant to the analysis but that were not included in it.

If late-breaking developments cannot be included in the analysis itself, they can at least be described. Readers can then evaluate the recommendations with these developments in mind.

13.24 If appropriate, specify the anticipated "shelf life" of the analysis and when or under what circumstances the recommendations should be reviewed.

Developments in medical information and technology may eventually render a decision analysis or a practice guideline obsolete. In fact, one concern about decision analyses and practice guidelines is whether they can be developed quickly enough to keep pace with rapidly changing technology (6). Specifying the circumstances under which an analysis should be reviewed helps put the analysis in context and, again, helps readers evaluate the recommendations.

13.25 Identify any clinical or administrative changes necessary to implement the recommendations and any social or behavioral factors that may nullify their effectiveness.

"Methods to implement and evaluate clinical practice policies lag behind the enthusiasm for setting them, and the obstacles that confound their adoption go unidentified or unsurmounted (6,13)."

Practice guidelines will be adopted more readily if they

- Are acceptable to health care providers
- Are comprehensible to health care providers
- Can be applied with some flexibility
- Can be applied easily within the health care setting
- Are developed by caregivers or those who practice medicine

Generally, health care providers are more likely to adopt clinical practice guidelines if 1) there are compelling incentives to do so, such as third-party payer insistence, reductions in malpractice insurance, or the opportunity to use adherence to the guidelines as defenses in malpractice cases, or 2) they are provided with prompt and regular feedback about how their practice compares with that of similar providers.

REFERENCES

1. **Richardson WS, Detsky AS.** Users' guide to the medical literature. VII. How to use a clinical decision analysis. A. Are the results of the study valid? The Evidence-Based Medicine Working Group. JAMA. 1995;273 (16):1292-5.
2. **The Evidence-Based Care Resource Group.** Evidence-based care: 2. Setting guidelines: how should we manage this problem? Can Med Assoc J. 1994;150 (9):1417-23.
3. **The Zitter Group.** Outcomes Backgrounder: An Overview of Outcomes and Pharmacoeconomics. San Francisco: The Zitter Group; 1994:1-56.
4. **Trobe JD, Fendrick AM.** The effectiveness initiative. I. Medical practice guidelines. Arch Ophthalmol. 1995;113:715-7.
5. **Leape LL.** Practice guidelines and standards: an overview. QRB Qual Rev Bull 1990;16(2): 42-9.
6. **Walker RD, Howard MO, Lambert MD, Suchinsky R.** Medical practice guidelines. West J Med. 1994;161(1):39-44.
7. **Naylor CD, Guyatt GH.** Users guide to the medical literature. X. How to use an article reporting variations in the outcomes of health services. JAMA 1996;275(7):554-8.
8. **Hayward RS for the Evidence-Based Medicine Working Group.** VIII. How to use clinical practice guidelines. A. Are the recommendations valid? The Evidence-Based Medicine Working Group. JAMA. 1995;274 (7):570-4.

9. **Ganiats TG.** Practice guidelines movement. West J Med. 1993;158(5):518-9.
10. **Crane VS, Gilliland M, Tuthill EL, Bruno C.** The use of a decision analysis model in multidisciplinary decision making. Hosp Pharm. 1991;26(4):309-25, 350.
11. **American Medical Association.** Attributes to Guide the Development of Practice Parameters. Chicago: American Medical Association; 1994:1-11.
12. **Hayward RS, Laupacis A.** Initiating, conducting and maintaining guidelines development programs. Can Med Assoc J. 1993; 148(4):507-12.
13. **Basinski SH.** Standards, guidelines and clinical policies. The Health Services Research Group. Can Med Assoc J.1992;146(6):833-7.
14. **Hayward RS, Wilson MC, Tunis SR, Bass EB, Rubin HR, Haynes RB.** More informative abstracts of articles describing clinical practice guidelines. Ann Intern Med.1993b; 118(9):731-7.
15. **Audet AM, Greenfield S, Field M.** Medical practice guidelines: current activities and future directions. Ann Intern Med. 1990; 113 (9):709-14.
16. **Schwartz WB, Gorry GA, Kassirer JP, Essig A.** Decision analysis and clinical judgment. Am J Med. 1973;55(3):459-72.
17. **Eddy DM.** Probabilistic reasoning in clinical medicine: problems and opportunities. In: Kahneman D, Slovic P, Tversky A, eds. Judgment Under Uncertainty: Heuristics and Biases. Cambridge, Cambridge University Press; 1982:249-67.
18. **Kassirer JP, Moskowitz AJ, Lau J, Pauker SG.** Decision analysis: a progress report. Ann Intern Med. 1987;106(2):275-91.
19. **Goel V.** Decision analysis: applications and limitations. The Health Services Research Group. Can Med Assoc J. 1992;147(4):413-7.
20. **Wilson MC, Hayward RS, Tunis SR, Bass EB, Guyatt GH.** Users' guides to the medical literature. VIII. How to use clinical practice guidelines. B. What are the recommendations and will they help you in caring for your patients? The Evidence-Based Medicine Working Group. JAMA. 1995;274(20): 1630-2.
21. **Eddy DM.** Designing a practice policy. Standards, guidelines, and options. JAMA. 1990; 263(22):3077-84.
22. **Laupacis A, Feeny D, Detsky AS, Tugwell PX.** How attractive does a new technology have to be to warrant adoption and utilization? Tentative guidelines for using clinical and economic evaluations. Can Med Assoc J. 1992;146(4):473-81.
23. **Pauker SG, Kassirer JP.** Decision analysis. N Engl J Med. 1987;316(5):250-8.
24. **Wasson JH, Sox HC, Neff RK, Goldman L.** Clinical prediction rules. Applications and methodological standards. N Engl J Med. 1985;313(13):793-9.

Chapter 14

CONSIDERING "PRIOR PROBABILITIES"

Reporting Bayesian Statistical Analyses

Bayesians deal with the probabilities of hypotheses, given a data set, whereas frequentists [those using classical hypothesis tests] deal with the probabilities of data sets, given a hypothesis.

R.J. LEWIS AND R.L. WEARS (1)

Most of the statistical analyses referred to in this book are based on what is called the "frequentist approach" or "classical hypothesis testing," which has been the most popular school of statistical thought since its introduction in the 1920s. However, an alternative school, called Bayesian statistics, is becoming increasingly popular among some medical researchers, and so we describe it briefly here. Because Bayesian analysis has not been commonly used in biomedical research (although Bayes' theorem is commonly used in diagnostic testing; ***see Guideline 10.13***), little is written about how to report this type of analysis. Thus, we suggest only a few guidelines.

A BRIEF DESCRIPTION OF BAYESIAN STATISTICS

Bayesian statistics is based on Bayes' theorem, which describes the mathematical relationships between the prior or "pre-trial" probability of an event and the posterior or "post-trial" probability of the event, given the implications of the trial data. Simply put, the Bayesian method begins with a set of expectations (the pre-trial probabilities) and then modifies these expectations on the basis of the data collected from a study to form a new set of expectations, called the post-trial probabilities (2).

The Bayesian approach is conceptually attractive because it models conventional decision making. Most decisions about the efficacy of a drug, for example, are made with some knowledge of how it has performed in the past. In most cases, experience or previous research indicates in general terms what the expected effect of the drug will be. As more information is obtained about the drug, these expectations are modified until such time as they are accepted as definitive. Bayesian statistics models this process explicitly.

In contrast, classical hypothesis testing is not easily understood. To begin with, hypothesis testing does not test directly whether a drug is effective. Rather, it assumes that the drug is *not* effective and produces a measure of the evidence in favor of this assumption (the P value). Only when the evidence is weak (that is, a small P value) does the researcher indirectly conclude that the drug is effective.

More precisely, what is actually tested is the **null hypothesis;** the hypothesis that the treatment and control groups are not different. If the evidence from the trial is strong enough to disprove the null hypothesis (that is, if the probability of finding a difference as large or larger than the one found, given that the null hypothesis of no difference is true, is, say, less than 5 times in 100), then the null hypothesis is usually rejected in favor of the **alternative hypothesis,** that the drug is more effective than placebo. However, there are many alternative hypotheses: such as those that hypothesize, say, a 5%, 7%, 10%, or 12% difference between the treatment and control groups. Only the hypothesis advanced by the researchers is usually mentioned, however. In contrast, the Bayesian approach gives the explicit probability that there is no difference between groups.

In addition, classical hypothesis testing does not incorporate previous knowledge about the drug. Every trial is structured to test the same hypothesis: the null hypothesis of no difference. So, no matter how much is known about the drug, the study still commences with the assumption that it either will have no effect (if compared to placebo) or that its effect will be no different that that of the drug to which it is being compared.

For example, suppose a study tested whether a new drug reduced coronary artery stenosis in humans. The researchers randomly assigned a sample of patients to either a treatment or a placebo control group, recorded baseline measurements of arterial diameters in both groups, administered the drug or placebo as indicated, and then took follow-up measurements of arterial diameters in both groups after several months. The difference in mean changes in arterial diameters between the groups was assessed statistically, and conclusions about the clinical value of the drug were then formulated.

If the researchers used classical hypothesis testing, they would first have formulated the null hypothesis of no difference and specified the conditions under which they could reject this hypothesis. In other words, they would have proceeded under the assumption that the drug would have no effect and that any difference between the means of the two groups was the result of chance. They would also specify that if the difference between the groups was greater than a specified amount, and that if the difference was likely to have occurred by chance under the null hypothesis less than, say, 5 times in 100, then they would reject the null hypothesis in favor of an alternative hypothesis, namely that the drug and not chance caused the difference between the groups. The results might be stated as "The medication reduced stenosis by 5% (95% CI = 3% to 7%), and this reduction was statistically significant at the 0.05 level ($P = 0.02$)."

If the researchers used Bayesian statistics, they would first have identified a distribution of pre-trial probabilities that the drug would have some effect. This prior probability (or simply, the "prior") might be estimated from reviews of published studies, pilot studies, or from expert opinion. Here, the prior might be stated as "there is a 60% probability that the drug will reduce coronary artery stenosis by a mean of 5%." Then the data from the study—the new information—would be used to update the prior—the existing information—to create the posterior or post-trial probability that the drug has an effect. Here, the results might be stated as: "We found an 83% probability that the drug reduces stenosis by 5% or more compared to placebo."

The primary and, for many, the overriding criticism of the Bayesian approach is that it is often difficult if not impossible to specify a convincing pre-trial probability distribution (1,3). In addition, few of the major statistical software packages include the capacity to perform Bayesian calculations, so applying the analysis requires extra effort. The advantages are that it is conceptually attractive, has results that are more easily interpreted clinically, and avoids the multiple analysis problem created in classical hypothesis testing by the interim analysis of accumulating data (generating many P values, which increases the probability of making a type I error ***(see Chapter 5)***.

The guidelines below are to be used in addition to those in Chapter 1 when reporting studies analyzed with Bayesian statistics.

14.1 Report the pre-trial probabilities and specify how they were determined.

The pre-trial probability distribution describes the likelihood that any of a range of treatment effects will occur **(Figure 14.1)**. Pre-trial probabilities may be derived from published studies, meta-analyses, pilot studies, or expert opinion, as is done in decision analysis ***(see Chapters 11 and 13)***.

However, if little reliable information is available on which to base the

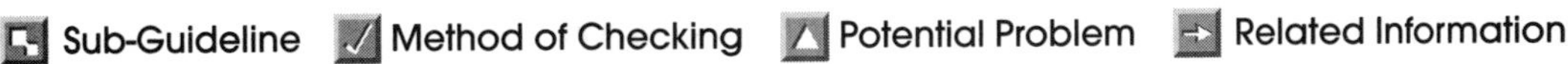
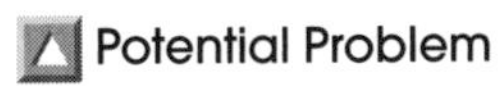
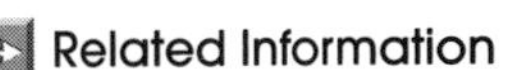

pre-trial probabilities (the priors), a "noninformative prior" can be specified, which simply means that the prior probability distribution is more or less flat; the range of expected outcomes is large. Lewis and Wears (1) report that "In most practical situations, the particular form of the prior information has little influence on the final outcome because it is overwhelmed by the weight of the experimental evidence."

Sometimes, researchers will perform "sensitivity analysis" on the prior probabilities; they will analyze the data with both a "skeptical" and an "enthusiastic" prior to assess the treatment effect under each condition.

14.2 Report the post-trial probabilities and their probability intervals.

The distribution of post-trial probabilities should have less variability as a result of the inclusion of the trial data (**Figure 14.1**).

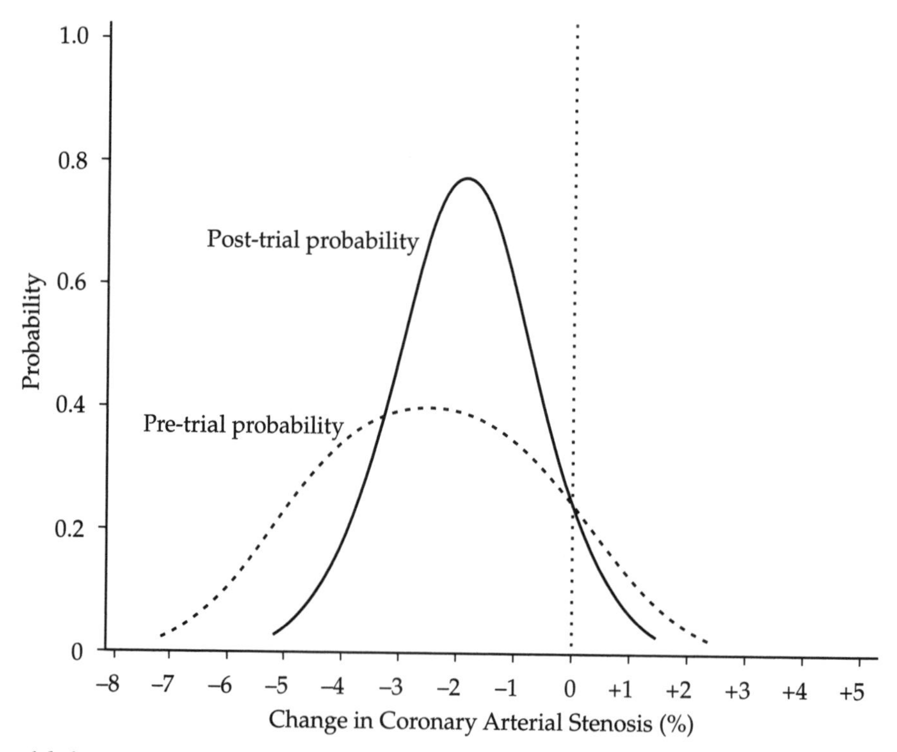

FIGURE 14.1 Hypothetical probability distributions for a Bayesian analysis. The pre-trial probability distribution (dashed line) shows a maximum prior probability of about 0.4 for a 2.5% decrease in coronary arterial stenosis. The post-trial probability distribution (solid line) reflects the new knowledge gained from the trial. The results of the trial have reduced the variation in the pre-trial probability distribution. Now, the maximum post-trial probability is estimated to be about 0.8 for a 2% decrease in coronary arterial stenosis.

The Bayesian *probability interval* or *credibility interval* (2) is analogous to the confidence interval of classical hypothesis testing. The probability interval indicates a range of results and their probabilities.

Graphical displays of the probability distributions, such as that shown in **Figure 14.1**, are also recommended (2,4).

14.3 Interpret the post-trial probabilities.

In Bayesian analyses, there is no arbitrary cutoff point between a negative and a positive study. (In contrast, in classical hypothesis testing, the arbitrary $P < 0.05$ is often taken to be a positive result and $P > 0.05$, a negative one.)

Bayesian analysis also gives the probability that the hypothesis of interest is true, unlike classical hypothesis testing, which gives only the probability of obtaining evidence as extreme or more extreme than that observed under the null hypothesis of no difference.

REFERENCES

1. **Lewis RJ, Wears RL.** An introduction to the Bayesian analysis of clinical trials. Ann Emerg Med. 1993;22(8):1328-36.
2. **Abrams K, Ashby D, Errington D.** Simple Bayesian analysis in clinical trials: a tutorial. Control Clin Trials. 1994;15:349-59.
3. **Jonson NE.** Everyday diagnostics—a critique of the Bayesian model. Med Hypotheses. 1991;34(4):289-95.
4. **Hughes MD.** Reporting Bayesian analyses of clinical trials. Stat Med. 1993;12(18):1651-63.

Chapter 15

FROM RESEARCH RESULTS TO DECISION-MAKING

Reporting Outcomes in Clinically Applicable Terms

Any reporting practice that impedes proper inference is inappropriate.

S. E. FIENBERG (1)

Most of the guidelines in this book are for documenting standard statistical procedures and analyses. Reporting the results of a study accurately and completely, however, does not ensure that they will be easily or appropriately interpreted for purposes of clinical decision-making. In this chapter, we identify six conventions for reporting outcomes in more clinically applicable terms.

15.1 Report the "clinical conclusions" of the research.

Many articles provide conclusions that focus on the science of the research rather than on the clinical implications of the research. In some cases, such as when one is testing a theory or replicating other research, this focus may be justified. Too often, however, the clinical implications of clinical research are not clearly identified. The article maintains a topic-based approach, which answers the questions posed by the researcher, and does not take a reader-based approach, which attempts to anticipate and respond to the questions of readers. The question that should be answered in most articles is "How will medicine be different as a result of this research?"

15.2 When applicable, make the patient the unit of reporting.

Many studies are designed to compare the mean values of two groups. If the difference between the means is large enough to be statistically significant, this fact will often be the only result reported. However, reporting that the mean insulin levels returned to normal after treatment says nothing about how many patients regained normal insulin levels. If the treatment caused insulin levels to decrease in some patients but caused them to increase in others in the same treatment group, the mean level would not reflect the change in individual patients. Thus, in addition to reporting the mean value for the group, reporting the number of patients whose condition improved or worsened after treatment can provide more useful information (2,3). (***See also Guideline 1.4.***)

15.3 Report confidence intervals for primary outcomes.

One of the purposes of scientific research is to obtain results that can be generalized to the larger population from which the sample was drawn. That is, the results of the study are often used to *estimate* the response that can be reasonably expected from administering the treatment to a similar group of patients. When it is appropriate to report results as estimates, it is also important to indicate the precision of the estimates. The measure of precision most commonly used in the medical literature is the confidence interval; in particular, the 95% confidence interval. Confidence intervals are explained in detail in **Chapter 3, Reporting Confidence Intervals.**

A common practice when comparing, say, two groups, is to give a summary value for each group and the P value for the difference between them. However, also reporting the actual difference between the groups with a confidence interval is often more useful. For example, compare the following presentations:

1. The complication rate of the control group was 32%, and that of the treatment group was 43% ($P = 0.02$).
2. The complication rate of the control group was 32%, and that of the treatment group was 43%, 11% higher (95% CI for the difference of 9% to 13%; $P = 0.02$).

The first presentation focuses on the fact that the difference between the groups is statistically significant. The second presentation focuses on the estimated effect of the treatment—an 11% increase in the complication rate—and the confidence interval indicates that the true rate is expected to range between 9% and 13%. The second presentation is preferred because it focuses on the size of the difference between the groups, not simply that there was a difference. The size of the difference is more clinically useful.

15.4 When applicable, include effort-to-yield measures.

Effort-to-yield measures (***see Guideline 12.18***) express results in terms of how many units of a resource need to be applied to produce one more unit

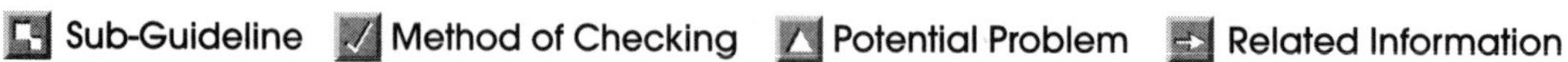

of outcome (4,5). Such measures are useful because they express the result in terms of the units under study, such as how many diagnostic tests will need to be performed to detect one additional case of disease or how much money will be required to prevent one additional case of substance abuse. Effort-to-yield measures are used frequently in economic evaluations, but they are quite useful for reporting the results of many other kinds of research.

In particular, the "number needed to treat," a common effort-to-yield measure, expresses a result in terms of the number of patients who will likely need to be treated to cure or prevent one additional case of the treatment under study. Because health care is delivered to individuals, the number needed to treat expresses results in terms that clinicians readily understand: patients. Alternative tests or treatments can also be more easily compared if both are reported with the same effort-to-yield measure. Effort-to-yield measures should also be presented with confidence intervals.

15.5 When applicable, describe the quality of life after treatment.

Too often, the results of medical research are limited to those biological or clinical changes that occur after treatment. Increasingly, as patients become more involved in their care, the quality of life after treatment—the degree of comfort, satisfaction, and peace of mind experienced by patients—has become an important consideration in accepting treatment (6) (***see also Guideline 9.13***).

Particularly in studies involving decision analysis or the development of clinical practice guidelines, a formal assessment of quality of life may be appropriate (***see also Guideline 12.12***). Informal assessments of quality of life, however, may also be valuable by focusing attention on the human implications of treatment. From the standpoint of applying research results to patient care, the technical success of a new type of surgery may be less important than the quality of life made possible by the new surgery.

15.6 When applicable, use a positive frame of reference.

"Framing" is a term that describes the reference points within which a result is presented. Different frames can promote different interpretations by changing the reference to which the result is compared. For example, describing a drinking glass as "half-full" may foster a different perception than describing the same glass as "half-empty."

A more pertinent example of framing is the fact that people form different opinions of a procedure described as having a 90% success rate (a positive frame) than they do to the same procedure when it is described as having a 10% failure rate (a negative frame). We recommend using the positive frame where possible. For the same reason, reporting survival rates may be preferable to reporting mortality rates.

A thorough discussion of how presenting information can influence readers' sense-making of a text is beyond the scope of this book. We simply wish to call attention to these important and often unaddressed processes. For an excellent review of the subject, see *Judgement Under Uncertainty: Heuristics and Biases* by Kahneman, Slovic, and Tversky (7).

REFERENCES

1. **Fienberg SE.** Damned lies and statistics: misrepresentations of honest data. In: Council of Biology Editors Editorial Policy Committee. *Ethics and policy in scientific publication.* Bethesda, MD: Council of Biology Editors; 1990:202-6.
2. **Felson DT, Anderson JJ, Meenan RF.** Time for changes in the design, analysis, and reporting of rheumatoid arthritis clinical trials. Arthritis Rheum. 1990;33(1):140-9.
3. **Moskowitz G, Chalmers TC, Sacks HS, Fagerstrom RM, Smith H.** Deficiencies of clinical trials of alcohol withdrawal. Alcohol Clin Exp Res. 1983;7(1):42-6.
4. **Laupacis A, Naylor CD, Sackett DL.** An assessment of clinically useful measures of the consequences of treatment. N Engl J Med. 1988; 318(26):1728-33.
5. **Laupacis A, Naylor CD, Sackett DL.** How should the results of clinical trials be presented to clinicians? [Editorial]. ACP Journal Club. 1992; (May/June):A-12-4.
6. **Redelmeier DA, Rozin P, Kahneman D.** Understanding patients' decisions. Cognitive and emotional perspectives. JAMA.1993;270:(1)72-6.
7. **Kahneman D, Slovic P, Tversky A, editors.** *Judgement Under Uncertainty: Heuristics and Biases.* City Cambridge University Press, 1982.

PART 2

GUIDE TO STATISTICAL TERMS AND TESTS

Statistics with plain English as a propellant are formidable missiles.

R. PEARL (1)

This Guide to Statistical Terms and Tests describes many of the more common statistical terms, tests, and concepts encountered in the medical literature. As is true of this book in general, these descriptions are intended to provide an overview of the entry, not necessarily a thorough explanation or a technically sophisticated definition. Fuller explanations for many entries are included in the text and can be located through the index. *(Entries are descriptions and not definitions per se.* ***Boldface*** *entries are listed in the Guide to Statistical Terms and Tests.)*

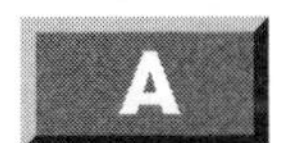

a priori

To perform in advance. An a priori hypothesis is one developed before the data are collected.

See also **post hoc.**

absolute (attributable) risk reduction (ARR)

The difference in risk between the exposed (or treatment) group and the unexposed (or control) group: Pc – Pt, where Pc is, say, the proportion of the control group experiencing the outcome of interest and Pt is the proportion of the treatment group experiencing the outcome of interest. For example, if the incidence of heart attack in men taking aspirin is 1.2% and the incidence in men treated with a placebo is 2.2%, then the ARR for men taking aspirin is 1% (2.2% – 1.2% = 1%), meaning that aspirin lowers the risk of heart attack by 1%. The inverse of the ARR [1/(Pc – Pt)] is the **number needed to treat (NNT),** that is, the number of patients that need to be treated to prevent one adverse event.

See **relative risk reduction** *and* **Guideline 12.18.**

actuarial method: *See* **life table method**

allocation concealment

In a randomized trial, a technique used to prevent selection bias by concealing the assignment sequence until the moment before allocation. Allocation concealment prevents study participants and personnel from predicting the assignment sequence. Allocation concealment is often combined with **masking,** in which group assignment remains concealed after assignment and is not intentionally disclosed until after the study is completed.

alpha (α) or **alpha level**

The probability of essentially accepting a difference as being statistically significant (actually, of rejecting the **null hypothesis**) when, in fact, the difference is the result of chance: the probability of making a **type I error.** The alpha level is the threshold of statistical significance that is established by the researcher. The smaller the probability, the lower the risk of making this type of error. Typical alpha levels are 0.05, 0.01, and sometimes even 0.001.

alpha-error: *See* **type I error**

alternative hypothesis (H_a)
An assertion that factors other than chance are responsible for a difference between groups. An alternative hypothesis is in opposition to the **null hypothesis** of, say, no difference between groups. If the null hypothesis can be rejected on the basis that the results are unlikely to be the result of chance, then the alternative hypothesis is more plausible. The **probability** that the difference is essentially the result of chance is given by the ***P* value**. The *P* value is then compared with the **alpha level** (for example, 0.05), which determines the point at which the researcher is willing to reject the null hypothesis and accept the alternative hypothesis. If the *P* value is less than the alpha level, the observed difference is essentially considered *not* to be the result of chance.

analysis of covariance (ANCOVA): *See* **ANCOVA**

analysis of variance (ANOVA): *See* **ANOVA**

ANCOVA (analysis of covariance; *pronunciation:* an-cova**)**
PURPOSE: To compare two or more groups on the **mean value** of a **response variable** while adjusting for **covariates** (additional variables).
RESPONSE VARIABLE: Continuous.
EXPLANATORY VARIABLE(S): Two or more groups and at least one covariate; ANCOVA models may also include other categorical and continuous explanatory variables (covariates).
RESULTS REPORTED: Two or more group means; the standard deviation for each mean; the actual ***P* value(s),** and the **test statistic(s);** results are often reported in a table.
See Chapter 8.

ANOVA (analysis of variance, *F* tests; *pronunciation:* an-nova)
PURPOSE: To compare three or more groups on the **mean value** of a **response variable.**
RESPONSE VARIABLE: Continuous.
EXPLANATORY VARIABLE(S): Three or more groups; ANOVA models may also include other categorical and continuous explanatory variables.
One-way ANOVA is applied for a single explanatory variable.
Two-way ANOVA is applied for two explanatory variables.
Multiway ANOVA is applied for three or more explanatory variables.
Randomized block ANOVA analyzes treatments that have been randomly assigned within "blocks" (of, say, a certain number of study participants) to ensure that each treatment is represented in each block.
Repeated-measures ANOVA compares three or more **matched** (or paired or

correlated) **groups** of **continuous data** to determine whether they differ significantly. For example, differences in the blood levels of five groups of participants tested every hour for 12 hours may be analyzed with repeated-measures ANOVA.

RESULTS REPORTED: Three or more group means; the standard deviations for each mean; the actual ***P* value(s),** and the **test statistics;** results are often reported in a table.

See Chapter 8.

anecdote; anecdotal

An unsupported observation, usually of a single case or occurrence. "Anecdotal evidence" is akin to hearsay evidence and is the weakest evidence of fact.

association, test of

A test used to assess the strength of a relationship between or among nominal variables. (As opposed to **correlation,** a term typically reserved for measures that assess the strength of a relationship between two ordinal or continuous variables.) If two or more variables are associated (or correlated), they tend to occur together. A test of association (such as the **chi-square test**) quantifies the strength of the relationship.

attributable risk (AR)

The probability, attributed to a certain characteristic, that an event or a particular outcome will occur when this characteristic is present. Usually used to calculate a **risk ratio,** which compares two or more risks.

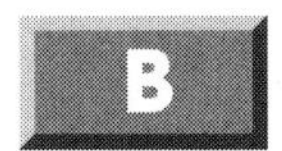

Bartlett's test

PURPOSE: To compare two or more groups on the **variability** of a **response variable.**

RESPONSE VARIABLE: Continuous.

EXPLANATORY VARIABLE(S): Two or more groups.

RESULTS REPORTED: The group variances (the standard deviations squared), the actual ***P* value,** and the **test statistic.**

baseline data

Data collected to describe the treatment and control groups at the start of a study, before treatment has been given. Between the groups, baseline data may be compared to determine whether the groups are similar or whether they are "unbalanced" on one or more variables. Within each group, the baseline data are often compared with the data collected after treatment to determine the effects of treatment.

Bayes' theorem; Bayesian statistics

A theory of statistics involving the concept of **prior probabilities, conditional probabilities,** and **posterior probabilities.** Bayes' theorem specifies the mathematical relationships among these three probabilities. Often used to analyze diagnostic test results. After Thomas Bayes (1702–1761), who developed the theory.

See Chapter 14.

Berkson-Gage method: *See* **life table method**

beta (β) or **beta level**

The probability of concluding that an observed difference is essentially the result of chance when, in fact, it is a real difference; the probability of making a **type II error.** The lower the probability, the better. The value of β is usually not reported; however, 1 –β is the **statistical power** of the test to detect a given difference if one truly exists. Typical values for β are 0.2, which indicates a statistical power of 0.8, and 0.1, which indicates a statistical power of 0.9. Researchers often conclude that, say, two groups are equivalent when differences between them are not statistically significant. If the samples are small, statistical power may be low, and such a conclusion might be wrong. That is, the difference might truly exist, but there may not be enough power to detect it. Larger samples have more statistical power, which means that true differences between groups are more likely to be detected.

See also **alpha.**

beta-error: *See* **type II error**

beta weight: *See* **regression coefficient**

bias

Systematic (as opposed to random) **error** in the conduct of a research study. Often encountered in sample selection and measurement.

bias, selection

The **systematic error** in sampling the population (for example, for a population of men, only men shorter than the interviewer were approached).

binomial test

PURPOSE: To compare two proportions.
RESPONSE VARIABLE: Categorical (expressed as a proportion).
EXPLANATORY VARIABLE(S): Two groups.
RESULTS REPORTED: The two proportions and the difference between them, the 95% **confidence interval** for the difference, the actual ***P* value,** and the **test statistic.**

binomial variable

A variable that has only two mutually exclusive alternatives, such as survival (survived or died) or sex (male or female).

biserial correlation: *See* **point biserial correlation**

blinded; blinding (a "blinded" study): *See* **masking**

blocking
A sampling technique, commonly used in **analysis of variance,** to control for confounding factors.

BMDP
A statistical software package commonly used to analyze biomedical data.

Bonferroni's correction or **adjustment**
A conservative adjustment for the **multiple testing problem.**
See Chapter 5.

Breslow's generalized Wilcoxon test: *See* **Wilcoxon's test**

box plot
A graphical display of the distribution of continuous data in which usually the middle 50% of the observations is indicated by a rectangle and vertical lines above and below the rectangle represent other portions of the range of the data. The median value is often drawn as a horizontal line within the rectangle.
See Figure 2.2, p 45.

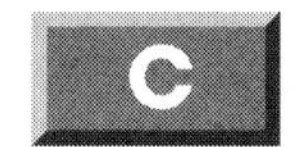

case-control study
A **retrospective study** in which the histories of people with the condition of interest are compared with the histories of a group of people without the condition. Also called a **chart study** because most are based on reviews of medical records.

case-series
A descriptive study in which characteristics of a group or series of patients are recorded and analyzed.

categorical data
Data that are either included in or excluded from a category, such as male or female, where gender is the categorical variable. Categorical data can be **nominal data** or **ordinal data,** as opposed to **continuous data** that can be placed along a continuum. Because data are classified into categories on the basis of a particular quality, categorical data are also referred to as **qualitative data.**

censored data
In survival analysis (*see* **time-to-event analysis**), response values that are unknown because the patient is still living or no longer being followed in the study. Sometimes called **right-censored data** because the time-to-event line is plotted from left to right and the event (usually death) has not yet occurred

when the analysis is performed. (**Left-censored data** are also possible but are much less common.) Authors should report how censored data were dealt with statistically.

See Chapter 9.

census

A data set collected from an entire population, not just from a sample of the population.

central limit theorem

An important theorem in statistics. States that the means of samples drawn even from markedly non-normally distributed populations will be approximately normally distributed for samples larger than 30.

central tendency, measures of

Statistics that describe the "center" of a distribution of values; a single value that best represents the bulk of the observations. The most common are the **mean,** the **median,** and the **mode.**

chart study

Research based on the analysis of a sample of medical records.

See **case-control study; retrospective study.**

chi-square test (χ^2, **Greek letter** χ; *pronunciation:* kigh-square)

A group of tests for **categorical data.**

See also Chapter 6.

chi-square contingency test (also called the **chi-square test of independence** or the **chi-square test of association):**

PURPOSE: To determine whether two attributes of the sample are independent or whether the presence of one is, in fact, associated with the presence of the other.

VARIABLES: Two categorical variables, neither of which is identified as an explanatory or a response variable.

RESULTS REPORTED: Two or more proportions, the actual ***P*** **value,** and the **test statistic.**

chi-square test for proportions:

PURPOSE: To determine whether the proportions or event rates of two or more groups are different.

RESPONSE VARIABLE: Categorical.

EXPLANATORY VARIABLE(S): Two or more groups.

RESULTS REPORTED: Two or more proportions, the actual ***P*** **value,** and the **test statistic.**

exact chi-square test: a chi-square test for proportions used with small samples

chi-square test for goodness-of-fit; the **chi-square test for homogeneity:**

PURPOSE: To determine whether the proportions or event rates from the groups differ from event rates known or estimated in advance.

RESPONSE VARIABLE: Categorical.
EXPLANATORY VARIABLE(S): Categorical.
RESULTS REPORTED: Two or more proportions, the actual ***P* value,** and the **test statistic.**

clinical practice guideline
A written plan that guides patient care decisions by identifying in advance the events and decisions expected during the treatment of a disease. Usually indicates optimal treatments and choices.
See also Chapter 13.

cluster analysis
A statistical technique for classifying subjects into coherent nominal categories. Cluster analysis is used to try to identify an appropriate categorization on the basis of similar characteristics. In contrast to **discriminate analysis,** where the categories are known before the analysis.

Cochran-Mantel-Haenszel test
PURPOSE: To compare two or more proportions while controlling for another categorical explanatory variable.
RESPONSE VARIABLE: Categorical.
EXPLANATORY VARIABLE(S): Two or more categorical explanatory variables
RESULTS REPORTED: The group proportions, the actual ***P* value,** and the **test statistic.**
Also called the **Mantel-Haenszel test.**

Cochran's Q
An extension of **McNemar's test** for three or more matched groups.

coefficient
A term used in statistical modeling, such as **regression analysis** or **analysis of variance;** refers to the weighting of factors in the model. A term also used in **correlation analysis** and in **confidence intervals.**

coefficient of determination (r^2)
The square of the **correlation coefficient.** In simple linear **regression analysis,** the proportion of the variation in the **response variable** that is explained by its relationship to the **explanatory variable.** For example, if the correlation between response variable A and explanatory variable B is $r = 0.8$, then the coefficient of determination $r^2 = 0.64$, which means that 64% of the variability in variable A can be attributed to its relationship to variable B.

coefficient of multiple determination (R^2)
The square of the **correlation coefficient.** In multiple **regression analysis,** the proportion of the variation in the **response variable** that is explained by its relationship to the **explanatory variables.** Not to be confused with r^2, or the **coefficient of determination** used in **simple regression analysis.**
See Chapter 7.

coefficient of variation (CV)

The **standard deviation** of a distribution divided by the **mean** multiplied by 100%. Used to measure relative variation. Useful for comparing the dispersions of several samples or of competing outcomes because it is expressed as a percentage.

See Guideline 2.11.

cohort

A group of persons who have characteristics in common and who are studied over a long period of time. A cohort study is a **longitudinal study.**

cohort, historical

A group of study participants characterized by archival data (medical records, family histories, and so on), as opposed to data collected **prospectively.**

colinearity

In **regression analysis,** the condition of two or more explanatory variables being correlated or not independent of one another.

See Guideline 7.15.

concurrent (parallel) controls

Study participants assigned to a control group and studied during the same period as the treatment group. Contrasts with **historical controls.**

conditional probability

The probability of event A computed under the assumption that another event, B, has occurred. Used frequently in **diagnostic testing, decision analysis,** and **Bayesian statistics.**

See Chapter 14.

confidence bands

In simple linear **regression analysis,** curves showing upper and lower confidence limits (usually 95% confidence limits) around the regression line.

See Figure 7.1, p 110.

confidence coefficient

A percentage indicating the degree of confidence the author has in an estimate. The 95% **confidence interval** has a confidence coefficient of 95.

confidence interval (CI)

An indication of the precision of an estimate of a population value. A 95% or a 99% confidence interval is typical. The range of the confidence interval is usually, but not always, symmetrical with respect to the estimate and is expressed in the same units as the estimate. Wider intervals indicate lesser precision; narrow intervals indicate greater precision.

confidence limits

The upper and lower bounds of the **confidence interval.**

confounding variable

An **explanatory variable** that is related to the **response variable** and that obscures or confounds the primary comparison.

contingency table

A table used to present data for analysis, especially with **chi-square (χ^2) tests.** Values are placed in the cells where the rows (r) and columns (c) intersect. A "2 × 2 table" has two rows, two columns, and four cells.

See Table 6.1, p 98.

continuous data

Data that are measured on a continuum of equal intervals and that can have fractions (for example, 2.35 kg). **Ordinal data** with 10 or more equally spaced categories and **discrete data** (counts of units that do not contain fractions, such as patients) are often analyzed as though they were continuous data.

contributory variable

An **explanatory variable.**

control group

A group of study participants who will receive standard treatment, no treatment, or **placebo** treatment. The results will then be compared with those of the participants in the experimental group who received the treatment under study.

controlled trial

A prospective study in which data are collected from one or more **treatment** and **control groups** under specified conditions. When participants are randomly assigned to groups, the trial is said to be a **randomized controlled trial.**

correlation

A relationship between two variables (usually ordinal or continuous) indicating that a change in one variable is often accompanied by a change in the other. **Association,** a more general term, is typically used to describe a relationship among categorical variables.

correlation coefficient (*r*)

A measure of the linear association between two variables. Varies between +1 (a perfect positive association: as one variable increases, the other also increases) and −1 (a perfect negative association: as one variable increases, the other decreases). A value of $r = 0$ indicates that the two variables are not associated or "co-related." **Kendall's rank-correlation coefficient** measures the linear relationship between two ordinal variables; **Pearson's product-moment correlation coefficient** measures the linear relationship between two approximately normally distributed continuous variables; and **Spearman's rank-order correlation coefficient** measures the linear relationship between two variables, one or both of which are markedly non-normally distributed continuous variables.

cost-benefit analysis

A form of economic evaluation that compares monetary costs to benefits expressed in dollars.

See Chapter 12.

cost-benefit ratio

A ratio of the cost of treatment to the benefit of treatment. Technically, both costs and benefits are expressed in dollars; however, the term is often used for any cost-outcome ratio.

See Chapter 12.

cost-effectiveness analysis

A form of economic evaluation that compares monetary costs to a measure of clinical effectiveness, such as years of life saved.

See Chapter 12.

cost-effectiveness ratio

A ratio of the cost of a treatment to clinical outcome, such as life-years extended or premature deaths avoided.

See Chapter 12.

cost-identification analysis

A type of economic evaluation used to determine the actual costs incurred in providing a service.

See Chapter 12.

cost-minimization analysis

A type of economic evaluation used to determine which options would provide equivalent care or service for the lowest cost.

See Chapter 12.

cost-of-illness analysis

A type of economic evaluation that estimates the total cost of a disease or disability, generally to a population or to a nation. Includes measures of lost productivity as well as treatment costs.

See Chapter 12.

cost-utility ratio

A ratio of the cost of a treatment to a utility, which is the product of a clinical outcome and a health status index. Common utilities are "well years" and **quality-adjusted life-years (QALYs).**

See Chapter 12.

covariate

A variable in a study. Sometimes used to mean an **explanatory variable** and sometimes a **confounding variable.** Used in **analysis of covariance (ANCOVA).**

Cox-Mantel test: *See* **log-rank test**

Cox proportional hazards regression analysis

PURPOSE: In **time-to-event analysis,** a procedure used to determine relationships between the time to the event (usually death) and the explanatory variables.

RESPONSE VARIABLE: Time from a starting point to the event of interest (usually death) or the last follow-up visit if the event has not occurred.

EXPLANATORY VARIABLE(S): Usually several categorical or continuous variables, or both.
RESULTS REPORTED: Proportion of subjects alive at certain times during the study, the actual ***P* value(s),** and the **test statistic(s) for each explanatory variable;** results are often reported in a table.
See Guideline 9.11.

criterion standard
The standard to which, say, the results of a new diagnostic test (called the **index** test) are compared to validate the test. The criterion standard is usually the most accurate measure (the best **reference** test) of the variable under study. The term is preferred to **gold standard,** a term whose meaning is generally limited to the Western world.

Cronbach's alpha
A measure of internal reliability or consistency of the items in a questionnaire. Ranges from 0 to 1 and indicates the degree of association among responses to questions pertaining to the same dimension (such as altruism or hostility) of the questionnaire.

cross-over study
A study design commonly used in pharmaceutical research in which each subject serves as his or her own control. After being assigned to, say, a treatment group for a period, and after a **wash-out period,** the participant will be "crossed-over" to the **control group** for a similar period.

cross-product ratio: *See* **odds ratio**

cross-sectional study
A survey or screening test administered at a single point in time.

Cutler-Ederer method: *See* **life table method**

cutpoint
A value used to separate a distribution into two components. Often used in diagnostic testing, where cutpoints separate the "normal" values from the "abnormal" values. Test results in the normal or acceptable range are termed *negative results;* results in the abnormal range are termed *positive results.*

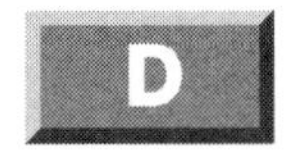

data
A collection of measurements or observations. "Data" is the plural of "datum." "Data are ..." is the correct expression.

data dredging
An informal term for the process of analyzing the results of a study in as many

ways as possible solely to find a statistically significant finding, which is then reported as though the finding were the purpose of the study. When acknowledged and directed by a scientific rationale, such analyses can appropriately be termed *exploratory*. Data dredging, however, is usually driven by nonscientific motives.

See Chapter 5.

decision analysis

A statistical approach to decision making that identifies the optimum alternatives, given various conditions and assumptions.

See Chapter 13.

decision tree

A flow chart for modeling a **decision analysis.** Consists of a starting point and outcomes, as well as branching points that are either chance nodes, which have biologically determined outcomes, or decision nodes, the outcomes of which are decided by patients and providers.

degrees of freedom (df)

The number of values free to vary when a statistic is computed. For example, the number of independent comparisons that can be made among individuals in a sample. A term commonly used in **hypothesis testing,** degrees of freedom are often reported as a subscript number or in parentheses after the related **test statistic.** For example, degrees of freedom should be reported with **Student's *t* test, analysis of variance** (the ***F* test**) for both the numerator and denominator of the *F* ratio, and the **chi-square test,** among others.

Delphi process

A consensus-building technique used in decision analysis and economic evaluations to establish the various assumptions, options, judgments, and numerical values used in the research.

dependent variable: *See* **response variable**

descriptive statistics

Numbers, such as **mean, median,** or **range,** that organize, summarize, or describe a data set.

df

Abbreviation for **degrees of freedom.**

diagnostic accuracy

A characteristic of a diagnostic test; the number of correct diagnoses divided by the number of diagnoses attempted, times 100%. A correct diagnosis may be either a **true-positive** result or a **true-negative** result.

See Table 10.1, p 156.

diagnostic test

A test ordered specifically either to establish the presence or identity of a disorder or to rule it out.

diagnostic yield

A term without a standard meaning sometimes used in diagnostic testing. In contrast to sensitivity, which is a characteristic of a diagnostic test (when computed from an appropriately designed study), and to the positive predictive value, which is a function of disease prevalence in a population and the sensitivity of the test, diagnostic yield is often used to describe what happened when the test was used in a given study. For example, a "low diagnostic yield" may mean that 1) relatively few of the test results were positive, 2) relatively few of the results could be interpreted, or 3) the number of **true-positive** results (when a second test was used as the criterion standard) was relatively low compared with the total number of results obtained. The term should be defined if it is to be used.

discounting

In **economic evaluations,** the practice of expressing future costs and benefits in current dollars. Also called **present value analysis.** Future costs and benefits are multiplied by a "discount factor" to convert them to current dollars.

See Guideline 12.19.

discrete data

Data that can be expressed only in whole numbers because fractions are not possible, as opposed to **continuous data,** which can be measured in fractions. For example, the number of surgeries performed is a discrete variable; "half-surgeries" is not a meaningful concept. Height is a continuous variable because it can be measured in progressively smaller units.

discriminate analysis

A statistical technique for identifying the distinguishing characteristics of nominal categories. Discriminate analysis is used to identify the combinations of variables that reveal differences among known categories, in contrast to **cluster analysis,** where the categories are not known before the analysis.

dispersion, measures of

Statistics that describe the variability of a distribution of values. The most common are the **variance,** the **standard deviation,** the **range,** and the **interquartile range.**

distribution

Typically refers to a frequency distribution: a set of ordered values and the frequencies with which they are observed; usually presented as a graph. That is, the range of values for the variable is plotted on the horizontal axis and the frequency with which each value is observed is plotted on the vertical axis. May also refer to a **probability** distribution of all possible values of a **test statistic** and their associated probabilities, from which ***P* values** are derived. Examples of such distributions include the binomial, the *t*, the *F*, the χ^2, the **Gaussian** or normal, the Uniform, the Weibull, and the **Poisson distributions.** There are many others.

dot chart
A general method of presenting categorical or continuous data in which a line of dots is used like a column or bar chart or like a **box plot.** Useful because it saves space and can be created on a word-processing program.
See Figure 2.3, p 46.

double-blind or **double-masked**
A study design in which neither the study participants nor the investigators are told to which group subjects have been assigned.

drop-out
A study participant who does not complete a study; someone who withdraws from a study. Knowing the characteristics of participants who drop out, as well as their reasons for dropping out, is important in determining the entire effects of the treatment. The drop-out rate of a study should be reported for this reason.

Duncan's multiple-range procedure: *See* **multiple (pairwise) comparison procedures**

Dunn's procedure: *See* **multiple (pairwise) comparison procedures**

Dunnett's procedure: *See* **multiple (pairwise) comparison procedures**

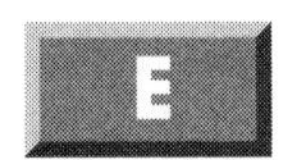

economic conversion
In **economic evaluations,** the process of expressing a clinical outcome or state of health in dollars or another numerical unit (for example, well years; **quality adjusted life-years**) so that treatments can be compared or ranked. Common economic conversions in medicine are the **human capital approach,** the **willingness-to-pay approach,** and the **indirect approach.**
See Guideline 12.11.

economic evaluation
Research that relates the costs (both direct and indirect) of a medical treatment to health outcomes (direct, indirect, and intangible). The most common types of analyses are **cost-identification analysis, cost-minimization analysis, cost-of-illness analysis, cost-benefit analysis, cost-effectiveness analysis,** and **cost-utility analysis.**
See Chapter 12.

effect size
The result of a study; expressed as the magnitude of a difference or the strength of a relationship. Commonly used in sample size estimation (which requires

knowing the smallest effect size that will be considered to be clinically important) and in **meta-analysis.**

effort-to-yield measure

An expression that relates the amount of resources needed to produce a unit change in outcome. For example, the **number needed to treat (NNT)** indicates how many patients must be treated with, say, aspirin, to prevent a heart attack in one person. Other measures include the cost per life saved or the number of procedures required to extend life by 5 years, for example.

See Guideline 12.18.

endpoint

The outcome of a study.

See **response variable.**

error

The difference between a measured, observed, or calculated value and the true value. Three types of errors are commonly encountered in scientific research:

Measurement error is the inherent variability of the measuring instrument: atomic clocks are more accurate than stop watches, which are more accurate than wall clocks.

Sampling error is the error inherent in measuring only a sample of the population.

Systematic error is a nonrandom or consistent source of **bias,** such as would occur if a blood gas monitor consistently reported results 10% below normal because it had been calibrated incorrectly.

error bars

On a chart or graph, vertical lines extending above and below a value, say, a mean score, to indicate dispersion of the data or the variability of the estimate. The value represented by the error bar should be identified: it may refer to the **standard deviation,** the **standard error** (usually the **standard error of the mean;** not preferred to the confidence interval), or the 95% **confidence interval** of the estimate.

See Figure 3.1, p 62.

error mean square (abbreviated out of order as MSE)

In **regression analysis,** a measure of the variation in the random error in the model. (The random error is the error not accounted for by the explanatory variables in the model.) Also called "residual mean square."

estimate

A value believed to represent the "true" value of a variable in a population. Usually derived from an "observed" or measured value in a sample. The "precision" of the estimate can be expressed with a **confidence interval.** A **point estimate** is a single value, such as a **mean.**

exact test

A form of hypothesis test typically used with statistical tests applied to unusually small samples.

exclusion criteria

The characteristics (such as a diagnosis, demographic feature, or clinical condition) that preclude enrollment in a research study. Contrasts with **inclusion criteria,** which are characteristics that are required for enrollment.

experimental group

The group of subjects receiving the treatment under study. In contrast to the **control group.** Also used to mean the "treatment group."

experimental study

A comparative study planned in advance of its conduct and that involves at least one intervention. The comparison may be between two or more groups or between pre- and post-intervention data from a single group.

explanatory study

A study conducted under tightly controlled conditions, as opposed to real-world conditions, to identify underlying biological processes. Usually used in contrast to a **pragmatic study,** which is designed to test the overall effectiveness of a treatment.

See Guideline 1.1.

explanatory variable

A variable believed to affect the response variable of a study; an **independent variable.** Also referred to as a **contributory variable, predictor variable, risk factor,** or **prognostic factor.** Usually indicated with X's (Y's indicate **response variables**).

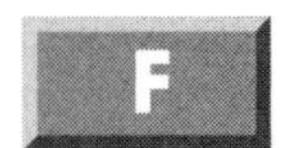

***F* test**

Same as one-way **ANOVA.**

PURPOSE: To compare three or more groups on the mean value of a response variable.

RESPONSE VARIABLE: Continuous.

EXPLANATORY VARIABLE(S): Three or more groups.

RESULTS REPORTED: The group means and standard deviations, the actual ***P* value,** and the **test statistic.**

See Chapter 8.

factor

An **explanatory variable.** A term commonly used in **analysis of variance.**

factor analysis

A statistical procedure used primarily to group related variables to reduce the number of variables needed to represent the data. Usually used to explain correlations among groups of variables or factors.

false-negative rate

The **probability** that a diagnostic test or procedure result will be negative when the disease is present. The false-negative rate is equal to 1 minus the sensitivity of the test.

See Table 10.1, p 156.

false-positive rate

The **probability** that a diagnostic test or procedure result will be positive when the disease is not present. The false-positive rate is equal to 1 minus the specificity of the test.

See Table 10.1, p 156.

Fisher's exact test

PURPOSE: To compare two or more proportions; it is used for small samples.

RESPONSE VARIABLE: Categorical (expressed as proportions).

EXPLANATORY VARIABLE(S): Two or more groups.

RESULTS REPORTED: The group proportions, the actual ***P* value,** and the **test statistic.**

Fisher's least-significant-difference (LSD) method: *See* **multiple (pairwise) comparisons procedures**

Fisher's *z* test

PURPOSE: To compare two groups on the **mean value** of a **response variable** (similar to **Student's *t* test**).

RESPONSE VARIABLE: Continuous.

EXPLANATORY VARIABLE(S): Two groups.

RESULTS REPORTED: The group means and the difference between them, the 95% **confidence interval** for the difference, the actual ***P* value,** and the **test statistic.**

follow-up period

The period of a clinical study after the treatment has been delivered but over which data are still being collected. Because some treatments and adverse side effects take time to appear, the length of a follow-up period can be important in determining the overall effectiveness of the treatment.

frequency polygon

A column chart or **histogram** in which the midpoints of the tops of each column are connected with lines.

Friedman's test

A nonparametric form of the **randomized block ANOVA test.**

PURPOSE: To compare three or more proportions or median values of the **response variable.**

RESPONSE VARIABLE: Categorical (commonly ordinal; it can be expressed as proportions or, if there are many categories, as medians).

EXPLANATORY VARIABLE(S): Three or more groups.

RESULTS REPORTED: The group proportions or medians, the actual ***P* value,** and the **test statistic.**

See **ANOVA.**

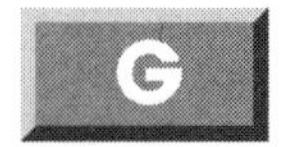

Gaussian distribution
A bell-shaped curve that is symmetrical about the mean.
See **standard normal distribution.**

gold standard: *See* **criterion standard**

goodness-of-fit
In model building, the relationship between a **regression** or an **ANOVA** equation (or model) and the data summarized by the equation. A model that "fits" the data well provides a better summary of the data than one that does not. Also seen as goodness-of-fit hypothesis tests, in which the observed values are compared with expected values taken from a known or theorized distribution (for example, the **chi-square goodness-of-fit test**).

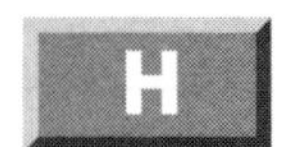

Hartley's test
PURPOSE: To compare two or more groups on the variability or dispersion of a **response variable.**
RESPONSE VARIABLE: Continuous.
EXPLANATORY VARIABLE(S): Two or more groups.
RESULTS REPORTED: The group **variances,** the actual ***P* value,** and the **test statistic.**

hazard function
A mathematical formula used to compute the probability that a participant will experience an event, typically death, after a certain point in time.

hazard ratio
A ratio of the risk of an event in one group to that of another when time-to-event is the primary response variable (that is, when some data may be **censored**). Sometimes called **risk ratios** or **relative risk.** A hazard ratio of 1 indicates that neither group is more at risk for the event (say, death) than the other. If the hazard ratio is, say, 5, then the group represented in the numerator is five times more likely to experience the event than the group represented in the denominator.

histogram
A type of column chart for displaying distributions of data. Histograms with many columns are often redrawn as **frequency polygons** or as smoothed **dis-**

tributions by connecting the tops of the columns and eliminating the columns themselves.

historical controls

An **historical cohort** of subjects used as a control group for comparison with an experimental group. In contrast to **concurrent (parallel) controls,** for whom data are collected at the same time as the treatment group.

homogeneity, test of

There are many tests of homogeneity; each has different applications.

PURPOSE: To compare two or more groups, usually on the variability of a response variable.

RESPONSE VARIABLE: Continuous or categorical.

EXPLANATORY VARIABLE(S): Two or more groups.

RESULTS REPORTED: The group **standard deviations** (or other summary statistics of interest), the actual ***P* value,** and the **test statistic.**

human capital approach (to economic conversion)

An **economic conversion** in which the cost of a medical condition is calculated as the earnings lost, both actual and potential, as a result of having a medical condition. Also called the "lost earnings" approach.

See Guideline 12.11.

hypothesis

A statement that will be accepted or rejected on the basis of the results of the study. For example: "The mean bacteria count of the treatment group equals the mean count of the control group" can be tested and supported by the data (the mean counts are equal) or not (the means are not equal; actually, that there is enough evidence to reject the assertion that they are equal).

hypothesis testing

A mathematical process of testing a **hypothesis** on the basis of evidence (data). A process in which a decision is made to accept or reject the **null hypothesis** of no difference on the basis of probabilities. Accepting the null hypothesis essentially means attributing the result to chance; rejecting the null hypothesis essentially means attributing the result to biological factors.

See also **type I and type II errors** *and Chapters 4 and 14.*

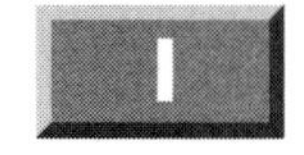

incidence

The rate with which *new* events or cases occur during a certain period of time. In contrast to **prevalence,** which is the rate at which existing events or cases are found at a given point or period in time.

inclusion criteria
The characteristics (such as a diagnosis, demographic feature, or clinical condition) that must be displayed by a study participant as a prerequisite for enrollment in a research study. Contrasts with **exclusion criteria,** which are characteristics that preclude enrollment.

independence; independent samples
Samples whose values are not affected by other samples. In contrast to **paired** or **matched samples,** in which the second value depends to some extent on the value of the first (such as testing the same subjects before and after an intervention), as well as on any experimental intervention.

independent variable: *See* **explanatory variable**

index test
The test under study, as opposed to the **reference test** to which it is validated, and the **criterion standard,** which is the reference test considered to be the most definitive.

indirect approach (to economic conversion)
An **economic conversion** in which the cost of a medical condition is determined from indirect measures, such as medical malpractice settlements, rather than from direct measures collected from surveys of patients or of a community.
See Guideline 12.11.

inferential statistics
Statistical procedures that infer (or estimate) the characteristics of a **population** from measurements of a **sample** of the population.

informed consent
A principle of biomedical research stating that study participants have the right to know the risks and benefits involved in participating in a research study, and that they may not be included in such studies without their explicit written consent. For manuscripts describing research on human subjects, most journals require a statement that informed consent was obtained from all subjects as a condition for publication.

intention-to-treat analysis
A primary strategy for analyzing the results of randomized controlled trials. Patients are analyzed with the group to which they were assigned, whether or not they completed the treatment given to the group. Medical necessity sometimes precludes patients from completing the trial as planned, but because patients may leave the study *because* of the treatment under study, the results are first analyzed on the basis of the intention-to-treat. Additional analyses are often performed to adjust for patients who do not complete the trial as planned.

interaction; interactive effect
Two explanatory variables interact when the effect of one variable on the

response variable depends on the value of the other variable. Compared with the **main effect,** which is the influence of a *single* explanatory variable on the response variable.

See Figure 7.3, p 118.

interclass correlation

A measure of association that deals specifically with multiple measurements or observations from each subject by multiple raters. Indicates the between-rater correlation. The correlation coefficient is a number that ranges from –1 (complete disagreement) to +1 (complete agreement).

interim analysis (of accumulating data)

A statistical analysis performed before the study is completed; may be associated with **stopping rules** and may create the **multiple testing problem.**

See Guidelines 5.7 and 5.8.

interquartile range

The range of values containing the central half of the observations; that is, the range between the 25th and 75th percentiles. Used with the **median** value (instead of the mean ± standard deviation) to report data that are markedly non-normally distributed.

inter-rater reliability

The degree of agreement among judges' or raters' evaluations. Often used in assessing the reliability of a diagnostic test.

interval data

A form of continuous data measured on an interval scale of equal intervals but without a true zero point. Scores on an interval scale can be meaningfully added and subtracted but not multiplied or divided. For example, temperature is indicated on an interval scale of degrees. However, 40 °C is not twice as hot as 20 °C. (To make such a statement, temperature measured on a "ratio" scale is needed. In this case, temperature measured in kelvins, a ratio scale that includes absolute zero, would be necessary.)

intervening variable: *See* **confounding variable**

interventional study

A study that tests the effects of an intervention, such as a new treatment; an **experimental study.** In contrast to an **observational study,** which is descriptive.

intraclass correlation

A measure of association that deals specifically with multiple measurements or observations from each study participant by a single rater. Indicates the within-rater correlation. The correlation coefficient is a number that ranges from –1 (complete disagreement) to +1 (complete agreement).

intra-rater reliability

The reproducibility of a judgment by a single judge on the same judgment task at different times.

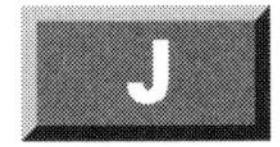

jackknife procedure

A method of validating a regression model by removing the data from one subject at a time and recalculating the model each time. The model changes each time a study participant is removed; the more similar the set of recalculated models, the more valid the full model.

See Guideline 7.7.

Kaplan-Meier curve

Typically, a graph of the percentage of a sample that has not yet experienced the event of interest (usually death) at different times during a follow-up period. The graph is not a smooth curve but a step function that drops from left to right as mortality increases. When used to indicate the probability of experiencing an event, the graph rises from left to right as the probability increases. Often accompanied by a **log-rank test** that compares two or more curves to determine whether they differ significantly.

See Figure 9.1, p 139.

Kaplan-Meier method (the **product-limit method)**

A statistical method used in **survival (time-to-event) analysis** to estimate the probability of experiencing an event, such as death (or of being event-free), at different times in the study.

kappa statistic

A measure of association that deals specifically with multiple measurements or observations from each subject. Measures agreement or classification accuracy within or between raters. Ranges from –1 to +1, where +1 is complete concordance, –1 is complete discordance, and 0 is no relationship among the judgments.

Kendall's rank-correlation coefficient, tau (τ)

A **correlation coefficient** used to assess the linear relationship between two ordinal or continuous variables. Ranges from –1 to +1, where +1 is perfect positive correlation, –1 is perfect negative correlation, and 0 is no correlation.

Kolmogorov-(Kolmogoroff)-Smirnov goodness-of-fit test

PURPOSE: To compare the distribution of values in a sample to a known distribution of values.

RESPONSE VARIABLE: Categorical or continuous.

EXPLANATORY VARIABLE(S): Just one group; there is no explanatory variable.

RESULTS REPORTED: Depends on the distribution of interest. Include the actual ***P* value** and the **test statistic.**

Kruskal-Wallis test

Nonparametric counterpart to **one-way analysis of variance (ANOVA).**
PURPOSE: To compare three or more groups on the median value of a **response variable.**
RESPONSE VARIABLE: Continuous (or discrete or ordinal with many levels).
EXPLANATORY VARIABLE(S): Three or more groups.
RESULTS REPORTED: The group **medians,** the actual ***P* value,** and the **test statistic.**

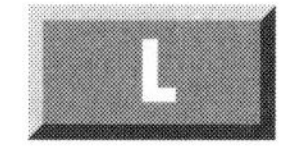

lead-time bias

A bias found in **time-to-event analyses** that leads to an overestimate of survival time. Occurs when the biological starting point of, say, an illness, does not correspond to the clinical starting point of a study for many of the participants. For instance, the median time from the biological onset of cancer to death may be the same in two groups, but if cancer was coincidentally reported earlier in its course in one group, this group would have a longer reported median survival time as a result of lead-time bias.

least-significant-difference (LSD) method: *See* **Fisher's least-significant-difference (LSD) method**

least-squares regression line

A statistically calculated line drawn through a group of points to minimize the distances (actually the sum of the squares of the distances) between each point and the line itself. The **regression** line used in linear **regression** is usually a least-squares line.

left-censored data: *See* **censored data**

level of significance

The **alpha level;** the probability of committing a **type I error** of wrongly concluding that the groups differ.

levels of measurement

A classification of how variables are measured based on the complexity of the classification. Common levels, from low to high complexity, are **nominal, ordinal,** and **continuous** levels. **Nominal** (for example, alive or dead, male or female) and **ordinal** (for example, low, medium, and high; satisfaction measured on a scale of from one to five) variables are "categorical" or "qualitative" variables because a particular quality is used to place the observation in one category or another. **Discrete data** are counts and are typically treated as continuous data. **Continuous data** are "quantitative" because they are usually measured rather than counted. It is helpful to know the levels of measurement of the explanatory and response variables because they help determine the statistical procedures used to analyze the data.

life table method

A statistical method for **time-to-event** (or **survival**) **analysis.** Same as the **actuarial life table method** and the **Berkson-Gage method.**

likelihood ratio, positive

A ratio comparing the probabilities of getting a positive diagnostic test result from diseased and nondiseased patients. The likelihood ratio for a positive test is sensitivity divided by the quantity 1 minus the specificity of the test. The likelihood ratio thus combines sensitivity and specificity into a single number. If the positive likelihood ratio is equal to 1, then patients with the disease are no more likely to have a positive test result than are patients without the disease. If the positive likelihood ratio is, say, 3.5, then those with the disease are 3.5 times more likely to have a positive test than those without. There are also negative likelihood ratios.

See Table 10.1, p 156.

linear regression: *See* **regression analysis**

log-rank test

PURPOSE: To compare two or more groups on the proportions of study participants alive (or event-free) at certain times during the study (usually comparing two or more survival curves).

RESPONSE VARIABLE: Time to an event (usually death) or to the last follow-up visit.

EXPLANATORY VARIABLE(S): Two or more groups.

RESULTS REPORTED: In **survival analysis,** the estimated proportion of participants in each group alive (or event-free) at certain times during the study, the actual ***P* value,** and the **test statistic.**

See Chapter 9.

logistic regression analysis: *See* **regression analysis**

longitudinal study

A study that follows patients over a period of time.

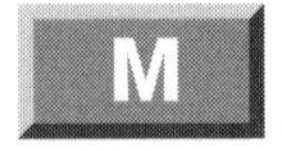

magnitude estimation technique

A method of assigning a **utility** or a quality-of-life measure to a medical condition. Respondents are asked to describe one alternative in terms of how undesirable it is when compared with another (for example, "Twice as bad").

See Guideline 12.12.

main effect

The influence of a single **explanatory variable** on the response variable. Contrasts with an **interactive effect,** in which two or more explanatory variables must be considered together in determining the effect on a single response variable.

Mann-Whitney *U* test: *See* **Wilcoxon's rank-sum test**

Mantel-Haenszel test: *See* **Cochran-Mantel-Haenszel test**

MANOVA

Multivariate (more than one response variable) **analysis of variance.**

Markov process

A technique commonly used to model complex **decision trees.**

See Guideline 13.9

masked; masking (a "masked" study)

The practice of preventing patients, caregivers, and even statisticians from knowing who is in the experimental group and who is in the control group. In a single-masked study, generally only the patients are masked. In a double-masked study, the patients and data collectors (the caregivers, investigators, or both) are masked, although the data evaluators (the investigators, biostatisticians, or both) are not. Although rare, in a triple-masked study, the patients, data collectors, and data evaluators are masked. The term *masking* is preferred to *blinding* to avoid confusion with the common meaning of the term *blinding.*

matched samples; matching: *See* **paired data**

McNemar's test for dependent proportions (*pronunciation: mack* ne mar)

PURPOSE: To compare proportions among two or more matched groups.

RESPONSE VARIABLE: Categorical (expressed as proportions).

EXPLANATORY VARIABLE(S): Two or more matched groups.

RESULTS REPORTED: The group proportions and the difference between them; the 95% **confidence interval** for the difference, the actual ***P* value,** and the **test statistic.**

Also called **Cochran's Q.**

mean; mean value

The arithmetic average value of a group of values. The mean is a common descriptive statistic best used to summarize the central tendency of approximately normally distributed data. In this use, it is usually accompanied by the **standard deviation,** which indicates the dispersion or variability of the data. When the data are approximately normally distributed, the mean is a useful **measure of central tendency.** When the data are markedly **non-normally distributed,** the **median** is preferred because it is unaffected by the magnitude of extreme values.

measure of association: *See* **association, test of**

measure of central tendency

Statistics that describe the "center" of a distribution of values; a single value that best represents the bulk of the observations. The most common measures of central tendency are the **mean,** the **median,** and the **mode.**

measure of dispersion

Statistics that describe the variability of a distribution of values. The most common measures of dispersion are the **variance,** the **standard deviation,** the **range,** and the **interquartile range.**

measurement error (bias)

Systematic error introduced as a result of variability in the measuring instrument.

See also **error.**

median; median value

The value that separates the highest 50% of the scores from the lowest 50%. Useful in describing the central tendency of **non-normally distributed data** because it is less influenced by **outlier** data (extreme values) that skew the distribution and that can have a disproportionate effect on the mean. The median is correctly used in conjunction with the **interquartile range** to summarize markedly non-normally distributed data.

median test

PURPOSE: To compare two groups on the median value of the response variable.
RESPONSE VARIABLE: Continuous.
EXPLANATORY VARIABLE(S): Two groups.
RESULTS REPORTED: The group **medians** and the difference between them, the 95% **confidence interval** for the difference, the actual ***P* value,** and the **test statistic.**

meta-analysis

A summary and statistical analysis of the results of several studies testing the same relationship. Combining the studies provides a larger sample for analysis and more statistical power. Used to increase the evidence for, or confidence in, a conclusion.

See Chapter 11.

mode

The most common of three or more values or measurements; the value with the highest frequency. Often used when a distribution is "bi-modal," indicating that it has two peaks rather than one.

model, statistical or **mathematical**

A mathematical equation that describes, to a greater or lesser degree, relationships between or among variables.

Monte Carlo simulation

A technique commonly used in **decision analysis** to generate expected probabilities for each outcome.

See Guideline 13.9.

multiple (pairwise) comparisons procedures

Any of several procedures or techniques used to determine which groups dif-

fer significantly after another more general test (such as **ANOVA**) has determined that significant differences exist among the groups. Examples include **Tukey's procedure,** the **Neuman-Keuls procedure, Duncan's multiple range procedure, Dunn's procedure, Dunnett's procedure, Scheffe's method, Bonferroni's correction,** and **Fisher's least-significant-difference method.** Used to prevent the errors that can arise from the **multiple testing problem.**
See Chapter 5.

multiple linear regression: *See* **regression analysis**

multiple logistic regression: *See* **regression analysis**

multiple looks
The **multiple testing problem.**

multiple regression analysis: *See* **regression analysis**

multiple testing problem
The problem that arises from performing a large number of statistical tests in a single study. If statistical significance is defined as $P < 0.05$, then a single test has less than 5 chances in 100 of being falsely significant. However, if, say, seven groups are compared two at a time, 21 tests will be required, which distorts the level of significance. That is, under these conditions, the chance that a single test will be significant (will have a P value less than 0.05) is now 0.66, or two in three. Authors should call attention to the possibility of the multiple testing problem and indicate how this problem was addressed.

multivariable analysis
Analyses that consider the effects of more than one **explanatory variable** on a *single* **response variable.**

multivariate analysis
Analyses that consider the effects of one or more **explanatory variables** on *more than one* **response variable.**

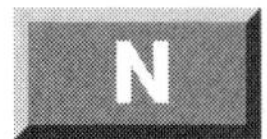

N
The number of study participants in the **population** of interest; contrasts with n, the number in a **sample** of a population. In common usage, although incorrect, the size of the overall sample in a study.

n
The number of study participants in a **sample** of the population of interest; contrasts with N, the number in the **population.** In common usage, although incorrect, the size of the individual groups or subsamples in a study.

negative predictive value

The **probability** that the disease is not present when the result of the test or procedure is negative. The value depends on the "pre-test incidence" of the disease, which should be reported with the negative predictive value.

See Table 10.1, p 156.

Neuman-Keuls procedure: *See* **multiple (pairwise) comparison procedures**

nominal data

Data that can be placed into categories that have no inherent ranking. For example: sex (male or female); blood type (A, B, AB, O); status (alive or dead). In contrast to **ordinal data,** which can be ranked in some ascending or descending order.

nomogram

A graphic device consisting of several lines marked off to scale and arranged in such a way that a straightedge connecting known values on two lines will indicate the size of an unknown value at the point of intersection with another line. Sometimes used in diagnostic testing to relate the **pre-test probability** (prevalence) and the likelihood ratio of a positive test to determine the **post-test probability** of disease (the positive predictive value).

See Figure 10.5.

non-normally distributed data

Data that do not conform to a symmetric, bell-shaped distribution; skewed data. Such data must be analyzed with **nonparametric statistical techniques** or must be **transformed** before using **parametric techniques.**

nonparametric statistics

A class of statistical techniques used to analyze data that do not conform to a known **parametric** distribution. For example, if data are markedly **non-normally distributed,** nonparametric statistical tests are appropriate. **Categorical data** are usually analyzed with nonparametric tests.

normally distributed data

Data that have a symmetrical, bell-shaped distribution where the **mean, median,** and **mode** are identical. The flatness or peakedness of the curve (that is, the variation of the data) may vary. Many statistical tests (called **parametric tests**) require that the data be normally distributed; authors should indicate whether they examined the normality of the distribution before continuing with statistical analysis.

See **Gaussian distribution.**

null hypothesis

The hypothesis being tested about a population. Typically, the statistical assumption that no true difference exists between, say, the mean values of two groups. If no actual difference exists between the two groups, small observed differences could be the result of chance. Larger differences will occur by chance less often, and at some point (usually when $P < 0.05$), the chance becomes so small that the null hypothesis is rejected in favor of the **alternative**

hypothesis that the groups are different. In practice, the null hypothesis is seldom presented; however, the **alternative hypothesis** should be detailed in the Introduction section of a scientific article.

number needed to treat (NNT)

The number of patients that must be treated to prevent a single occurrence of the outcome of interest. For example, if 33 persons must be treated with hypertensive medications for 5 years to prevent one heart attack, the NNT is 33 at 5 years. The **NNT** is the inverse of the **absolute risk reduction (ARR).**

See Guideline 12.18.

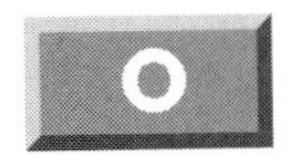

observational study

A descriptive study, in contrast to an **experimental study.**

odds

The probability that an event will occur divided by the probability that it will *not* occur. If the *probability* of an event occurring is P, the *odds* of the event occurring are equal to $P/(1 - P)$. For example, if the probability of recovery is 0.3, then the odds of recovering are 0.3/0.7 = 0.43. Whereas the ***probability*** of drawing a diamond from a deck of cards is one in four (13/52 = 1/4 = 0.25), the ***odds*** of drawing a diamond are one in three (0.25/1 – 0.25 = 1/3 = 0.33).

odds ratio

A ratio of the odds of an event in one group to those of another, where **odds** is the **probability** that an event will occur divided by the probability that it will not occur. Used in retrospective, **case-control** studies as an estimate of relative risk, where the groups are defined on the basis of an outcome (say, the presence or absence of lung cancer) and the interest is in determining the effects of a risk factor (such as smoking). An odds ratio of one indicates that smokers and nonsmokers were equally likely to develop lung cancer. If the odds ratio is, say, three, then smokers are three times more likely to develop lung cancer than nonsmokers.

See Guideline 7.25.

one-tailed (one-sided) test (or **directional test**)

A condition for a hypothesis test, specified before data are collected, as an alternative to a **two-tailed test.** Used, for example, when the "direction of the difference" between two groups is known in advance or when differences observed in the opposite direction are not of interest or are not possible. For instance, a drug may increase the length of long bones but it will not decrease it. A study of changes in bone length is thus not concerned with the probability that bones will be *shorter* at the end of the study, only the probability that they will be *longer.* A one-tailed test is probably appropriate in this circumstance. If the bones could plausibly be *either* shorter *or* longer is of interest, a two-tailed test would be appropriate. The minimum difference required for statistical significance is slightly less for a one-tailed test than for a two-tailed test. The two-tailed test is more conservative and it is also more common. Authors should specify whether the statistical test was one- or two-tailed and should justify the use of a one-tailed test.

operational definition
A definition based on measurable or observable criteria. For example, depression might be operationally defined as a certain score on a survey about depression.

ordinal data
Categorical data that can be placed into categories ranked in order by some criterion. For example, "high, medium, or low;" "none, mild, moderate, or severe." Ordinal data are sometimes referred to as **semiquantitative data.**

outcome or **outcome variable**
The event of interest; the **response variable.**

outlying values ("outliers")
Values so extreme that they appear not to be part of the distribution. Often few in number, they can distort the **mean** value. The **median** value is not affected by the magnitude of these values, however, and should be used to report data with outliers.

"overfitting"
A term used to describe a statistical model with too many explanatory variables. Such models are said to "overfit" the data.

oversampling: *See* **stratification**

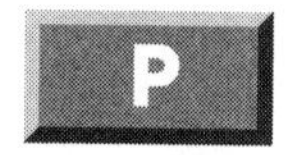

***P* value**
A probability value; the probability that an outcome would occur essentially by chance. *P* values range from one (absolutely certain) to zero (absolutely impossible). A *P* value equal to or less than an **alpha level** of, say, 0.05 is said to be "statistically significant," meaning that the observed outcome is not likely to be the result of chance. Results do not "approach" significance or "trend toward significance." They either are or are not significant according to the alpha level established by the researcher. Some authorities refer to findings significant at the 0.05 level as "significant" and those at the 0.01 level as "highly significant," but this practice is not encouraged. Statistical significance essentially indicates only the probability under the null hypotheses that the outcome occurred by chance: it *does not* indicate the strength or the clinical importance of the association. Also, sometimes groups are tested to confirm that they *do not* differ significantly; for example, *P* greater than 0.05 can be a desirable result.

Report actual *P* values ($P = 0.35$), as opposed to threshold values ($P < 0.05$).
Both the *Council of Biology Editors Scientific Style and Format*, 6th edition, and the *AMA Manual of Style*, 8th edition, state that the symbol *P* should be presented in upper-case and italic type.

paired data; paired tests
Observations that are paired or matched with other observations; that is, observations that are dependent on or related to one another. For example, blood pressure readings from the same patient before and after exercise, or the weight of two patients matched for age and height. Paired data are treated differently (with paired tests) because the second value is related to or similar to the first. In contrast, data from **independent samples** are assumed not to be related.

paired *t* test
PURPOSE: To compare two matched groups on the **mean value** of the **response variable;** actually, to compare the mean of the changes or differences of all of the matched pairs to zero.
RESPONSE VARIABLE: Continuous.
EXPLANATORY VARIABLE(S): TWO MATCHED GROUPS.
RESULTS REPORTED: The group means, the **mean** and **standard deviation** of the changes or differences between the pairs, the 95% **confidence interval** for the mean of the changes or differences between the pairs, the actual ***P* value,** and the **test statistic.**

pairwise comparison: *See* **multiple (pairwise) comparison procedures**

parallel controls: *See* **concurrent controls**

parameter
A numerical characteristic of a **population,** such as a mean or standard deviation; usually denoted by a Greek letter. As opposed to a **statistic,** which is a numerical characteristic of a **sample** of the population and which is usually denoted by a Roman letter. Statistics are used to estimate parameters. The term *parameter* is often used incorrectly to mean a "factor" or "variable." Variables are measured, whereas parameters are estimated.

parametric statistics or **tests**
A class of statistical tests used to analyze data that conform to a known distribution (often the normal distribution). The characteristics of the distribution or "parameters" are known (hence "parametric"), whereas **nonparametric statistics** are used when the characteristics or "parameters" are unknown. **Categorical data** are often analyzed with nonparametric tests.

Pearson's chi-square test: *See* **chi-square test**

Pearson's product-moment correlation coefficient (*r*)
A measure of the strength of the linear relationship between two ("bivariately normally distributed") continuous variables. The coefficient, *r*, is a number that ranges between –1 and +1.
See Guideline 6.12.

person-trade-off technique
A method of assigning a **utility** or a quality-of-life measure to a medical condition. Respondents are asked to choose between helping a group of patients with condition X or a group with condition Y.
See Guideline 12.12.

pharmacoeconomics
The description and analysis of the cost of drug therapy to health care systems and society.

phi coefficient (pronounced *"fee"*)
A measure of the strength of an **association** between nominal variables, phi is a number that ranges between –1 and +1. Similar to a **correlation coefficient** used for continuous variables.

placebo
A biologically inactive substance or condition used in medical research to simulate the treatment under study but that presumably has no biological effect. Pertains to the "placebo effect," in which participants' beliefs about being treated alter their perceptions (and sometimes even their physiological reactions) during a study.
See also **sham surgery; vehicle.**

point biserial correlation coefficient
A measure of the relationship between a continuous variable and a categorical variable with two levels.

point estimate
An estimate of an unknown population value **(parameter)** from a known sample value **(statistic)**. A point estimate is often accompanied by a confidence interval, such as a 95% **confidence interval.**

point multiserial correlation coefficient
A measure of the relationship between a continuous variable and a categorical variable with three or more levels.

Poisson distribution
A probability distribution used to detsermine the probability of rare events in large samples or to model random events. After Simeon Denis Poisson (1781–1840) who first characterized the distribution.

population
In the statistical use of the term, the group of subjects from which the sample is drawn and to which the results can be generalized. The size of the population is usually indicated by N (upper-case en); n (lower-case en) usually indicates the size of samples drawn from the population. The common use of the term is broader. For example, "all leukemia patients in the world" is a population in the common use of the term, but only if every leukemia patient in the world has a chance of being included in the sample would this group be considered a population in the statistical sense. In reality, "all the leukemia

patients seen at this institution" is the statistical population, even though generalizations to all leukemia patients in the world may be made on the basis of the study.

positive predictive value
The probability that the disease is present when the test or procedure is positive. The value depends on the "pre-test incidence" of the disease, which should be reported with the positive predictive value.
See Table 10.1, p 156.

post hoc (analysis)
A term meaning "after the fact." A post-hoc analysis is an analysis not specified before the data are collected and may, in fact, be suggested by the data. Contrasts with **a priori.**

post-test odds
In diagnostic testing, the **odds** that a subject has the disease after the results of a diagnostic test are known; similar to **predictive values** and **posterior probabilities.**
See also **Bayes' theorem.**

posterior probability
In diagnostic testing, the conditional probability that the disease is present when the test is positive (the **positive predictive value**) or that the disease is not present when the test is negative (the **negative predictive value**).
See also **Bayes' theroem.**

power, statistical
The probability of finding a specified difference when one truly exists; the probability of correctly rejecting the null hypothesis. In **prospective** clinical studies, power should be specified in the design phase of the study and reported in the Materials and Methods under how the sample size was determined. It should be high: values of 0.8 or 0.9 are standard choices. Power is directly related to sample size; the larger the sample, the greater the power. Power is equal to 1 minus beta, where **beta** is the probability of making a **type II error.**

practice parameters
The American Medical Association's term for **clinical practice guidelines.**

pragmatic study
A study conducted under real-world conditions, as opposed to tightly controlled conditions, to determine the effectiveness of a treatment. Usually used in contrast to an **explanatory study**, which is designed primarily to identify underlying biological relationships.

predictive value: *See* **negative predictive value; positive predictive value**

predictor variable
An **explanatory variable.** A term used mainly in **regression analysis.**

present value analysis: *See* **discounting**

pre-test odds
In diagnostic testing, the **odds** that a study participant has the condition before the results of a diagnostic test are known; similar to disease **prevalence** and **prior probabilities.**
See **Bayes' theorem.**

prevalence
The proportion or rate of persons in a **population** who have a condition at any given time. Contrasts with **incidence,** which is the rate at which new cases of the condition occur.

primary comparison
The major purpose of the study. Most studies involve comparing two or more groups in some way: to each other, to a standard value, or to themselves over time. The primary comparison, then, is the comparison of interest, the relationship between the major explanatory variables and the major response variable.

principal components analysis
A statistical procedure used to group related variables to help summarize data. Similar to **factor analysis.**

prior probability ("priors")
In diagnostic testing, the **probability** that the disease is present before the test is administered; the disease **prevalence.**

probability
A number between zero and one, indicating how likely an event is to occur. When added together, the probabilities of all alternatives in a given situation equal one, assuming the alternatives are mutually exclusive. For example, if the probability of a patient being male is 0.6, than the probability of the patient being female is 0.4.

product-limit method (Kaplan-Meier method): *See* **Kaplan-Meier method, survival analysis**

prognostic factor
An **explanatory variable.**

proportional hazards regression: *See* **Cox proportional hazards regression analysis**

prospective study
A study that is planned in advance of data collection. Considered to be more reliable than **retrospective** or **cross-sectional studies** because potentially confounding variables can be better controlled when the study question is known before data are collected.

protocol
A procedure; a set of instructions or directions for performing a task. A protocol for data collection or measurement, for example, can help reduce bias by reducing subjectivity from certain aspects of the process.

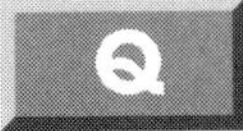

QALY (quality-adjusted life-year)
An outcome measure often used in **cost-utility studies.** The quality of life for a condition is represented as a number between 0 (indifference between life and death) and 1 (robust health). The number of years a patient might spend in this condition is then determined. The product of these two numbers is expressed in QALYs.
See also **utility.**

qualitative data
Data that fit into categories on the basis of attributes that they either have or do not have. **Nominal** and **ordinal data** are **qualitative data.** In contrast to **quantitative** or **continuous data.**

quality-of-life measure
A numerical index that indicates the quality of a person's life; used to compare the outcomes of various treatments on a common index; used especially in economic evaluations and in decision analyses.
See Guideline 12.12

quantitative data
Data that are measured on a numerical scale of equal intervals. **Interval** and ratio data are **quantitative data.** In contrast to **qualitative** or **categorical data.**

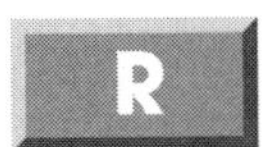

random assignment
The process of assigning study participants to experimental or control groups at random such that each participant has an equal **probability** of being assigned to any given group. Such a method of assignment helps to prevent bias in a study and is usually based on a series of random numbers from a special table or generated by a computer. **Random assignment** is not the same as "haphazard assignment."

random sample
A sample chosen with as little bias as possible. A simple random sample is a sample in which every member of the population has an equal chance of being included in the sample.

randomization; randomized
Less preferred terms for **random assignment.** The term *randomized* is acceptable in the phrase "randomized controlled trial." However, patients are not randomized; they are randomly assigned.

randomized controlled trial

An **experimental study** in which participants are randomly assigned to a treatment or a control group. In contrast to **retrospective** and **cross-sectional studies** and to **prospective studies** without **random assignment.**

range

The distance between the highest and the lowest value of a distribution.

rank-sum test (ranked-sum test): *See* **Wilcoxon's rank-sum test**

rate

The number of cases occurring per unit population or per unit time. For example, the mortality rate from motor vehicle accidents might be 0.03% (2.94 deaths per 10000 people).

receiver operating characteristics (ROC) curve

A graphic device for summarizing the diagnostic accuracy of a test whose interpretation depends on a cutpoint on a continuum of test scores. A graph in which the Y axis represents sensitivity (the proportion of **true-positive** results) and the X axis represents 1 minus the specificity (or the proportion of **false-positive** results). As the decision threshold of the test is varied (that is, as the cutpoint that separates healthy patients from ill patients is changed), the sensitivity and specificity of the test also change. These values are plotted and joined to produce the ROC curve.

See Figure 10.3, p 160, and Guideline 10.10.

reference test

The diagnostic test to which an **index test** is compared in determining its characteristics.

See **criterion standard.**

referral filter bias

Bias introduced when the patients recruited for a study are not typical of those with the condition under study because of the way in which they have come to the researchers' attention. For example, a study done at a county hospital may draw from a different population than a large, private tertiary-care facility.

registry

A database, usually of a particular patient type or study population.

regression analysis

A class of procedures for predicting the value of a **response variable** when the value of one or more **explanatory variables** is known.

See Chapter 7 and Guideline 9.11.

simple linear regression analysis

PURPOSE: To predict the value of a single **response variable** from a given value of a single **explanatory variable.**

RESPONSE VARIABLE: Continuous.

EXPLANATORY VARIABLE(S): One continuous variable.

RESULTS REPORTED: The regression equation, the coefficient of determination

(r^2), the 95% **confidence interval** for the slope of the regression line, the actual ***P* value,** and the **test statistic;** results are sometimes presented graphically with the associated **scatter plot.**

See Figure 7.1, p 110.

multiple linear regression analysis

PURPOSE: To predict the value of a single **response variable** from a combination of **explanatory variables.**

RESPONSE VARIABLE: Continuous.

EXPLANATORY VARIABLE(S): Two or more continuous or categorical variables.

RESULTS REPORTED: Results are usually reported in a table giving the details of the model.

See Table 7.1, p 115.

simple logistic regression analysis

PURPOSE: To predict the value of a single **response variable** from a given value of a single **explanatory variable.**

RESPONSE VARIABLE: Categorical.

EXPLANATORY VARIABLE(S): One continuous or categorical variable.

RESULTS REPORTED: The regression equation, the **odds ratio,** the 95% **confidence interval** for the **odds ratio,** the actual ***P* value,** and the **test statistic.**

See Table 7.2, p 120.

multiple logistic regression analysis

PURPOSE: To predict the value of a single **response variable** from a combination of explanatory variables.

RESPONSE VARIABLE: Categorical.

EXPLANATORY VARIABLE(S): Two or more continuous or categorical variables.

RESULTS REPORTED: Results are usually reported in a table giving the details of the model.

See Table 7.3, p 124.

regression coefficient

A number in a regression equation associated with a variable. Sometimes called a **beta weight.**

regression equation

The statistical model that results from **regression analysis.**

regression to the mean

The tendency of extreme values to become less extreme (to "approach the mean" value) on subsequent measurements. (Not related to regression analysis, per se.)

relative risk (RR) or **risk ratio:** *See* **risk ratio**

relative risk reduction (RRR)

The reduction in risk to the treatment or unexposed group expressed as a percentage, [(Pc – Pt)/Pc] × 100%, where Pc is the proportion of the control or unexposed group experiencing the outcome of interest and Pt is the proportion of the treatment or exposed group experiencing the outcome of interest. If the incidence of nausea in men with esophageal reflux disease who take omeprazole is 1.2% and the incidence in men given another drug is 2.2%, then the RRR for men taking omeprazole is 45% [(2.2% – 1.2%)/2.2% = 45%].

See Guideline 12.18 and **absolute (attributable) risk reduction**.

reliability

The ability of a measure (such as a diagnostic test) to reproduce the same results under the same conditions. Contrasts with **validity,** which is the ability of a test to measure what it is supposed to measure.

repeated-measures analysis of variance: *See* **ANOVA**

residual

In **regression analysis,** the difference between an observed value and a predicted value.

See Figure 7.1, p 110.

residual standard deviation

In regression analysis, the square root of the **error mean square (MSE).** Also called the **root mean square.** A measure of variability of the data.

response variable

The outcome or endpoint; the **dependent variable.** Usually indicated with Y's, not X's.

See **explanatory variable.**

retrospective study

A study conducted after data have already been collected, often for another purpose. Specific types include **case-control** or **chart studies.**

right-censored data: *See* **censored data**

risk

The probability that an event or a particular outcome will occur, usually expressed as a percentage.

risk factor

An **explanatory variable.** The term is typically used in **logistic regression** and **survival analyses.**

risk ratio (relative risk)

A ratio of the risk of an event in one group to that of another, where risk is the probability that an event or a particular outcome will occur, usually expressed as a percentage. Used in prospective and observational studies, where the groups are defined in advance (say, vegetarians versus meat eaters) and the event (colon cancer) may or may not occur. A risk ratio of 1 indicates that neither group is more at risk for the event than the other. If the risk ratio is, say, 4.5, then meat eaters are 4.5 times more likely to develop colon cancer than are vegetarians.

robust

An adjective used to describe a statistical test that provides the same conclusion even when its underlying assumptions are not strictly met. For example, **Student's *t* test** is often described as a robust test because in some cases either of the two data groups compared can be somewhat asymmetrically distributed (skewed) without affecting the conclusion of the test.

ROC analysis: *See* **receiver operating characteristics (ROC) curve analysis**

root mean square: *See* **residual standard deviation**

sample
The portion of a **population** about which information is actually obtained.

sampling error
The difference between the sample value and the true population value resulting solely from the fact that only a sample of the population has been measured.

SAS
Statistical Analysis Software, a computer software package commonly used to perform statistical analyses in the biomedical sciences.

scatter plot or **scatter diagram**
A graph of data from two continuous variables, usually associated with **correlation** and **simple linear regression analysis.** So-called because the data are "scattered" on the graph.
See Figures 6.1, 6.2, and 7.1 (pp 94 and 110, respectively).

Scheffe's procedure (*pronunciation:* **sh-fays**)**:** *See* **multiple (pairwise) comparison procedures**

screening test
A test performed on apparently healthy, asymptomatic people to identify those who may be at risk for a given disorder. Contrasts with **diagnostic test.**

SD
Abbreviation for **standard deviation.**

selection bias
A systematic error in choosing a sample. For example, a sample of names from a phone book is biased against people who do not have phones, people who do not have phones listed in their names, and people who have unlisted numbers.

SEM
Abbreviation for **standard error of the mean.**

semiquantitative data: *See* **ordinal data**

sensitivity

The **probability** that a test result will be positive when the disease is present. The proportion of **true-positive** results; the proportion of diseased patients who have a positive test. Usually expressed as a percentage. Contrasts with **specificity.**

See Table 10.1, p 156.

sensitivity analysis

A method often used in **meta-analysis, economic evaluations,** and **decision analyses** for assessing the effects of key assumptions or values on the final result. The assumptions are varied over their range of values to determine their effect on the result. Large differences in effects indicate that the analysis is "sensitive" to the assumption. One-way sensitivity analysis varies one variable at a time. Two-way sensitivity analysis varies two at a time, and so forth.

See Guidelines 11.17, 12.20, and 13.15.

sham surgery

In animal research, a surgical procedure that presumably causes the same degree of trauma to the animal as does the surgery under study but that otherwise does not interfere with or modify the animal's anatomy or physiology. The surgical equivalent of a **placebo** treatment.

sign test

PURPOSE: To compare two proportions.

RESPONSE VARIABLE: Categorical (expressed as proportions).

EXPLANATORY VARIABLE(S): Two groups.

RESULTS REPORTED: The group proportions, the difference between them, the **95% confidence interval** for the difference, the ***P*** **value,** and the **test statistic.**

signed-rank test: *See* **Wilcoxon's signed-rank test**

significance, statistical: *See* **alpha level; Introduction**

Contrasts with "clinical importance."

skewed data or **distribution**

An asymmetrical frequency distribution. Skewed distributions with longer right tails are said to be positively skewed; those with longer left tails are negatively skewed. Data that are markedly **non-normally distributed.** When the **mean** and **median** differ markedly, the data are probably skewed.

slope (of a regression line)

In simple linear regression analysis, the amount of change in the **response variable** for each unit change in the **explanatory variable.**

Spearman's rank-order correlation coefficient (Spearman's rho)

Assesses the linear relationship between two continuous variables that are not necessary normally distributed. As do all **correlation coefficients,** Spearman's rho ranges from –1 (a perfect negative correlation) to +1 (a perfect positive correlation).

specificity

The **probability** that a test result will be negative when the disease is not present. The proportion of **true-negative** results; the proportion of nondiseased patients who have a negative test result. Usually expressed as a percentage. Contrasts with **sensitivity.**

See Table 10.1, p 156.

SPSS

Statistical Package for the Social Sciences, a computer software package commonly used to perform statistical analyses, especially in the social and medical sciences.

standard deviation (SD)

A measure of the dispersion or variability of a set of values. Defined mathematically, it is the square-root of the **variance** of these observations. By definition, approximately 68% of the values in the **normal distribution** (or bell-shaped curve) fall within one standard deviation on either side of the mean. If the standard deviation exceeds one-half the mean (and when negative values are not possible), the data are not normally distributed.

standard error (of the estimate)

A measure of the precision of an estimate. Whereas the **standard deviation** is a measure of dispersion of the values around the mean in a single sample, the standard error can be thought of as a measure of dispersion of point estimates from several samples taken from the same population.

standard error of the difference (SE_{diff})

A measure of the dispersion of the possible differences between samples of two **populations,** usually the differences between the means of the **samples.** Used in **Student's *t* test.**

standard error of the mean (SEM) ($SE_{\bar{x}}$)

A measure of the dispersion of a distribution of the means of all possible samples from the same **population.** When the distribution of sample means is normally distributed, the observed sample mean ± 1 SEM includes about 68% of the possible sample means. Thus, the mean ± 1 SEM defines about a 68% **confidence interval** for the true population mean.

The SEM is often used inappropriately as a descriptive statistic (in the form of a mean ± the SEM), instead of the standard deviation (SD). Because the SEM is smaller than the SD, this incorrect presentation makes the measurements look more "precise" because the data appear to vary less. When reporting the precision of an estimate of a mean, most authorities prefer the 95% confidence interval, which is usually the range defined by the mean ± about two times the SEM.

standard error of the proportion (SEp)

A measure of the precision of an estimated proportion.

standard gamble technique

A method of assigning a **utility** or a quality-of-life measure to a medical con-

dition. Respondents are asked to chose between two alternatives that have different stated probabilities of occurrence.
See Guideline 12.12.

standard normal distribution
A special type of normal distribution in which the mean is 0 and the standard deviation is 1. Useful for comparing the scores from two or more different but normal distributions through what is known as a z **transformation,** where a z **score** is expressed in units of **standard deviation.**

standardized score (*z* score; standard score; standard deviate score): *See* ***z* score**

statistic
A numeric characteristic of a **sample,** for example, a **mean** or a **range.** In contrast with a **parameter,** which is a numerical characteristic of a **population.** A statistic is an estimate of a parameter.

statistical overview
A **meta-analysis.**
See Chapter 11.

statistical power: *See* **power, statistical; beta (β)** or **beta level**

statistical significance: *See* **significance, statistical**

stopping rules
A set of statistical criteria applied during an **interim analysis** of study data to determine whether the results are so clear that the study should be stopped to avoid putting patients at risk unnecessarily. If the study is stopped too soon (after too few participants have completed the study), its statistical power may be unacceptably low. If the study is allowed to continue, participants may be put at risk needlessly and resources may be used unnecessarily.

stratification; stratified sampling
A method of sampling in which a **population** is first divided into subgroups on the basis of one or more characteristics thought to affect the outcome and then sampling from the subgroups. (This process is sometimes referred to as **oversampling** because some subgroups may need to be sampled more heavily than others to obtain the desired number of subjects.) Stratified sampling allows researchers to balance important characteristics between experimental and control groups to reduce bias and to permit the analysis of important subgroups.

Student-Neuman-Keuls procedure (Neuman-Keuls procedure): *See* **multiple (pairwise) comparison procedures**

Student's *t* test
PURPOSE: To compare two groups on the **mean value** of a **response variable.**
RESPONSE VARIABLE: Continuous.
EXPLANATORY VARIABLE(S): Two groups.

RESULTS REPORTED: The group **means** and **standard deviations,** the difference between the means, the 95% **confidence interval** for the difference, the actual ***P* value,** and the **test statistic.** (Developed by William Gossett, a student of Karl Pearson, and published under the pseudonym "Student.")

systematic error
A nonrandom or consistent source of error; bias.

surrogate endpoint
A study outcome believed to be related to a disease state but that is not the disease. For example, the point at which a patient with amyotrophic lateral sclerosis is switched to mechanical ventilation to prevent death by suffocation may be used as a surrogate endpoint for death in a study examining the time between the onset of symptoms and "death."

survival analysis: *See* **time-to-event analysis**

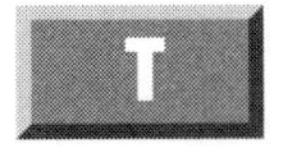

***t* test** *See:* **Student's *t* test**

test statistic
A number, computed from the data, that is compared with the associated probability distribution to determine the ***P* value** for the comparison in question. The statistic is associated with a statistical test that uses it and that sometimes has the same name (for example, the *F* statistic is associated with the ***F* test**).

threshold analysis
A technique used in **decision analysis** and **economic evaluations** to determine the "break even" point of a variable; that is, the value at which the variable no longer affects the outcome. Used to help assess the importance of the variable in the overall analysis.

time horizon
The period over which the findings of a study are expected to pertain. In economic evaluations and decision analyses, the period over which the costs and benefits of a treatment accrue.
See Guideline 12.9.

time-to-event analysis
Statistical procedures for analyzing the time between a given starting point and a given event (usually death) where there are **censored** observations; that is, when the event has not occurred in some subjects. **Survival analysis** is the most common form of time-to-event analysis used in medicine.
See **Kaplan-Meier curve; Kaplan-Meier method; Cox proportional hazards regression analysis; log-rank test.**

time-trade-off technique
A method of assigning a **utility** or a quality-of-life measure to a medical condition. Respondents are asked to choose between living X years with a given quality of life and imminent death. The number of years and the quality of life are varied until respondents are as likely to choose one option as they are another.
See Guideline 12.12.

transformed data
Data that are mathematically converted to approximately conform to a known distribution. Often used to create a more **normal distribution** from markedly **non-normally distributed data.** Common transformations in medical science are the logarithmic transformation, the reciprocal transformation, the square-root transformation, and the exponential transformation.

trial
An experiment or **protocol,** as in a "clinical trial."

true-negative rate
In diagnostic testing, the **specificity** of the test. The number of negative test results in nondiseased participants divided by the number of participants who do not have the disease.

true-positive rate
In diagnostic testing, the **sensitivity** of the test. The number of positive test results in diseased participants divided by the number of participants who have the disease.

Tukey's procedure: *See* **multiple (pairwise) comparison procedures**

two-tailed (two-sided) test
A condition for a hypothesis test, specified before data are collected, as an alternative to a **one-tailed test.** A two-tailed test does not assume that the direction of the difference between, say, two values (larger or smaller) is known in advance. Two-tailed tests are more conservative and more common.

type I error (α; alpha)
Rejecting the **null hypothesis** when it should be accepted; wrongly attributing a difference to biology when, in fact, it is the result of chance. The **probability** of making this error is set by the researcher before the experiment is conducted; it is the **alpha level** and is typically set at 0.05 or 0.01. Using a legal metaphor, the probability of type I error can be thought of as the probability of "convicting an innocent defendant."

type II error (β; beta)
Accepting the null hypothesis when it should be rejected; wrongly attributing a difference to chance when, in fact, it is the result of biology. The higher the **statistical power** (defined as 1 minus beta), the lower the **probability** of making a **type II error.** Setting the **statistical power** at 0.8 means that type II error will likely be avoided 80% of the time. Using a legal metaphor, the probability

of type II error is the probability of "letting a guilty defendant go free" (often because the sample was too small; that is, not enough "evidence" was collected to obtain a "conviction").

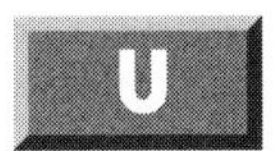

***U* test:** *See* **Wilcoxon's rank-sum test**

uncensored data
In survival analysis, data that are "complete" in that the event of interest (usually death) has occurred and that the time between the intervention and the event is known. Contrasts with **censored data,** which statistically must be treated differently because the event of interest has not yet occurred.

univariate analysis
In general, the first step in building a mathematical model, as in **regression analysis** or **ANOVA.** Each variable is assessed individually (hence, "univariate") for its effect on the outcome; those that have statistically significant effects are then selected for possible inclusion in the model itself.

unpaired data; unpaired tests
Data that are independent of one another; the tests for comparing such data. In contrast to **paired data** or **tests.**

utility
A measure of patient desirability or preference for various states of health and illness. The measure is usually a number ranging from 0 (indifference between life and death) to 1 (robust health). End-stage renal disease, for example, may be assigned a utility of 0.2, indicating an undesirable condition. Utilities can be measured in several ways. The most common in medicine are rating scales, the **standard gamble technique,** the **magnitude estimation technique,** the **time-trade-off technique,** and the **person trade-off technique.**
See Guideline 12.12.

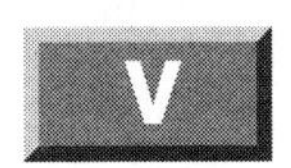

validity
The degree to which a measurement reflects the "true" value of what is being measured.
See **reliability.**

variance
The degree of dispersion of data about the mean. The square root of the vari-

ance is the **standard deviation.** For bell-shaped curves, the larger the variance, the flatter the distribution curve; the smaller the variance, the more peaked the curve.

variance components analysis
The process of isolating the sources of variability in the outcome variable.

vehicle
A solution for delivering a medication. Sometimes, the vehicle alone will be injected as a **placebo.**

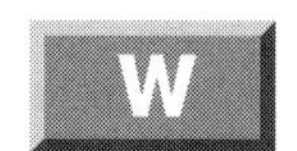

Wald's statistic
Test statistics used in many situations in many statistical tests; commonly used as approximate **chi-square test** statistics.

wash-out period
In drug studies, especially **cross-over studies,** a time during which patients are not given drugs that might interfere with an upcoming experiment. That is, the drugs they have been taking are allowed to "wash out" of their systems to avoid the possibility that the "old" drug will interfere with the "new" drug.

Wilcoxon's rank-sum test
Same as the **Mann-Whitney *U* test** and the ***U* test.** Sometimes presented as the rank-sum test. The nonparametric form of **Student's *t* test.**
PURPOSE: To compare two groups on the **median value** of the **response variable.**
RESPONSE VARIABLE: Continuous (discrete or ordinal with many categories).
EXPLANATORY VARIABLE(S): Two groups.
RESULTS REPORTED: The group medians, the difference between them, the 95% **confidence interval** for the difference, the ***P* value,** and the **test statistic.**

Wilcoxon's signed-rank test
A nonparametric form of the **paired *t* test** for comparing two samples.
PURPOSE: To compare two matched groups on the **median value** of the **response variable;** actually, to compare the median of the changes or differences of the matched pairs with zero.
RESPONSE VARIABLE: Continuous (discrete or ordinal with many categories)
EXPLANATORY VARIABLE(S): Two matched groups.
RESULTS REPORTED: The group medians, the median of all the changes or differences between the pairs, the 95% **confidence interval** for the median of the changes or differences between the pairs, the actual ***P* value,** and the **test statistic.**

Wilcoxon's test

(Differs from **Wilcoxon's rank-sum test** and **Wilcoxon's signed-rank test.** Also called Breslow's generalized Wilcoxon test.)

PURPOSE: To compare two or more groups on the proportions of subjects alive (or event-free) at certain times during the study (usually compares two or more survival curves).

RESPONSE VARIABLE: Time to an event (usually death) or to the last follow-up visit.

EXPLANATORY VARIABLE(S): Two or more groups.

RESULTS REPORTED: In survival analysis, the proportion of subjects in each group alive (or event-free) at certain times during the study, the actual ***P* value,** and the **test statistic.**

See Chapter 9.

willingness-to-pay approach

An **economic conversion** in which the cost of a medical condition is calculated on the basis of how much people are willing to pay to avoid having the condition.

See Guideline 12.11.

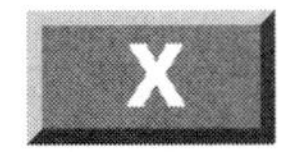

χ

The Greek letter chi, pronounced "kigh." Often seen as χ^2 to designate the **chi-square test** or **statistic.**

X

The notation for the explanatory variable(s) typically used in **regression analysis** and **ANOVA equations.**

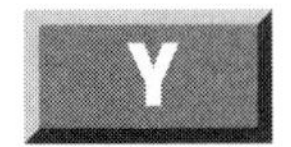

Y

The notation for the response variable typically used in **regression analysis** and **ANOVA** equations.

Yates' correction for continuity

A correction for a **chi-square test** to compensate for using a continuous probability distribution (the chi-square distribution) to estimate probabilities for categorical data.

Z

***z* score**

The distance between a value and the **mean** of a distribution expressed as the number of standard deviations from the mean. Example: $z = 2.4$ indicates that the value is 2.4 standard deviations above the mean. Also called the **standardized score** or the "standard normal deviate."

***z* test:** *See* **Fisher's *z* test**

***z* transformation**

The process of creating a "standardized score" by calculating the ***z* score** for a point on a distribution so that the point's value can be presented in units of standard deviations.

See also ***z* score.**

zzz

Sound made by most people after only a short period of reading *any* book on statistics.

REFERENCE

1. **Pearl R.** Introduction to Medical Biometry and Statistics. Philadelphia: WB Saunders, 1941.

Part 3

An Unannotated, Referenced List of the Guidelines

This section provides a quick reference to all of the guidelines, listed by chapter and unencumbered by the annotations and examples that fill the rest of the book. References that support or explain the importance of each guideline are also cited here for readers wishing more information about the topic. The name-date citation system is used to help readers identify authors who have contributed to the subject of statistical reporting and who may be known by name and reputation. References are cited by first author only. Complete bibliographic information for each reference is included in the book's bibliography.

Chapter 1
Asking Questions and Finding Answers: Reporting Research Designs and Activities

GUIDELINES ADDRESSED IN THE INTRODUCTION

1.1 **State the purpose of the study. Identify the relationships that were studied and the reasons for studying them.**
Altman 1983, Berry 1987, Cho 1994, Cooper 1989, Elenbaas 1983b, Evans 1984, Gardner 1983, Gardner 1986b, Gardner 1990, Goodman 1994a, Grant 1989, Haynes 1990, JAMA 1993, Journal of Hypertension 1992, Lionel 1970, Marks 1988, Morris 1988, Murray 1988, Murray 1991b, Pocock 1987, Squires 1990, Tyson 1983, Walker 1986

1.2 **If the study was designed to test one or more a priori hypotheses, state the hypotheses.**
Ad Hoc Working Group 1987, Bracken 1989, Cooper 1989, Goodman 1994a, Grimes 1992, Haynes 1990, Journal of Hypertension 1992, Murray 1991b

1.3 **State how the original data may be obtained for reanalysis and the format in which the data are stored.**
Bailar 1988, Mosteller 1979, Mosteller 1980, Stoto 1990

GUIDELINES ADDRESSED IN THE MATERIALS AND METHODS

The Study Focus

1.4 Specify the observational or experimental unit(s) of interest.
Altman 1991, Badgley 1961, Bailar 1988, Elenbaas 1983b, Evans 1989, Gartland 1988, Gore 1992, Gotzsche 1989, Hujoel 1992, Vaisrub 1985

1.5 Describe the population studied and to which the results are to be generalized.
Ambroz 1978, Badgley 1961, Bailar 1988, Chalmers 1981, Evans 1984, Fienberg 1990, Gardner 1983, Gartland 1988, Gifford 1969, Haynes 1981, Leis 1986, Lionel 1970, Mahon 1964, Marks 1988, Morris 1988, Sackett 1981, Sonis 1994, Squires 1990, Tyson 1983, Walker 1986, Yancy 1990, Zelen 1983

1.6 Provide operational definitions for all explanatory variables (independent variables, contributory variables, risk factors, predictive variables, or prognostic factors) and all response variables (dependent variables, endpoints, or outcomes).
Altman 1983, Badgley 1961, Berry 1987, Bland 1985, Bracken 1989, Christensen 1977, Cooper 1989, Elenbaas 1983b, Evans 1984, Evans 1989, Felson 1990, Gardner 1986b, Gardner 1990, Gartland 1988, Goodman 1994a, Gotzsche 1989, Grant 1989, Grimes 1992, Haynes 1990, Hemminki 1981, JAMA 1993, Koes 1995, Laupacis 1994, Marks 1987, Marks 1988, Meinert 1984, Moher 1994, Morris 1988, Moskowitz 1983, O'Brien 1981c, Squires 1990, Tugwell 1981, Tyson 1983, Vaisrub 1985, Vrbos 1993

1.7 Specify the minimum change or difference in the response variable(s) that is considered to be clinically important.
Andersen 1992, Braitman 1991, Chalmers 1981, Felson 1990, Freiman 1978, Grimes 1992, JAMA 1993, Liberati 1986, Marks 1988, Moher 1994, Raju 1992, Reed 1981, Simon R 1985, Sonis 1994, Tyson 1983, Weiss 1983

1.8 Indicate whether the study was approved by the appropriate Institutional Review Board(s) and whether animal subjects were treated according to approved guidelines.
Altman 1982, Bracken 1989, Cooper 1989, Evans 1984, Evans 1989, Garcia 1993, Gotzsche 1989, Grant 1989, Hemminki 1981, Mosteller 1979, Mosteller 1980

The Study as Planned

1.9 **Describe the study design.**
Altman 1981, Altman 1983, Altman 1990, Anonymous 1987, Berry 1987, Bracken 1989, Cho 1994, Gelber 1992, Goodman 1994a, Gore 1992, Gotzsche 1989, Haynes 1990, JAMA 1993, Juhl 1977, Lionel 1970, Morris 1988, Squires 1990, Vrbos 1993, Weiss 1983, Zelen 1983

1.10 **Describe fully the treatment under study and the protocol under which it was administered.**
Altman 1983, Ambroz 1978, Berry 1987, Bland 1985, Chalmers 1981, Christensen 1977, Evans 1984, Gardner 1986b, Gardner 1990, Gelber 1992, Grant 1989, Grimes 1992, Haynes 1990, Hemminki 1981, Koes 1995, Leis 1986, Liberati 1986, Morris 1988, O'Brien 1981c, Sackett 1981, Sonis 1994, Squires 1990, Tyson 1983, Zelen 1983

1.11 **If the groups are to be paired, report the criteria and rationale for the pairing.**
Bracken 1989, Gore 1992, JAMA 1993, Journal of Hypertension 1992, Murray 1991b, Peterson 1991, Weiss 1983, White 1979

1.12 **Describe any potential confounding variables and the methods used to control for them.**
Cho 1994, Vrbos 1993

1.13 **Identify the study setting and the source of the study participants.**
Bland 1985, Gardner 1983, Gardner 1986a, Gardner 1986b, Gardner 1990, Goodman 1994a, Grant 1989, Haynes 1990, Leis 1986, Lionel 1970, O'Brien 1981c, Squires 1990, Tugwell 1981, Walker 1986

1.14 **Specify how the sample size was determined. If the sample size was determined in combination with a power calculation, give the details of the calculation.**
Bracken 1989, Cho 1994, Gore 1992, Gotzsche 1989, Grant 1989, Grimes 1992, JAMA 1993, Journal of Hypertension 1992, Liberati 1986, Marks 1988, Meinert 1984, Moher 1994, Moskowitz 1983, Murray 1991a, Murray 1991b, Pocock 1987, Reed 1981, Rochon 1994, Schultz 1994, Sheehan 1980, Squires 1990, Tyson 1983, Vaisrub 1985, Vrbos 1993, Weiss 1983, Young 1983

1.15 **Specify the sampling technique.**
Altman 1983, Bailar 1988, Bland 1985, Bracken 1989, Cooper 1989, Gore 1992, Grant 1989, Haynes 1981, Hemminki 1981, JAMA 1993, Liberati

1986, Lionel 1970, Mahon 1964, Marks 1988, Morris 1988, Stoto 1990, Vaisrub 1985, Walker 1986, White 1979, Zelen 1983

1.16 **Give the inclusion and exclusion criteria for the study.**
Altman 1981, Altman 1983a, Ambroz 1978, Badgley 1961, Bailar 1988, Bland 1985, Bracken 1989, Chalmers 1981, Cho 1994, Christensen 1977, Cooper 1989, DerSimonian 1982, Feinstein 1969, Gardner 1986b, Gardner 1990, Gartland 1988, Gelber 1992, Goodman 1994a, Gore 1992, Grant 1989, Grimes 1992, Haynes 1990, Hemminki 1981, Horwitz 1979, International Committee 1991, Koes 1995, Leis 1986, Lionel 1970, Moskowitz 1983, Sonis 1994, Squires 1990, Tyson 1983, Vaisrub 1985, Vrbos 1993, Walker 1986

1.17 **Describe the circumstances under which informed consent was obtained.**
Bracken 1989, Grant 1989

1.18 **Specify how study participants were assigned to experimental groups (treatment or control groups).**
Altman 1982, Altman 1983a, Altman 1990, Ambroz 1978, Avram 1985, Bailar 1988, Berry 1987, Bland 1985, Christensen 1977, Cruess 1989, DerSimonian 1982, Elenbaas 1983b, Garcia-Cases 1993, Gardner 1986b, Gardner 1990, Gelber 1992, Gifford 1969, Goodman 1992, Goodman 1994a, Gore 1977, Gotzsche 1989, Grant 1989, Grimes 1991, Grimes 1992, Hemminki 1981, Horwitz 1979, International Committee 1991, JAMA 1993, Journal of Hypertension 1992, Koes 1995, Liberati 1986, MacArthur 1984, Mahon 1964, Marks 1988, Meinert 1984, Moher 1994, Moskowitz 1983, Mosteller 1979, Mosteller 1980, Murray 1988, Murray 1991b, Oxman 1992, Ross 1951, Sackett 1981, Schoolman 1968, Schultz 1994, Schulz 1995a, Squires 1990, Stoto 1990, Tyson 1983, Vaisrub 1985, Vrbos 1993, Weiss 1983, White 1979, Zelen 1983, Zivin 1976

1.19 **Specify the technique of masking (blinding), if applicable.**
Altman 1981, Altman 1983, Altman 1990, Ambroz 1978, Bailar 1988, Berry 1987, Bland 1985, Chalmers 1981, Cho 1994, Christensen 1977, Cooper 1989, DerSimonian 1982, Garcia-Cases 1993, Gardner 1986b, Gardner 1990, Gifford 1969, Goodman 1994a, Gore 1992, Gotzsche 1989, Grant 1989, Grimes 1991, Grimes 1992, Haynes 1990, Hemminki 1981, Horwitz 1979, International Committee 1991, JAMA 1993, Journal of Hypertension 1992, Koes 1995, Mahon 1964, Meinert 1984, Mosteller 1980, Murray 1991b, Rochon 1994, Sonis 1994, Squires 1990, Tugwell 1981, Tyson 1983, Vaisrub 1985, Vrbos 1993

1.20 **Describe fully any placebo medications, sham procedures or surgeries (in animal studies), or alternative or concomitant treatments received by control groups.**
Gotzsche 1989, Grant 1989, Guyatt 1993, Hemminki 1981, Koes 1995, Leis 1986, Lionel 1970, Moskowitz 1983, Rochon 1994

1.21 **Describe the methods of data collection or measurement.**
Altman 1983, Anonymous 1986, Anonymous 1987, Walker 1986

1.22 **Describe the planned nature and duration of follow-up efforts.**
Anonymous 1986, Bailar 1988, Berry 1987, Bland 1985, Bracken 1989, DerSimonian 1982, Evans 1984, Gardner 1986b, Gardner 1990, Gartland 1988, Gelber 1992, Haynes 1990, JAMA 1993, Laupacis 1992, Liberati 1986, O'Brien 1981c, Oxman 1992, Simon R 1985, Squires 1990, Tugwell 1981, Tyson 1983

1.23 **Describe any quality-control methods used to ensure completeness and accuracy of data collection.**
Anonymous 1986, Cooper 1989, Gelber 1992, Gotzsche 1989, Haynes 1981, Rochon 1994, Simon R 1985, Walker 1986, Zelen 1983

1.24 **Describe the administrative structure of multicenter trials.**
Meinert 1984

Statistical Methods

1.25 **Describe the comparisons to be made and the statistical procedures to be used for making them.**
Altman 1981, Altman 1982, Altman 1983, Altman 1991, Bailar 1988, Berry 1987, Chalmers 1981, Elenbaas 1983a, Fienberg 1990, Finney 1992, Garcia-Cases 1993, Gardner 1986a, Gardner 1986b, Gardner 1990, Gartland 1988, Goodman 1994a, Gore 1992, Gotzsche 1989, Hayden 1983, International Committee 1991, JAMA 1993, Lionel 1970, Meinert 1984, Moher 1994, Morris 1988, Mosteller 1980, Murray 1991b, Savitz 1992, Shott 1985, Sonis 1994 , Squires 1990, Vrbos 1993, Wainapel 1985

1.26 **State whether the statistical analysis will be on the basis of intention-to-treat.**
Altman 1991, Gotzsche 1989, Grant 1989, Grimes 1992, Guyatt 1993, Hampton 1981, Koes 1995, Liberati 1986, Murray 1991a, Salzberg 1985, Schulz 1995a, Simon R 1985, Stoto 1990, Zelen 1983

1.27 **Described any planned interim analyses and any stopping rules for the study.**
Geller 1987, Grant 1989, Murray 1991a, Murray 1991b, Simon R 1985

1.28 **Specify any procedures used to control for the multiple testing problem.**
Anonymous 1986, Avram 1985, Bracken 1989, Cruess 1989, Felson 1984, Felson 1990, Gelber 1992, Goodman 1994a, Gotzsche 1989, Grant 1989, Haines 1981, Healy 1992, JAMA 1993, Journal of Hypertension 1992, Lee 1980, MacArthur 1984, Mills 1993, Moskowitz 1983, Murray 1991a, Murray 1991b, O'Fallon 1978, Pocock 1987, Salsburg 1985, Schor 1966, Simon R 1985, Smith 1987, Vaisrub 1985, Walker 1986, White 1979, Yusuf 1991, Zivin 1976

1.29 **Report the levels of alpha (α) and beta (β) (or statistical power, $1 - \beta$).**
Freiman 1978, Goodman 1992, Moher 1994, Rochon 1994

1.30 **Report whether statistical tests were one- or two-tailed.**
Altman 1983, Altman 1991, Bailar 1988, Cooper 1989, Elenbaas 1983a, Elenbaas 1983b, Feinstein 1974, Gotzsche 1989, JAMA 1993, MacArthur 1984, Marks 1987, Marks 1988, Moher 1994, Moher 1994, Mosteller 1979, Mosteller 1980, Peace 1989, Salsburg 1985, Vaisrub 1985

1.31 **Identify the statistical package or program used to analyze the data.**
Altman 1983, Altman 1991, Bailar 1988, Committee on Data 1977, Concato 1993, International Committee 1991, Iverson 1983, Marks 1987, Prihoda 1992

GUIDELINES ADDRESSED IN THE RESULTS

The Study as Conducted

1.32 **Specify the beginning and ending dates of the data collection period and give the reasons for selecting those dates.**
Badgley 1961, Bailar 1988, Chalmers 1981, Gifford 1969, Grant 1989, Grimes 1992, Leis 1986, Liberati 1986, Lionel 1970, Sonis 1994

1.33 **When possible, provide a schematic summary of the study showing the number and disposition of participants at each stage.**
Hampton 1981, Squires 1990, Zelen 1983

1.34 **When appropriate, describe the subjects who were eligible and available but who were not approached to participate in the study.**
Ad Hoc Working Group 1987, Bailar 1988, Chalmers 1981, Cooper 1989, Evans 1984, Gardner 1986a, Gardner 1986b, Gardner 1990, Gore 1992, Grant 1989, Grimes 1992, Hampton 1981, Meinert 1984, Moskowitz 1983, O'Brien 1981c, Sonis 1994 , Walker 1986

1.35 **When appropriate, describe the subjects who were evaluated for participation but who did not meet the inclusion criteria.**
Chalmers 1981, Leis 1986

1.36 **Describe the subjects who were approached but who declined to participate in the study.**
Bracken 1989, Leis 1986, Rochon 1994

1.37 **Describe the participants who were enrolled in the study but who did not complete it (the withdrawals or "drop-outs").**
Ad Hoc Working Group 1987, Altman 1991, Badgley 1961, Chalmers 1981, Christensen 1977, Elenbaas 1983b, Evans 1984, Gardner 1986b, Gardner 1990, Goodman 1994a, Gore 1992, Gotzsche 1989, Grant 1989, Grimes 1992, Hemminki 1982, Journal of Hypertension 1992, Juhl 1977, Koes 1995, Leis 1986, Meinert 1984, Mills 1993, Moskowitz 1983, Schulz 1995a, Simon R 1985, Sonis 1994 , Squires 1990, Vrbos 1993, Zelen 1983

1.38 **Describe the participants who completed the treatment but who were lost to follow-up.**
Gore 1992, Grimes 1992, Gross 1988, Guyatt 1993, Haynes 1990, Journal of Hypertension 1992, Laupacis 1994, Leis 1986, Liberati 1986, Simon R 1985, Vaisrub 1985, Zelen 1983

1.39 **Describe the actual nature and duration of follow-up efforts.**
Anonymous 1986, Bailar 1988, Berry 1987, Bland 1985, Bracken 1989, DerSimonian 1982, Evans 1984, Gardner 1986b, Gardner 1990, Gartland 1988, Gelber 1992, Haynes 1990, JAMA 1993, Laupacis 1992, Liberati 1986, O'Brien 1981c, Oxman 1992, Simon R 1985, Squires 1990, Tugwell 1981, Tyson 1983

1.40 **Describe the participants who completed the course of treatment and the follow-up examinations.**
Goodman 1994a, Gotzsche 1989, Grant 1989, Haynes 1981, Hemminki 1981

1.41 **Indicate how representative the sample is of the population of interest.**
Altman 1982, Altman 1990, Anonymous 1977, Anonymous 1986, Avram 1985, Badgley 1961, Bailar 1988, Berry 1987, Chalmers 1981, Cho 1994, Cooper 1989, Elenbaas 1983b, Evans 1984, Evans 1989, Gardner 1986b, Gelber 1992, Gelber 1992, Bland 1985, Gore 1992, Marks 1987, Morris 1988, Sackett 1981, Sonis 1994

1.42 **Indicate the similarities and differences between the control group(s) and the experimental group(s) at baseline.**
Cho 1994, Gore 1992, Gotzsche 1989, Grant 1989, Grimes 1992, Hemminki 1981, Koes 1995, Levine 1994, Liberati 1986, Lionel 1970, Meinert 1984, Moskowitz 1983, Mosteller 1979, O'Brien 1981c, Rochon 1994, Ross 1951, Schultz 1994, Simon R 1985, Squires 1990, Vaisrub 1985, White 1979

1.43 **Indicate whether allocation concealment and masking (blinding) were successful.**
Gotzsche 1989, Grant 1989, Hemminki 1981, Hemminki 1982, International Committee 1991, Moskowitz 1983, Schultz 1995a, Schultz 1995b

1.44 **For observations based on judgments, provide a measure of consistency or agreement among the evaluators.**
Brown 1985, Cooper 1989, Koes 1995, Sackett 1983, Simon R 1985

Study Outcomes

1.45 **Present the results of the study.**
Altman 1981, Chalmers 1981, Haynes 1990, Sackett 1981, Sonis 1994

1.46 **Report absolute (and relative, if desirable) changes or differences for all primary endpoints.**
Goodman 1994b, Forrow 1992

1.47 **Report (95%) confidence intervals for changes or differences in the primary endpoints.**
Ad Hoc Working Group 1987, Altman 1980b, Altman 1983, Ambroz 1978, Anonymous 1987, Badgley 1961, Bailar 1988, Berry 1987, Bland 1985, Bourne 1987, Braitman 1991, Browner 1986, Bulpitt 1987, Cooper 1989, Council of Biology Editors 1983, Eisenhart 1968, Evans 1989, Fienberg 1990, Gardner 1986a, Gardner 1986b, Gardner 1988, Gardner 1990, Gelber 1992, Goodman 1994a, Gore 1981, Gore 1992, Gotzsche 1989, Grant 1989, Guyatt 1993, Haynes 1990, JAMA 1993, Jewett 1991, Journal of Hyper-

tension 1992, Liberati 1986, Marks 1987(4), Marks 1988, Morgan 1989, Morris 1988, Murray 1989, Murray 1991b, Pocock 1987, Rochon 1994, Rothman 1986, Savitz 1994, Shott 1985, Simon R 1985, Simpson 1988, Squires 1990, Sumner 1992, Vaisrub 1985, Walker 1986, Wulff 1973, Yancy 1990

1.48 **Report actual *P* values for all primary analyses.**
Altman 1983, Bailar 1988, Braitman 1991, Bulpitt 1987, Bulpitt 1987, Chalmers 1981, Cooper 1989, Gibbons 1975, Gore 1992, Gore 1992, Haynes 1990, Haynes 1990, JAMA 1993, Journal of Hypertension 1992, Mainland 1984, Mosteller 1980, Murray 1989, Murray 1991b, Pocock 1987, Rochon 1994, Salsburg 1985, Sonis 1994 , Sumner 1992

1.49 **Whenever possible, present the main findings of the study in figures or tables.**
Altman 1983, Braitman 1991, Connett 1994, Cooper 1989, Godfrey 1985, Goodman 1994a, Journal of Hypertension 1992, Morris 1988, Murray 1988, Murray 1991b, Walker 1986

1.50 **When feasible, report statistical findings with enough detail to allow subsequent reanalysis or meta-analysis.**
Council of Biology Editors 1983, International Committee 1991

1.51 **Report any potential confounding or interactive effects.**
Bracken 1989, Koes 1995

1.52 **Indicate the degree to which study participants adhered to the protocol and explain any exceptions or deviations from the protocol.**
Altman 1983, Gelber 1992, Goodman 1994a, Gotzsche 1989, Grant 1989, Grimes 1992, Liberati 1986, Meinert 1984, Moskowitz 1983, Reizenstein 1983, Reizenstein 1983, Rochon 1994, Tyson 1983, Vrbos 1993, Zelen 1983

1.53 **Report all potential treatment-related side effects and adverse events.**
American Journal of Clinical Oncology 1986, Bailar 1988, Berry 1987, Chalmers 1981, DerSimonian 1982, Elenbaas 1983b, Garcia-Cases 1993, Gardner 1986b, Gartland 1988, Gelber 1992, Goodman 1994a, Gotzsche 1989, Grant 1989, Grimes 1992, Hemminki 1982, International Committee 1991, Liberati 1986, Moskowitz 1983, Reiffenstein 1968, Rochon 1994, Sonis 1994 , Squires 1990

1.54 **Describe the treatment of outlying values.**
Altman 1983, Gotzsche 1989, Shott 1985, Stoto 1990

1.55 **Account for all observations and explain any missing data.**
Cho 1994, Connett 1994, Gifford 1969, Gotzsche 1989, Grant 1989, Guyatt 1993, Journal of Hypertension 1992, Meinert 1984, Sackett 1981, Simon R 1985, Stoto 1990, Vaisrub 1985, Walker 1986

1.56 **Report any anecdotal evidence or observations that might contribute to a more accurate or complete understanding of the study or its results.**

GUIDELINES ADDRESSED IN THE DISCUSSION (COMMENT)

1.57 **Discuss the implications of the primary analyses first.**
Meinert 1984

1.58 **Distinguish between clinical importance and statistical significance.**
Bracken 1989, Jamart 1992

1.59 **Discuss the results in the context of the published literature.**
Bracken 1989, Goodman 1994a, Grant 1989, Iverson 1983, Laupacis 1994, Simon R 1985

1.60 **Discuss the generalizability of the results.**
Bracken 1989, Goodman 1994a, Grant 1989, Iverson 1983, Laupacis 1994, Simon R 1985

Limitations of the Study

1.61 **Discuss any weaknesses in the research design or problems with data collection, analysis, or interpretation.**
Altman 1983, Bailar 1988, Elenbaas 1983b, Goodman 1984, Gore 1992, Journal of Hypertension 1992, Mainland 1984, Meinert 1984, Mosteller 1980, Murray 1991b, Savitz 1992, Stoto 1990

Conclusions

1.62 **Limit conclusions to those supported by the results of the study.**
Badgley 1961, Berry 1987, Bracken 1989, Cho 1994, Elenbaas 1983b, Evans 1984, Fienberg 1990, Gardner 1986a, Gardner 1986b, Gardner 1990, Goodman 1994a, Gore 1992, Gotzsche 1989, Grant 1989, Haynes 1990, Lionel 1970, Meinert 1984, Morris 1988, O'Fallon 1978, Schor 1966, Squires 1990, Stoto 1990, Tyson 1983, Vaisrub 1985, Vrbos 1993, White 1979

1.63 **List the conclusions of the study and describe their implications.**
Ad Hoc Working Group 1987, Bracken 1989, Cooper 1989, Grant 1989, Haynes 1990

Chapter 2
Summarizing Data: Reporting Data and Descriptive Statistics

NUMERICAL PRECISION

2.1 **Report all numbers with the appropriate degree of precision.**
Altman 1980b, Altman 1981, Altman 1982, Altman 1983, Bailar 1988, Council of Biology Editors 1983, Ehrenberg 1977, Ehrenberg 1981, Eisenhart 1968, Finney 1992, Iverson 1983, Journal of Hypertension 1992, Murray 1988, Murray 1991b, Sumner 1992

REPORTING PERCENTAGES

2.2 **When reporting percentages, always give the numerators and denominators of the calculations.**
Altman 1983, Bailar 1988, Evans 1984, Evans 1989, Mainland 1936

2.3 **When the sample size is *greater* than 100, report percentages to no more than one decimal place. When sample size is *less* than 100, report percentages in whole numbers. When sample size is less than, say, 20, consider reporting the actual numbers rather than percentages.**
Altman 1983, Evans 1989, Journal of Hypertension 1992, Murray 1991b, Sumner 1992

2.4 **When reporting changes in data as percent change, use the formula: [(Final Value – Initial Value)/Initial Value] × 100%.**

SUMMARIZING CATEGORICAL DATA

2.5 **Specify the denominators of rates, ratios, proportions, and percentages.**
Bailar 1988, Evans 1989, Goodman 1994a, Vaisrub 1985, Walker 1986

2.6

If continuous data have been separated by "cutpoints" into ordinal categories, give the cutpoints and the rationale for choosing them.
Brown 1985, Vaisrub 1985

SUMMARIZING CONTINUOUS DATA

2.7

Provide appropriate measures of central tendency and dispersion when summarizing data that have a continuous distribution.
Altman 1983, Altman 1990, Badgley 1961, Bunce 1980, Committee on Data 1977, Cooper 1989, Elenbaas 1983a, Elenbaas 1983b, Feinstein 1976, Feinstein 1987, Felson 1984, Gore 1977, Gore 1992, Marks 1987(4), Murray 1991b, O'Brien 1981c, Schultz 1994

2.8

Do not summarize continuous data with the mean and the standard error of the mean (SEM).
Altman 1980b, Altman 1983, Altman 1990, Avram 1985, Brown 1985, Bunce 1980, Cruess 1989, Ehrenberg 1977, Elenbaas 1983a, Feinstein 1976, Feinstein 1987, Gardner 1986b, Glantz 1980, Goodman 1992, Hall 1982b, Hayden 1983, Jamart 1992, MacArthur 1984, Mantha 1992, Morgan 1989, Murray 1991b, Oliver 1989, Weech 1974, Yancy 1990

SUMMARIZING NORMALLY DISTRIBUTED DATA

2.9

Use the mean and standard deviation only when describing approximately normally distributed data.
Altman 1980b, Altman 1983, Brown 1982, Brown 1985, Cooper 1989, Evans 1989, Feinstein 1976, Feinstein 1987, Goodman 1992, Haines 1981, Hall 1982a, Hall 1982b, Iverson 1983, Jamart 1992, Journal of Hypertension 1992, Kanter 1994, Murray 1988, Murray 1991b, O'Brien 1981a, Oliver 1989, Simpson 1988, Sumner 1992, Vaisrub 1985, Wainapel 1985, Weech 1974, Yancy 1990

2.10

Use the "±" symbol only when presenting the mean and standard deviation of a distribution and only for approximately normally distributed data. Identify the meaning of the interval (that is, the standard deviation) at first use.
Altman 1981, Altman 1983, Bailar 1988, Brown 1985, Eisenhart 1968, Evans 1989, Feinstein 1976, Feinstein 1987, Gardner 1975, Gardner 1983, Iverson 1983, Journal of Hypertension 1992, Murray 1991b, Oliver 1989, Salsburg 1985, White 1979

2.11 **When comparing the variability of two or more sets of normally distributed data, use the coefficient of variation instead of the standard deviation.**
Feinstein 1987

SUMMARIZING NON-NORMALLY DISTRIBUTED DATA

2.12 **Describe markedly non-normally distributed (skewed) data with the median and range or interquartile range (or other interpercentile range).**
Altman 1980b, Altman 1983, Brown 1982, Evans 1989, Feinstein 1974, Feinstein 1976, Feinstein 1987, Gardner 1986a, Gore 1977, Iverson 1983, Journal of Hypertension 1992, Murray 1991b, O'Brien 1981a, Sumner 1992, Weech 1974, White 1979

REPORTING PAIRED DATA

2.13 **Report paired observations together.**
Altman 1983, Healy 1992, Journal of Hypertension 1992, Murray 1991b

REPORTING TRANSFORMED DATA

2.14 **Indicate whether and how markedly non-normally distributed data were transformed into an approximately normal distribution.**
Altman 1983, Fienberg 1990, Gardner 1975, Gardner 1986a, Journal of Hypertension 1992, Murray 1991b

2.15 **If data have been transformed, convert the units of measurement back to the original units for reporting.**
Altman 1983, Gardner 1986a

SUMMARIZING DATA FROM SMALL SAMPLES

2.16 **If appropriate, present all the data when the number of observations is small or when descriptive statistics would be misleading.**
Altman 1983, Braitman 1991, Gore 1992, Hayden 1983, Journal of Hypertension 1992, Mainland 1984, Mike 1982, Murray 1991b, O'Fallon 1978, Shott 1985

2.17 **Avoid using percentages to summarize small samples.**
Altman 1983, Evans 1989

Chapter 3
Generalizing from a Sample to a Population: Reporting Estimates and Confidence Intervals

CONFIDENCE INTERVALS WITH INFERENTIAL FUNCTIONS

3.1 **Provide confidence intervals for all primary comparisons, whether the results are positive (statistically significant) or negative (statistically nonsignificant).**
See references for Guideline 1.47

3.2 **Report the upper and lower values of the confidence interval. Use the "±" format only in tables to save space and only when the confidence interval is symmetrical.**
Altman 1983, Bulpitt 1987, Eisenhart 1968, Feinstein 1976, Journal of Hypertension 1992, Sumner 1992

CONFIDENCE INTERVALS WITH DESCRIPTIVE FUNCTIONS

3.3 **Report (95%) confidence intervals for all estimates of population characteristics that are of primary interest.**
See references for Guideline 1.47

3.4 **Report the upper and lower values of the confidence interval. Use the "±" format only in tables to save space and only when the confidence interval is symmetrical.**
See references for Guideline 3.2

Chapter 4
Comparing Groups: I. Reporting *P* Values

GUIDELINES ADDRESSED IN THE INTRODUCTION

4.1 **State the hypothesis being tested.**
Bailar 1988, Marks 1987(4), Murray 1991b, Sheehan 1980, White 1979, Yancy 1990

GUIDELINES ADDRESSED IN THE METHODS

4.2 **Specify the minimum difference between the groups that is considered to be clinically important.**
See references for Guideline 1.7

4.3 **Specify the alpha (α) level: the probability below which findings will be considered to be "statistically significant."**
Ad Hoc Working Group 1987, Anonymous 1987, Badgley 1961, Bourne 1987, Cruess 1989, Freiman 1978, JAMA 1993, Marks 1988, Moher 1994, Moskowitz 1983, Mosteller 1979, Schor 1966

4.4 **If applicable, for primary comparisons, report the details of an *a priori* power calculation.**
Altman 1982, Ambroz 1978, Bailar 1986, Berry 1987, Bland 1985, Bourne 1987, Bracken 1989, Chalmers 1981, Christensen 1977, DerSimonian 1982, Emerson 1983, Evans 1984, Felson 1990, Freiman 1978, Gardner 1986b, Glantz 1993, Gore 1992, Gotzsche 1989, Grant 1989, Haines 1981, Hall 1982b, Hemminki 1981, Hujoel 1992, Huth 1982, Iverson 1983, JAMA 1993, Jewett 1991, Liberati 1986, MacArthur 1984, Mainland 1984, Marks 1987, Marks 1988, Meinert 1984, Moher 1994, Moskowitz 1983, Mosteller 1979, Mosteller 1980, Murray 1988, O'Fallon 1978, Prihoda 1992, Reed 1981, Rochon 1994, Sheehan 1980, Simon 1985, Simon 1986, Stoto 1990. Elenbaas 1983b, Sumner 1992, Tugwell 1981, Tyson 1983, Vaisrub 1985, Young 1983, Zelen 1983

4.5 **Identify the statistical test used for each comparison.**
Altman 1980b, Altman 1981, Altman 1982, Altman 1983, Altman 1990, Anonymous 1987, Avram 1985, Bailar 1988, Berry 1987, Committee on Data 1977, Cooper 1989, Cruess 1989, DerSimonian 1982, Elenbaas 1983a, Evans 1984, Feinstein 1974, Feinstein 1976, Felson 1984, Fienberg 1990,

Gardner 1983, Gardner 1990, Goodman 1992, Gore 1992, Gotzsche 1989, Grant 1989, Haines 1981, Hall 1982a, Hayden 1983, Hemminki 1981, Hujoel 1992, Huth 1982, International Committee 1991, Iverson 1983, Journal of Hypertension 1992, Kanter 1994, Liberati 1986, Lionel 1970, MacArthur 1984, Marks 1987(4), Moher 1994, Moskowitz 1983, Mosteller 1979, Mosteller 1980, Murray 1988, Murray 1991b, Oliver 1989, Prihoda 1992, Schor 1966, Simon 1985, Tyson 1983, Vrbos 1993, White 1979, Zelen 1983

4.6 **Cite a reference for complex or uncommon statistical tests used to analyze the data.**
Altman 1983, Bailar 1988, Cooper 1989, Council of Biology Editors 1983, DerSimonian 1982, Finney 1992, Gardner 1983, Grant 1989, Iverson 1983, Iverson 1983, Kanter 1994

4.7 **If appropriate for the test, specify whether the test is one- or two-tailed. Justify the use of one-tailed tests.**
Altman 1983, Altman 1991, Bailar 1988, Cooper 1989, Elenbaas 1983a, Elenbaas 1983b, Feinstein 1974, Gotzsche 1989, JAMA 1993, Kanter 1994, MacArthur 1984, Marks 1987, Marks 1988, Moher 1994, Mosteller 1979, Mosteller 1980, Peace 1989, Salsburg 1985, Vaisrub 1985

4.8 **Specify whether the test is for unpaired or paired data (that is, whether it is for independent or matched samples).**
Altman 1980a, Altman 1982, Altman 1983, Brown G 1985, Elenbaas 1983a, Feinstein 1974, Gore 1977, Gotzsche 1989, Haines 1981, Hall 1982c, Journal of Hypertension 1992, Kanter 1994, Lionel 1970, Mosteller 1979, Murray 1988, Shott 1985, White 1979

4.9 **Reference the statistical packages or programs used to analyze the data.**
Altman 1983, Altman 1991, Bailar 1988, Committee on Data 1977, Concato 1993, International Committee 1991, Iverson 1983, Marks 1987, Prihoda 1992

GUIDELINES ADDRESSED IN THE RESULTS

4.10 **Report the results of all primary analyses first.**
Altman 1981, Bailar 1986, Felson 1990, Liberati 1986, Mills 1993

4.11 **Report any outlying values and how they were treated in the analysis.**
Altman 1983, Gotzsche 1989, Shott 1985, Stoto 1990

4.12 **Confirm that the assumptions of the test have been met.**
Altman 1981, Altman 1982, Altman 1983, Anonymous 1977, Anonymous 1987, Avram 1985, Berry 1987, Cooper 1989, Cruess 1989, Elenbaas 1983a, Evans 1984, Fienberg 1990, Gardner 1983, Glantz 1993, Gore 1977, Gore 1992, Gotzsche 1989, Haines 1981, Hall 1982a, Hall 1982c, Hoffman 1976, Iverson 1983, Jamart 1992, Journal of Hypertension 1992, Kanter 1994, Lionel 1970, MacArthur 1984, Marks 1987, Murray 1988, Murray 1991b, Rennie 1978, Savitz 1992, Schoolman 1968, Schor 1966, Shott 1985, Stoto 1990, Sumner 1992, White 1979, Zivin 1976

4.13 **Report absolute (and relative, if desirable) changes or differences for all primary endpoints.**
Goodman 1994b, Forrow 1992

4.14 **Report (95%) confidence intervals for changes or differences in the primary endpoints.**
Ad Hoc Working Group 1987, Altman 1980b, Altman 1983, Ambroz 1978, Anonymous 1987, Badgley 1961, Bailar 1988, Berry 1987, Bland 1985, Bourne 1987, Braitman 1991, Browner 1986, Bulpitt 1987, Cooper 1989, Council of Biology Editors 1983, Eisenhart 1968, Evans 1989, Fienberg 1990, Gardner 1986a, Gardner 1986b, Gardner 1988, Gardner 1990, Gelber 1992, Goodman 1994a, Goodman 1994b, Gore 1981, Gore 1992, Gotzsche 1989, Grant 1989, Guyatt 1993, Haynes 1990, JAMA 1993, Journal of Hypertension 1992, Kanter 1994, Liberati 1986, Marks 1987, Marks 1988, Morgan 1989, Morris 1988, Murray 1989, Murray 1991b, Pocock 1987, Rochon 1994, Rothman 1986, Shott 1985, Simon R 1985, Simpson 1988, Squires 1990, Sumner 1992, Vaisrub 1985, Walker 1986, Wulff 1973, Yancy 1990

4.15 **Give the actual *P* value, to two significant digits, whether or not the value is statistically significant.**
Altman 1983, Bailar 1988, Braitman 1991, Bulpitt 1987, Chalmers 1981, Connett 1994, Cooper 1989, Gibbons 1975, Goodman 1994b, Gore 1992, Haynes 1990, JAMA 1993, Journal of Hypertension 1992, Mainland 1984, Mosteller 1980, Murray 1989, Murray 1991b, Pocock 1987, Rochon 1994, Salsburg 1985, Sumner 1992

4.16 **Report the value of the test statistic.**
Altman 1983, Chalmers 1981, Cooper 1989, Gardner 1986a, Haines 1981, Journal of Hypertension 1992, Liberati 1986, MacArthur 1984, Moskowitz 1983, Mosteller 1980, Murray 1991b, Rochon 1994, Salzberg 1985, Sumner 1992

4.17 **For primary comparisons, specify the degrees of freedom (df) of the test, if applicable.**
Cooper 1989, Cruess 1989, Feinstein 1974, Finney 1992, Gardner 1986a, Gore 1977, JAMA 1993, MacArthur 1984

GUIDELINES ADDRESSED IN THE DISCUSSION

4.18 **Distinguish between clinical importance and statistical significance.**
Altman 1981, Altman 1982, Altman 1983, Altman 1991, Bailar 1988, Bracken 1989, Braitman 1991, Brown G 1985, Committee on Data 1977, Concato 1993, Council of Biology Editors 1983, Diamond 1983, Elenbaas 1983a, Elenbaas 1983b, Evans 1984, Evans 1989, Fleiss 1986, Gardner 1986a, Gibbons 1975, Gifford 1969, Gotzsche 1989, Haines 1981, Iverson 1983, Jekel 1977, Journal of Hypertension 1992, Mainland 1984, Moher 1994, Murray 1988, Murray 1989, Murray 1991a, Murray 1991b, O'Brien 1981d, Reizenstein 1983, Sackett 1981, Schor 1981, Sheehan 1980, Simon 1986, Smith 1987, Squires 1990, Sumner 1992, Vaisrub 1985, Vrbos 1993, Walter 1995

4.19 **For differences that are *clinically* important but not *statistically* significant, report the observed difference, the (95%) confidence interval for the difference, and the actual *P* value of the comparison.**

Chapter 5 Comparing Groups: II. The Multiple Testing Problem

5.1 **Indicate whether any accommodations were made for multiple testing. If so, describe the accommodation.**
Anonymous 1986, Avram 1985, Bracken 1989, Cruess 1989, Felson 1984, Felson 1990, Gelber 1992, Goodman 1992, Goodman 1994a, Gotzsche 1989, Grant 1989, Haines 1981, Healy 1992, JAMA 1993, Journal of Hypertension 1992, Lee 1980, MacArthur 1984, Mills 1993, Moskowitz 1983, Murray 1991a, Murray 1991b, O'Fallon 1978, Pocock 1987, Salsburg 1985, Schor 1966, Simon R 1985, Smith 1987, Vaisrub 1985, Walker 1986, White 1979, Yusuf 1991, Zivin 1976

ESTABLISHING GROUP EQUIVALENCY

5.2 **Report the clinical values used to assess group equivalence at baseline. Do not rely on *P* values to establish equivalence.**
Altman 1990, Diamond 1983, Freiman 1978, Gore 1992, Gotzsche 1989, Grant 1989, Guyatt 1993, Hall 1982b, Hemminki 1981, Journal of Hypertension 1992, Lee 1980, Liberati 1986, Mainland 1984, Murray 1991b, Pocock 1987, Schultz 1994, Sumner 1992

MULTIPLE PAIRWISE COMPARISONS OF TREATMENT GROUPS

5.3 **Specify the multiple comparison procedure used to identify which pairs of groups most influence the overall statistical significance of a group comparison.**
Altman 1982, Avram 1985, Felson 1984, Godfrey 1985, Jamart 1992, Kanter 1994, Murray 1988, Murray 1991a, Pocock 1987, Prihoda 1992, Salzberg 1985, Smith 1987, Sumner 1992, Vrbos 1993, White 1979, Yusuf 1991

SECONDARY (RETROSPECTIVE OR POST-HOC) ANALYSES

5.4 **Differentiate between primary analyses and secondary (retrospective or post-hoc) analyses.**
Abramson 1992, Altman 1983, American Journal of Clinical Oncology 1986, Bracken 1989, Chalmers 1981, Diamond 1983, Elenbaas 1983b, Evans 1989, Godfrey 1985, Goodman 1992, Grant 1989, Haines 1981, Haynes 1990, JAMA 1993, Jamart 1992, Journal of Hypertension 1992, Lee 1980, Liberati 1986, MacArthur 1984, Mills 1993, Mosteller 1979, Murray 1991b, Naylor 1992, Oxman 1992, Pocock 1987, Schoolman 1968, Smith 1987, Stoto 1990, Vaisrub 1985, Walker 1986, Weiss 1983, Yusuf 1991

SUBGROUP ANALYSES

5.5 **Specify how the subgroups were identified and the rationale for analyzing them.**
Murray 1991a, Oxman 1992, Pocock 1987, Simon R 1985, Yusuf 1991

MULTIPLE ENDPOINTS

5.6 **Identify the primary endpoints or outcomes of interest before beginning the study.**
Hemminki 1981, Murray 1988, Pocock 1987, Smith 1987, Weiss 1983

INTERIM ANALYSES OF ACCUMULATING DATA

5.7 **Report all interim analyses of accumulating data and give the rationale for the analyses.**
Altman 1991, American Journal of Clinical Oncology 1986, Ashby 1993, Chalmers 1981, Geller 1987, Grant 1989, Haines 1981, Jamart 1992, Journal of Hypertension 1992, McPherson 1974, Murray 1988, Murray 1991a, O'Brien 1981a, Pocock 1987, Simon R 1985, Zelen 1983

5.8 **Report the statistical criteria for stopping the study and indicate whether these criteria were developed before the study began.**
Anonymous 1986, Ashby 1993, Freiman 1978, Geller 1987, Liberati 1986, Pocock 1987, Zelen 1983

5.9 **Identify to whom the results of the interim analyses were reported.**
Geller 1987

COMPARING GROUPS AT MULTIPLE TIME POINTS

5.10 **If groups were compared at multiple time points, specify the statistical procedure used for the comparisons and what adjustments were made for multiple comparisons.**

Chapter 6
Testing for Relationships: Reporting Association and Correlation Analyses

MEASURES AND TESTS OF ASSOCIATION: RELATIONSHIPS BETWEEN TWO CATEGORICAL VARIABLES

6.1 **Describe the association of interest.**

6.2 Identify the variables used in the association and summarize each with descriptive statistics.

6.3 Identify the test of association used.

6.4 Indicate whether the test was one- or two tailed. Justify the use of one-tailed tests.

6.5 State that the assumptions of the test have been met.

6.6 Report the actual *P* value of the test.

6.7 For associations of primary interest, report the value of the test statistic and the degrees of freedom.

CORRELATION ANALYSIS: (LINEAR) RELATIONSHIPS BETWEEN TWO CONTINUOUS VARIABLES

6.8 Describe the relationship of interest.

6.9 Identify the variables used in the comparison and summarize each with descriptive statistics.

6.10 Identify the correlation coefficient used.

6.11 State that the assumptions of the test have been met.

6.12 Report the value of the correlation coefficient.

6.13 Report the actual *P* value of the correlation.

6.14 For primary comparisons, report the (95%) confidence interval for the correlation coefficient, whether or not the coefficient is statistically significant.

6.15 For primary comparisons, include a scatter plot of the data.
Altman 1980b, Altman 1983, Cooper 1989, Feinstein 1976, Journal of Hypertension 1992, Murray 1991b, Schoolman 1968, Yancy 1990

Chapter 7
Analyzing Multiple Variables: I. Reporting Regression Analyses

SIMPLE LINEAR REGRESSION ANALYSIS: PREDICTING ONE CONTINUOUS RESPONSE VARIABLE FROM ONE CONTINUOUS EXPLANATORY VARIABLE

7.1 **Describe the relationship of interest or the purpose of the analysis.**

7.2 **Identify the variables used in the comparison and summarize each with descriptive statistics.**

7.3 **Confirm that the assumptions of simple linear regression analysis were met and state how each was checked.**

7.4 **Report the linear regression equation.**

7.5 **Report the actual *P* value and the (95%) confidence interval for the regression coefficient of the explanatory variable.**
Elenbaas 1983a

7.6 **Report the coefficient of determination (r^2).**
Feinstein 1976, Godfrey 1992

7.7 **Specify whether the model was validated.**
Concato 1993

7.8 **Report how any outlying data were treated in the analysis.**
Concato 1993, Cruess 1991

7.9 **For primary comparisons, include a scatter plot of the data, the regression line, and the (95%) confidence interval (or prediction bands) of the regression line.**
Altman 1980a, Altman 1981, Altman 1983, Feinstein 1976, Godfrey 1992, Gore 1992, Journal of Hypertension 1992, Murray 1991b, O'Brien 1981b, Yancy 1990

7.10 **Name the statistical package or program used in the analysis.**
Concato 1993

MULTIPLE LINEAR REGRESSION ANALYSIS: PREDICTING ONE CONTINUOUS RESPONSE VARIABLE FROM TWO OR MORE EXPLANATORY VARIABLES

7.11 **Describe the relationships of interest or the purpose of the analysis.**

7.12 **Identify the variables used in the comparison and summarize each with descriptive statistics.**

7.13 **Confirm that the assumptions of multiple linear regression analysis have been met and state how each was checked.**

7.14 **Specify how the explanatory variables that appear in the final model were chosen.**
Concato 1993

7.15 **Specify whether all potential explanatory variables were assessed for colinearity (nonindependence).**
Concato 1993

7.16 **Specify whether the explanatory variables were tested for interaction.**
Concato 1993, Kaufman 1986

7.17 **Report the multiple linear regression equation or summarize the equation in a table. Include the number of observations in the analysis and the associated standard error, *P* value, and (95%) confidence interval for each coefficient in the equation.**
Altman 1980b, Altman 1983, Avram 1985, Committee on Data 1977, Concato 1993, Cooper 1989, Feinstein 1976, Godfrey 1992, Lee 1993, Marks 1987, Palmas 1993

7.18 **Give the coefficient of multiple determination (R^2).**
Feinstein 1976, Marks 1987

7.19 **Specify whether the model was validated.**

7.20 **Report how any outlying data were treated in the analysis.**

7.21 **Name the statistical package or program used in the analysis.**
Concato 1993

SIMPLE LOGISTIC REGRESSION ANALYSIS: PREDICTING ONE (BINARY) CATEGORICAL RESPONSE VARIABLE FROM ONE EXPLANATORY VARIABLE

7.22 Describe the relationship of interest or the purpose of the analysis.

7.23 Identify the variables used in the comparison and summarize each with descriptive statistics.

7.24 Confirm that the assumptions of simple logistic regression analysis were met and state how each was checked.

7.25 Summarize the logistic regression equation in a table. Include the number of observations in the analysis, the coefficient of the explanatory variable, and the associated standard error, the odds ratio, the (95%) confidence interval of the odds ratio, and the *P* value.

7.26 Specify whether the model was validated.

7.27 Report how any outlying data were treated in the analysis.

7.28 Name the statistical package or program used in the analysis.
Concato 1993

MULTIPLE LOGISTIC REGRESSION ANALYSIS: PREDICTING ONE (BINARY) CATEGORICAL RESPONSE VARIABLE FROM TWO OR MORE EXPLANATORY VARIABLES

7.29 Describe the relationships of interest or the purpose of the analysis.

7.30 Identify the variables used in the comparison and summarize each with descriptive statistics.

7.31 Confirm that the assumptions of multiple logistic regression analysis have been met and state how each was checked.

7.32 Specify how the explanatory variables that appear in the final model were chosen.

7.33 Specify whether the potential explanatory variables were assessed for correlation or association.

7.34 **Specify whether the independent variables were tested for interaction.**

7.35 **Summarize the multiple logistic regression equation in a table. Include the number of observations in the analysis, the coefficients of the explanatory variables, the associated standard errors, the odds ratios, the 95% confidence intervals for the odds ratios, and the actual *P* values.**
Altman 1980b, Altman 1983, Avram 1985, Committee on Data 1977, Concato 1993, Cooper 1989, Feinstein 1976, Godfrey 1992, Lee 1993, Marks 1987, Palmas 1993

7.36 **Specify whether the model was validated.**

7.37 **Report how any outlying data were treated in the analysis.**

7.38 **Name the statistical package or program used in the analysis.**
Concato 1993

Chapter 8
Analyzing Multiple Variables: II. Reporting Analysis of Variance (ANOVA)

GUIDELINES ADDRESSED IN THE INTRODUCTION

8.1 **Describe the relationships of interest or the purpose of the analysis.**

GUIDELINES ADDRESSED IN THE METHODS

8.2 **Identify the variables used in the comparison and summarize each with descriptive statistics.**

8.3 **Identify the type of analysis used.**

GUIDELINES ADDRESSED IN THE RESULTS

8.4 **Confirm that the assumptions of the analysis have been met.**

8.5 **Report the results of the ANOVA in a table.**

8.6 **Specify whether the explanatory variables were tested for interaction and how these interactions were treated.**

8.7 **Report the actual *P* value for each explanatory variable.**

8.8 **Provide an assessment of the goodness-of-fit of the ANOVA model to the data.**

8.9 **Specify whether the model was validated.**

8.10 **Report how any outlying data were treated in the analysis.**

8.11 **Name the statistical package or program used in the analysis.**
Concato 1993

Chapter 9
Assessing Time-to-an-Event as an Endpoint: Reporting Survival Analyses

9.1 **Describe the relationship to be studied and the reasons for studying it.**

9.2 **Describe the clinical characteristics of the population under study.**
Feinstein 1969

9.3 **Specify the starting time that marks the beginning of the analysis.**
Feinstein 1969

9.4 **Specify the nature of any censored data.**
Feinstein 1969, Mosteller 1980, Zelen 1983

9.5 **Specify the statistical methods used to estimate the survival rate.**

9.6 **Confirm that the requirements of survival analysis have been met.**
Reznick 1989

9.7 **For each group, give the estimated survival rate at appropriate follow-up times, with confidence intervals, and the number of participants at risk of death at each time.**
Altman 1983, Journal of Hypertension 1992, Liberati 1986, Murray 1991b, Simon R 1986

9.8 **When indicated, present the full results in a graph or table.**

9.9 **Specify the statistical methods used to compare two or more survival curves.**

9.10 **When comparing two or more survival curves with hypothesis tests, report the actual *P* value of the comparison.**

9.11 **Report the regression model used to assess the associations between explanatory variables and the survival rate.**

9.12 **Report a measure of risk for each explanatory variable.**

9.13 **Describe the quality of life for survivors.**
Feinstein 1969

Chapter 10 Determining the Presence or Absence of Disease: Reporting the Characteristics of Diagnostic Tests

PURPOSE OF THE TEST

10.1 **Identify the purpose of the test.**
Guyatt 1986, Haynes 1981, Sox 1986, Wald 1989

10.2 **Specify the stage of the condition (disease) for which the test is appropriate.**
Altman 1983, Begg 1987, Begg 1991, Felson 1990, Gehlbach 1993, Guyatt 1986, Haynes 1981, Jaeschke 1994a, Metz 1978, Ransohoff 1978, Reid 1995, Riegelman 1989, Sox 1986

10.3 **Explain the meaning or clinical meaning of a positive test result.**
Arroll 1988, Begg 1991, Gehlbach 1993, Griner 1981, Guyatt 1986, Haynes 1981, Metz 1978, Mills 1993, Riegelman 1989, Sheps 1984, Sox 1986, Wald 1989

CHARACTERISTICS OF THE TEST

10.4 **Describe the biological principle on which the test is based.**

10.5 **Report the validity of the index test that is under study and the reference test to which it was validated.**
Arroll 1988, Begg 1987, Begg 1991, Cooper 1988, Gehlbach 1993, Guyatt 1986, Haynes 1981, Jaeschke 1994a, Metz 1978, Reid 1995, Riegelman 1989, Sheps 1984, Sox 1986

10.6 **Report the reliability of the test.**
Begg 1987, Cooper 1988, Haynes 1981, Jaeschke 1994a, Reid 1995, Riegelman 1989

10.7 **Explain the meaning of equivocal results and how such results were incorporated into the calculation of the test's characteristics.**
Begg 1987, Begg 1988b, Begg 1991, Reid 1995, Simel 1987

10.8 **Report the diagnostic sensitivity and specificity of the test, including the associated (95%) confidence intervals.**
AMA 1994, Arroll 1988, Cooper 1988, Gehlbach 1993, Goodman 1994a, Griner 1981, Guyatt 1986, Haynes 1990, Metz 1978, Reid 1995, Riegelman 1989, Schor 1966, Sheps 1984, Sox 1986, Wald 1989

10.9 **Report the positive and negative likelihood ratios of the test.**
Guyatt 1986, Irwig 1994, Jaeschke 1994a, Sackett 1983, Sox 1986, Wald 1989

10.10 **When a diagnostic test is an essential part of the research, and when its interpretation depends on a cutpoint on a continuum, illustrate its characteristics with a receiver operating characteristics (ROC) curve.**
AMA 1994, Begg 1991, Cooper 1988, Gehlbach 1993, Goodman 1994a, Griner 1981, Guyatt 1986, Haynes 1990, Metz 1978

10.11 **When a test is an essential part of the research, report the number and proportion of patients with and without the disease who were tested to determine the specificity and sensitivity.**
Haynes 1981, Riegelman 1989, Schor 1966

CLINICAL APPLICATION OF THE TEST

10.12 **Describe how the test is to be administered.**
Arroll 1988, Haynes 1981, Jaeschke 1994a, Sheps 1984

10.13 **Report the positive and negative predictive values of the test, as well as the prevalence of the disease associated with these values.**
Altman 1980c, Altman 1982, Altman 1983, AMA 1994, Arroll 1988, Cooper 1988, Diamond (for examples), Gehlbach 1993, Goodman 1994a, Griner 1981, Guyatt 1986, Haynes 1990, Jaeschke 1994b, Riegelman 1989, Sheps 1984, Stoto 1990, Wald 1989

10.14 **When reporting the use of two or more diagnostic tests in combination, indicate the order in which the tests were given, the characteristics of each, and the contribution of each test to the final result.**
Begg 1987, Haynes 1981, Riegelman 1989, Wald 1989

CONSIDERATIONS IN ADOPTING THE TEST

10.15 **Present other pertinent information about the test.**
Begg 1987, Guyatt 1986, Nierenberg 1988

10.16 **Describe the human, financial, and physical resources necessary to offer the test in a given setting.**

10.17 **Describe the medical costs and benefits of adopting the test.**
Begg 1987, Begg 1988b, Guyatt 1986, Wald 1989

10.18 **Describe the financial costs and benefits of adopting the test.**
Begg 1991, Guyatt 1986, Neuhauser 1975, Wald 1989

10.19 **Describe how the test compares with similar tests.**
Begg 1987, Guyatt 1986, Wald 1989

Chapter 11
Combining the Results of Several Studies: Reporting the Results of Meta-Analyses

GUIDELINES ADDRESSED IN THE INTRODUCTION

11.1 **State the purpose of the study. Identify the relationship that was studied and the reasons for studying it.**
AMA 1994, Dickersin 1992, Guyatt 1995, Henry 1992, Light 1984, Simes 1990, Wilson 1992

11.2 **Describe the population(s) studied and to which the results are to be generalized.**
AMA 1994, Simes 1990

GUIDELINES ADDRESSED IN THE METHODS

11.3 **State whether the research was guided by a written protocol.**
Andersen 1992, Wilson 1992

11.4 **Provide operational definitions for the explanatory and response variables (the outcomes or endpoints).**
Dickersin 1992, Jones 1992, Light 1984, Simes 1990, Wilson 1992

11.5 **Report the minimum difference in the response variable that is considered to be clinically important.**
Andersen 1992

11.6 **Report the period of time covered by the literature search.**
AMA 1994

11.7 **Describe in detail the information sources and search strategies used to find the studies to be analyzed.**
AMA 1994, Andersen 1992, Dickersin 1992, Felson 1992, Guyatt 1995, Henry 1992, Jones 1992, Kassirer 1992, Simes 1990, Wilson 1992

11.8 **State the measures taken to reduce and identify publication bias.**
Dickersin 1990, Dickersin 1992, Felson 1992, Jones 1992, Light 1984, Moher 1995, Wilson 1992

11.9 **Report the criteria used for including or excluding studies from the meta-analysis.**
AMA 1994, Andersen 1992, Dickersin 1992, Felson 1992, Guyatt 1995, Henry 1992, Jones 1992, Kassirer 1992, Light 1984, Simes 1990, West 1993, Wilson 1992

11.10 **Describe the criteria used in extracting the data from the studies. Include a measure of inter-extracter reliability to establish the consistency of extraction.**
AMA 1994, Dickersin 1992, Felson 1992, Henry 1992, Jones 1992, Kassirer 1992, Wilson 1992

11.11 **Describe the statistical analyses used to analyze the data.**
Dickersin 1992, Jones 1992, Kassirer 1992, Simes 1990

GUIDELINES ADDRESSED IN THE RESULTS

11.12 **Provide a summary measure, with a confidence interval, of the estimated size and direction of the effect of the treatment.**
AMA 1994, Kassirer 1992, Wilson 1992

11.13 **Summarize the results of the individual studies and of the meta-analysis in a graph or a table.**
Dickersin 1992, Simes 1990, Wilson 1992

11.14 **State the statistical power of the analysis.**
Andersen 1992

11.15 **Provide an assessment of the quality of each study included in the analysis.**
Dickersin 1992, Felson 1992, Guyatt 1995, Henry 1992, Jones 1992, Moher 1995, West 1993, Wilson 1992

11.16 **List the studies excluded from the meta-analysis and the reason for their exclusion.**
Andersen 1992

11.17 **Test important choices and assumptions with sensitivity analysis to determine whether their impact on the result is warranted.**
AMA 1994, Andersen 1992, Jones 1992, Simes 1990, Wilson 1992

GUIDELINES ADDRESSED IN THE DISCUSSION

11.18 **Discuss the variability (or "heterogeneity") of the results of the individual trials.**
AMA 1994, Andersen 1992, Dickersin 1992, Guyatt 1995, Henry 1992, Kassirer 1992, Light 1984, Moher 1995, Simes 1990, Wilson 1992

11.19 **Discuss the populations represented in the meta-analysis and the generalizability of the results of the meta-analysis to other populations.**
Andersen 1992, Dickersin 1992, Kassirer 1992, Wilson 1992

11.20 **Discuss the implications of the results.**
AMA 1994, Guyatt 1995, Wilson 1992

Chapter 12
Weighing the Costs and Consequences of Treatment: Reporting the Results of Economic Evaluations

GUIDELINES ADDRESSED IN THE INTRODUCTION

12.1 **State the purpose of the study. Identify the treatments that were studied and the reasons for studying them.**
Eddy 1992, Hillman 1995, Lee 1991, Maynard 1990, Stoddart 1984b, Warner 1989

12.2 **State the type of economic evaluation undertaken.**
Adams 1992, Hall 1990, Kupersmith 1994, Lee 1991, Zitter 1994

12.3 **State the perspective of the designers of the evaluation.**
Adams 1992, Evans 1990b, Ganiats 1991, Hall 1990, Hillman 1991, Hillman 1995, Kupersmith 1994, Laupacis 1992, Maynard 1990, Phelps 1991, Stoddart 1984b, Udvarhelyi 1992, Warner 1989, Weinstein 1977, Weinstein 1990, Zitter 1994

12.4 **Identify who funded the study and describe the relationship between the researchers and the funding agent.**
Hillman 1991, Hillman 1995

GUIDELINES ADDRESSED IN THE METHODS

12.5 **Describe the treatments being compared and give the reasons for comparing them.**
Adams 1992, Detsky 1990, Ganiats 1991, Hall 1990, Hillman 1991, Hillman 1995, Kupersmith 1994, Lee 1991, Mason 1993, Maynard 1990, Stoddart 1984b, Warner 1989

12.6 **Verify the clinical effectiveness of each treatment being evaluated.**
Detsky 1990, Hall 1990, Mason 1993, Stoddart 1984a, Stoddart 1984b

12.7 **Describe any pilot studies undertaken in preparation for the primary study.**
Hillman 1991, Hillman 1995

12.8 **State whether the study was conducted according to a written protocol.**
Hillman 1991, Hillman 1995

12.9 **Identify the "time horizon" over which the costs and benefits of the treatments are expected to accrue.**
Detsky 1990, Hall 1990, Hillman 1995, Kupersmith 1994, Maynard 1990

12.10 **Identify the key assumptions and value judgments used in the evaluation.**
Adams 1992, Hillman 1991, Hillman 1995, Kassirer 1994, Kupersmith 1994, Stoddart 1984b, Udvarhelyi 1992

12.11 **Identify the types of costs included in the evaluation (and important costs that were not included) and state how these costs were determined.**
Adams 1992, Bulpitt 1990, Ganiats 1991, Hall 1990, Hillman 1991, Hillman 1995, Laupacis 1992, Lee 1991, Mason 1993, Maynard 1990, Stoddart 1984b, Udvarhelyi 1992, Warner 1989, Weinstein 1977

12.12 **Identify the outcomes (benefits) of the treatments being compared and how these outcomes were determined.**
Adams 1992, Eddy 1992, Ganiats 1991, Hall 1990, Kaplan 1993, Laupacis 1992, Lee 1991, Maynard 1990, Nord 1992, Stoddart 1984a, Udvarhelyi 1992, Warner 1989

12.13 **Report any mathematical model used to compare costs and outcomes.**
Kassirer 1994, Kupersmith 1994

12.14 **Describe the sources of data and the methods of data collection.**
Hillman 1991, Hillman 1995, Kupersmith 1994, Stoddart 1984b

GUIDELINES ADDRESSED IN THE RESULTS

12.15 **Report the individual and aggregate costs for each treatment. Establish that the costs were identified fully, measured well, and valued appropriately.**
Adams 1992, Bulpitt 1990, Evans 1990b, Ganiats 1991, Hillman 1995, Kupersmith 1994, Laupacis 1992b, Mason 1993, Maynard 1990, Stoddart 1984b, Udvarhelyi 1992, Weinstein 1990

12.16 **Report the individual and aggregate outcomes for each treatment. Establish that the outcomes were identified fully, measured well, and valued appropriately.**
Adams 1992, Ganiats 1991, Hall 1990, Hillman 1995, Kupersmith 1994, Laupacis 1992b, Maynard 1990, Phelps 1991, Stoddart 1984b, Udvarhelyi 1992

12.17 **Report both average and incremental cost-outcome ratios for each treatment.**
Adams 1992, Detsky 1990, Ganiats 1991, Hall 1990, Hillman 1995, Laupacis 1992, Lee 1991, Maynard 1990, Phelps 1991, Stoddart 1984b, Udvarhelyi 1992, Warner 1989, Weinstein 1977, Weinstein 1990

12.18 **Provide a measure of "therapeutic effort to clinical yield" (an effort-to-yield ratio) for each treatment.**
AMA 1994, Brett 1989, Guyatt 1995, Laupacis 1988, Laupacis 1992b, Naylor 1992

12.19 **State the method of discounting used to adjust for costs and benefits that accrue during different time periods.**
Adams 1992, Bulpitt 1990, Detsky 1990, Evans 1990a, Ganiats 1991, Hall 1990, Hillman 1995, Kupersmith 1994, Laupacis 1992, Lee 1991, Mason 1993, Maynard 1990, Stoddart 1984b, Udvarhelyi 1992, Warner 1989, Weinstein 1977, Weinstein 1990

12.20 **Test important choices and assumptions with sensitivity analysis to determine their impacts on the result.**
Adams 1992, Detsky 1990, Eddy 1992, Ganiats 1991, Hillman 1991, Hillman 1995, Kupersmith 1994, Laupacis 1992, Lee 1991, Mason 1993, Maynard 1990, Stoddart 1984b, Stoto 1990, Udvarhelyi 1992, Warner 1989, Weinstein 1977

GUIDELINES ADDRESSED IN THE DISCUSSION

12.21 **Discuss the generalizability of the results.**
Ganiats 1991, Hillman 1995, Stoddart 1984b, Warner 1989

12.22 **Describe the distributional effects of the alternative treatments, including the types and number of people who stand to benefit and to lose.**
Adams 1992, Detsky 1990, Kupersmith 1994, Laupacis 1992, Lee 1991, Stoddart 1984b

12.23 **Discuss the feasibility of implementing the treatment.**
Bulpitt 1990, Detsky 1990, Ganiats 1991, Stoddart 1984b, Warner 1989

12.24 **Discuss the limitations of the study.**
Adams 1992

Chapter 13
Considering Medical Risks and Patient Preferences: Reporting Decision Analyses and Clinical Practice Guidelines

GUIDELINES ADDRESSED IN THE INTRODUCTION

13.1 **State the question under study. Specify the diagnosis and the patient population of interest and, if appropriate, the providers and the setting involved and the time horizon over which the analysis is to be applied.**
AMA 1994, Crane 1991, Hayward 1993a, Hayward 1993b, Hayward 1995, Oxman 1994, Richardson 1995, Sonenberg 1993, Wasson 1996, Wilson 1995

13.2 **Indicate why the analysis was undertaken.**
Wilson 1995

13.3 **State the perspective from which the analysis was conducted.**
Goel 1992, Hayward 1993a, Kassirer 1987, Richardson 1995

13.4 **Identify the persons, groups, or both, who developed, funded, or have endorsed the practice guideline.**
AMA 1994, Hayward 1993a, Oxman 1994

GUIDELINES ADDRESSED IN THE METHODS

13.5 **Identify the decisions and implications under study: the starting point, branching points, and outcomes that were considered in the analysis.**
AMA 1994, Crane 1991, Goel 1992, Hayward 1993a, Hayward 1993b, Hayward 1995, Oxman 1994, Wasson 1996

13.6 **Describe the criteria used to include, exclude, combine, or otherwise evaluate the data used in the analysis.**
AMA 1994, Goel 1992, Hayward 1993a, Hayward 1995, Oxman 1994

13.7 **Describe the methods used to identify and collect the data on which the analysis is based.**
Crane 1991, Hayward 1993a, Hayward 1993b, Hayward 1995, Oxman 1994

13.8 **State how utilities (patient values or preferences) for different alternatives or outcomes were determined.**
Goel 1992, Hayward 1993a, Hayward 1993b, Hayward 1995, Kaplan 1993, Oxman 1994, Testa 1996

13.9 **Identify the statistical techniques and the associated statistical package or program used in the analysis.**
Kassirer 1987, Pauker 1987, Wasson 1996

13.10 **Identify the major assumptions and areas of potency, variability, and uncertainty in the analysis.**
Eddy 1992, Hayward 1993a

GUIDELINES ADDRESSED IN THE RESULTS

13.11 **Report the estimated probability for each alternative of each chance node, as well as the misclassification rate at each alternative.**
Goel 1992, Hayward 1993b, Hayward 1995, Oxman 1994, Swartz 1973

13.12 **Report the estimated probability of each alternative of each decision node.**
Goel 1992, Hayward 1993b, Hayward 1995, Oxman 1994, Swartz 1973

13.13 **Report the utility measure for each outcome and for each decision node, if applicable.**
Eddy 1990b, Goel 1992, Hayward 1995, Pauker 1987, Richardson 1995

13.14 **When possible and appropriate, illustrate the analysis with a decision tree.**
Goel 1992, Pauker 1987, Richardson 1995, Swartz 1973

13.15 **Report any sensitivity analyses used to test the assumptions.**
Crane 1991, Goel 1992, Hayward 1993a, Hayward 1995, Kassirer 1987, Wilson 1995

GUIDELINES ADDRESSED IN THE DISCUSSION

13.16 **State the recommendations and the conditions under which the alternatives at each decision node are and are not appropriate.**
AMA 1994, Hayward 1995, Oxman 1994

13.17 **Indicate the strength of the recommendations and the flexibility with which the decision analysis or practice guideline can be applied.**
AMA 1994, Eddy 1990, Ganiats 1993, Guyatt 1995, Hayward 1993b, Hayward 1995, Walker 1994, Wilson 1995

13.18 **Identify any dissenting opinions or disagreements among the guideline developers.**
Oxman 1994

13.19 **Describe any evaluation or validation process to which the decision analysis or practice guideline was subjected.**
Basinski 1992, Hayward 1993a, Hayward 1993b, Hayward 1995, Oxman 1994, Walker 1994, Wasson 1996, Wilson 1995

13.20 **Indicate the similarities and differences of the decision analysis or practice guideline to other analyses or guidelines covering similar content areas.**
AMA 1994

13.21 **Describe the expected benefits, problems, and costs that may affect patients if the recommendations are implemented.**
Hayward 1993a, Wasson 1996

13.22 **Give the dates of the most recent evidence considered in the analysis.**
AMA 1994, Hayward 1993a, Hayward 1995

13.23 **Identify in-progress or recent developments that may be relevant to the analysis but that were not included in it.**
AMA 1994, Hayward 1993a, Hayward 1995

13.24 **If appropriate, specify the anticipated "shelf life" of the analysis and when or under what circumstances the recommendations should be reviewed.**
AMA 1994, Walker 1994

13.25 **Identify any clinical or administrative changes necessary to implement the recommendations and any social or behavioral factors that may nullify their effectiveness.**
Basinski 1992, Walker 1994, Wasson 1996

Chapter 14
Considering "Prior Probabilities": Reporting Bayesian Statistical Analyses

14.1 **Report the pre-trial probabilities and specify how they were determined.**
Lewis 1993

14.2 **Report the post-trial probabilities and their probability intervals.**
Hughes 1993, Lewis 1993

14.3 **Interpret the post-trial probabilities.**
Lewis 1993

Chapter 15
From Research Results To Decision-Making: Reporting Outcomes in Clinically Applicable Terms

15.1 **Report the "clinical conclusions" of the research.**

15.2 **When applicable, make the patient the unit of reporting.**
Felson 1990, Moskowitz 1983

15.3 **Report confidence intervals for primary outcomes.**
See references for Guideline 3.1

15.4 **When applicable, include effort-to-yield measures.**
AMA 1994, Brett 1989, Guyatt 1995, Laupacis 1988, Laupacis 1992b, Naylor 1992

15.5 **When applicable, describe the quality of life after treatment.**
Feinstein 1969, Redelmeier 1993

15.6 **When applicable, use a positive frame of reference.**
Kahneman 1982

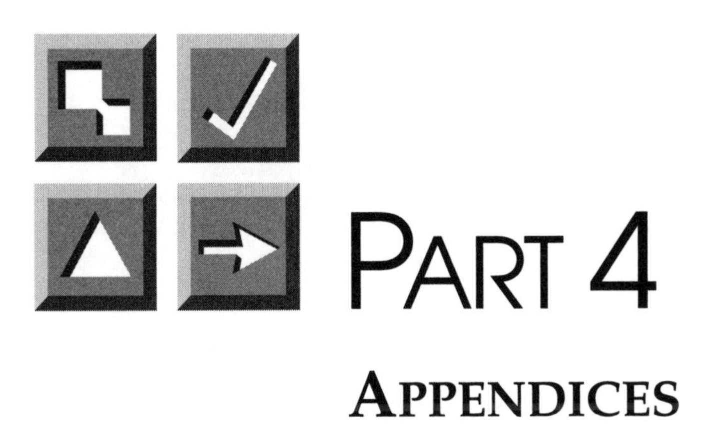

PART 4

APPENDICES

Appendix 1

Checklists For Reporting Clinical Trials

Shortly before this book went into production, *JAMA* published a special communication titled "Improving the Quality of Reporting of Randomized Controlled Trials: The CONSORT Statement" (1). The CONSORT (*CON*solidated *S*tandards *O*f *R*eporting *T*rials) Statement is a checklist for reporting randomized controlled clinical trials and is a synthesis of guidelines proposed by the Asilomar Working Group on Recommendations for Reporting Clinical Trials in the Biomedical Literature (2,3) and the SORT (*S*tandards *O*f *R*eporting *T*rials) group (4). The checklist is similar to others proposed in the literature over the past 30 years (5–40).

However, the CONSORT checklist differs from others in that it is intended to be used for the "structured reporting" of research studies. That is, the items on the checklist are to appear as subheadings in the published article, which will prevent the omission of important information and will aid readers in evaluating the study.

As of January 1997, *JAMA* will require authors submitting manuscripts for publication to include all the information on the CONSORT checklist and to indicate on the checklist the manuscript page number on which the guideline is addressed (an idea first proposed by Douglas Altman in 1990) (41). The checklist will be sent to reviewers but will not be published. Other journals may also adopt this requirement.

The CONSORT checklist uses subheadings different than those we propose here and fewer "descriptors," or what we have called guidelines. These subheadings and descriptors are reprinted in Table A1.1, along with our guideline numbers in parentheses that correspond to each descriptor. Our suggested subheadings and guidelines are also given for comparison.

TABLE A1.1 Relationship between the CONSORT Statement* Checklist and "Reporting Research Designs and Activities," Chapter 1 of *How To Report Statistics in Medicine*.† (Numbers in parentheses are the guideline numbers in this book.)

Headings, Subheadings, and Descriptors from the CONSORT Statement

Title: Identify the study as a randomized trial
Abstract: Use a structured format
Introduction:

- State prospectively defined hypothesis, clinical objectives, and planned subgroup or covariate analyses (1.1, 1.2)

Methods:

Protocol: Describe

- Planned study population, together with inclusion/exclusion criteria (1.5, 1.16)
- Planned interventions and their timing (1.10)
- Primary and secondary outcome measure(s) and the minimum important difference(s); indicate how the target sample size was projected (1.6, 1.7, 1.14)
- Rationale and methods for statistical analyses, detailing main comparative analyses and whether they were completed on an intention-to-treat basis (1.25, 1.26)
- Prospectively designed stopping rules (if warranted) (1.27)

Assignment: Describe

- Unit of random assignment (e.g., individual, cluster geographic) (1.4)
- Method used to generate the allocation schedule (1.18)
- Method of allocation concealment and timing of assignment (1.18)
- Method used to separate the generator from the executor of assignment (1.18)

Masking (Blinding):

- Describe mechanism (e.g., capsules, tablets); similarity of treatment characteristics (e.g., appearance, taste); allocation schedule control (location of code during trial and when broken); and evidence for successful blinding among participants, person doing the intervention, outcome assessors, and data analysts (1.18, 1.19, 1.20, 1.43)

Results:

Participant Flow and Follow-up:

- Provide a trial profile (a figure) summarizing participant flow, numbers and timing of random assignment, interventions, and measurements for each randomly assigned group (1.33)

Analysis:

- State estimated effect of intervention on primary and secondary outcomes measures, including a point estimate and measure of precision (confidence interval) (1.45, 1.47)
- State results in absolute numbers when feasible (e.g., 10/20, not 50%) (1.46)
- Present summary data and appropriate descriptive and inferential statistics in sufficient detail to permit alternative analyses and replication (1.50)
- Describe prognostic variables by treatment group and any attempt to adjust for them (1.45, 1.51)
- Describe protocol deviations from the study as planned, together with the reasons (1.52)

Comment:

- State specific interpretation of the study findings, including sources of bias and imprecision (internal validity) and discussion of external validity, including appropriate quantitative measures when possible (1.60, 1.61)
- State general interpretations of the data in light of the totality of the available evidence (1.59)

Headings, Subheadings, and Guidelines from "Reporting Research Designs and Activities"

Introduction (1.1 to 1.3)

Materials and Methods:

- **The Study Focus** (1.4 to 1.8)
- **The Study as Planned** (1.9 to 1.24)
- **Statistical Methods** (1.25 to 1.31)

Results:

- **The Study as Conducted** (1.32 to 1.44)
- **Study Outcomes** (1.45 to 1.56)
- **Discussion (Comment)** (1.57 to 1.60)
- **Limitations of the Study** (1.61)
- **Conclusions** (1.62, 1.63)

---

* Begg C, Cho M, Eastwood S, Horton R, Moher D, Oklin I, et al. Improving the quality of reporting of randomized controlled trials: The CONSORT Statement. JAMA. 1996;276(8):637-9. Copyright 1996, American Medical Association.

† Lang T, Secic M. How To Report Statistics in Medicine: Annotated Guidelines for Authors, Editors, and Reviewers. Philadelphia: American College of Physicians, 1997.

REFERENCES

1. **Begg C, Cho M, Eastwood S, Horton R, Moher D, Olkin I, et al.** Improving the quality of reporting of randomized controlled trials: The CONSORT Statement. JAMA 1996;276: 637-9.
2. **Working Group on Recommendations for Reporting Clinical Trials in the Biomedical Literature.** Call for comments on a proposal to improve reporting clinical trials in the biomedical literature: a position paper. Ann Intern Med. 1994;121:894-5.
3. **The Asilomar Working Group on Recommendations for Reporting Clinical Trials in the Biomedical Literature.** Checklist of information for inclusion in reports of clinical trials. Ann Intern Med. 1996;124(8): 741-3.
4. **The Standards of Reporting Trials Group.** A proposal for structured reporting of randomized controlled trials. JAMA. 1994;272: 1926-31. Erratum: JAMA 1995; 273:776.
5. **Altman DG, Gore SM, Gardner MJ, Pocock SJ.** Statistical guidelines for contributors to medical journals. Br Med J. 1983;286: 1489-93.
6. **Anonymous.** Methodologic guidelines for reports of clinical trials [Editorial]. Am J Clin Oncol. 1986;9:276.
7. **Bailar JC, Mosteller F.** Guidelines for statistical reporting in articles for medical journals. Ann Intern Med. 1988;108:266-73.
8. **Berry G.** Statistical guidelines and statistical guidance. Med J Australia. 1987;146:408-9.
9. **Bland JM, Jones DR, Bennett S, Cook DG, Haines AP, MacFarlane AJ.** Is the clinical trial evidence about new drugs statistically adequate? Br J Clin Pharmacol. 1985;19:155-60.
10. **Chalmers TC, Smith H, Blackburn B, Silverman B, Schroeder B, Reitman D, et al.** A method for assessing the quality of a randomized control trial. Control Clin Trials. 1981; 2:31-49.
11. **Cho MK, Bero LA.** Instruments for assessing the quality of drug studies published in the medical literature. JAMA. 1994;272:101-4.
12. **Christensen E, Juhl E, Tygstrup N.** Treatment of duodenal ulcer. Randomized clinical trials of a decade (1965 to 1974). Gastroenterology. 1977;73:1170-8.

13. **DerSimonian R, Charette LJ, McPeek B, Mosteller F.** Reporting on methods in clinical trials. N Engl J Med. 1982;306(22):1332-7.
14. **Elenbaas JK, Cuddy PG, Elenbaas RM.** Evaluating the medical literature, part III: results and discussion. Ann Emerg Med. 1983; 12:679-86.
15. **Gardner MJ, Altman DG, Jones DR, Machin D.** Is the statistical assessment of papers submitted to the British Medical Journal effective? Br Med J. 1983;286:1485-8.
16. **Gardner MJ, Machin D, Campbell MJ.** Use of checklists in assessing the statistical content of medical studies. Br Med J. 1986;292: 810-2.
17. **Goodman SN, Berlin J, Fletcher SW, Fletcher RH.** Manuscript quality before and after peer review and editing at Annals of Internal Medicine. Ann Intern Med. 1994; 121:11-21.
18. **Gore SM, Jones G, Thompson SG.** The Lancet's statistical review process: areas for improvement by authors. Lancet. 1992;340: 100-2.
19. **Gotzsche PC.** Methodology and overt and hidden bias in reports of 196 double-blind trials of nonsteroidal antiinflammatory drugs in rheumatoid arthritis. Control Clin Trials. 1989; 10:31-56.
20. **Grant A.** Reporting controlled trials. Br J Obstet Gynecol. 1989;96:397-400.
21. **Grimes DA, Schulz KF.** Randomized controlled trials of home uterine activity monitoring: a review and critique. Obstet Gynecol. 1992;79:137-42.
22. **Guyatt GH, Sackett DL, Cook DJ.** Users' guide to the medical literature. II. How to use an article about therapy or prevention. A. Are the results of the study valid? JAMA. 1993;270:2598-601.
23. **Haynes RB, Mulrow C, Huth E, Altman DG, Gardner MJ.** More informative abstracts revisited. Ann Intern Med. 1990;113:69-76.
24. **Horwitz RI, Feinstein AR.** Methodologic standards and contradictory results in case-control research. Am J Med. 1979;66:556-64.
25. **Koes BW, Bouter LM, van der Heijden G JMG.** Methodological quality of randomized clinical trials on treatment efficacy in low back pain. Spine. 1995;20:228-35.
26. **Liberati A, Himel HN, Chalmers TC.** A quality assessment of randomized control trials of primary treatment of breast cancer. J Clin Oncol. 1986; 4:942-51.
27. **Lionel NDW, Herxheimer A.** Assessing reports of therapeutic trials. Br Med J. 1970;3: 637-40.
28. **Mahon WA, Daniel EE.** A method for the assessment of reports of drug trials. Can Med Assoc J. 1964;90:565-9.
29. **Marks RG, Dawson-Saunders EK, Bailar JC, Dan BB, Verran JA.** Interactions between statisticians and biomedical journal editors. Stat Med. 1988;7:1003-11.
30. **Meinert CL, Tonascia S, Higgins K.** Content of reports on clinical trials: a critical review. Control Clin Trials. 1984;5:328-47.
31. **Morris RW.** A statistical study of papers in the Journal of Bone and Joint Surgery [Br] 1984. J Bone Joint Surg [Br]. 1988;70-B:242-6.
32. **Murray GD.** Statistical guidelines for the British Journal of Surgery. Br J Surg. 1991;78: 782-4.
33. **Raskob GE, Lofthouse RN, Hull RD.** Methodological guidelines for clinical trials evaluating new therapeutic approaches in bone and joint surgery. J Bone Joint Surg. 1985;67-A:1294-7.
34. **Rochon PA, Gurwitz JH, Cheung MC, Hayes JA, Chalmers TC.** Evaluating the quality of articles published in journal supplements compared with the quality of those published in the parent journal. JAMA 1994;272:108-13.
35. **Sonis J, Joines J.** The quality of clinical trials published in the Journal of Family Practice, 1974-1991. J Fam Pract. 1994;39:225-35.
36. **Squires BP.** Statistics in biomedical manuscripts: what editors want from authors and peer reviewers. Can Med Assoc J. 1990;142: 213-4.
37. **Tyson JE, Furzan JA, Reisch JS, Mize SG.** An evaluation of the quality of therapeutic studies in perinatal medicine. J Pediatrics. 1983;102:10-3.
38. **Vrbos LA, Lorenz MA, Peabody EH, McGregor M.** Clinical methodologies and incidence of appropriate statistical testing in orthopaedic spine literature: are statistics misleading? Spine. 1993;18(8):1021-9.

39. **White SJ.** Statistical errors in papers in the British Journal of Psychiatry. Br J Psychiatr. 1979;135:336-42.

40. **Zelen M.** Guidelines for publishing papers on cancer clinical trials: responsibilities of editors and authors. J Clin Oncol. 1983;1: 164-9.

41. **Altman DG, Dore CJ.** Randomisation and baseline comparisons in clinical trials. Lancet. 1990;335:149-53.

Appendix 2

Mathematical Symbols and Notation

Mathematical symbols are usually presented in italic type. Greek letters usually refer to characteristics of a population, and Roman letters usually refer to characteristics of a sample. Boldface terms in this appendix are described in Part 2: Guide to Statistical Terms and Tests.

α Greek letter **alpha**. *See* **alpha level** and **alpha error**

β Greek letter **beta**. *See* **beta** and **power, statistical (1 – β)**

F statistic *See* ***F* test** and **ANOVA**

H_0 **Null hypothesis** (pronounced *H not*)

H_a, H_1 **Alternative hypothesis**

P **Probability**

r **Pearson's product-moment correlation coefficient**

ρ **Spearman's rho,** a **correlation coefficient**

r^2 **Coefficient of determination**

σ Greek letter **sigma.** Standard deviation (SD) of a distribution of values for a characteristic of a *population.*

s **Standard deviation** of a distribution of values for a characteristic of a *sample* of a population

t statistic *See* **Student's *t* test**

τ **Kendall's tau,** a **correlation coefficient**

μ Greek letter **mu.** The mean value of a distribution of values for a characteristic of a population; micro (10^{-6}).

U statistic *See* **Wilcoxon's rank-sum test**

u (Lower-case letter u.) In draft manuscripts, often used in place of the Greek letter mu (μ), a character not available in some word-processing programs

χ^2 **Chi-square,** after the Greek letter chi (pronounced *kigh*). *See* **chi-square test.**

$\overline{x}$ The mean value of a distribution of values for a characteristic of a *sample* of a population (pronounced *x-bar*). Should be presented with an overbar.

Appendix 3

Rules for Presenting Numbers in Text

The rules listed here are abbreviated from the *Scientific Style and Format: The CBE Manual for Authors, Editors, and Publishers,* 6th edition, (Cambridge: Cambridge University Press; 1994), and the *AMA Manual of Style, 8th edition.* (Chicago: American Medical Association; 1989). These two styles are identical, except where indicated.

NUMBERS AS WORDS OR NUMERALS

AMA Manual of Style

Spell out the numbers one through nine and use numerals for numbers 10 and up, except:

- When reporting units of measurement, times, and dates: 2 mL, not two mL; 1996, not nineteen hundred ninety-six.
- When beginning a sentence: Fifteen days ago, not 15 days ago.
- When comparing similar quantities: the sample included 15 people with type A blood, 12 with type B, and 3 with type AB.
- When reporting consecutive numerical expressions in which two classes of numbers must be differentiated: five, 72-kg men, not 5, 72-kg men.
- When reporting large numbers in general expressions: a hundred; several thousand.

CBE Style Manual

All numbers should be expressed as numerals except:

- When beginning a sentence.
- When reporting consecutive numerical expressions in which two classes of numbers must be differentiated (see above).
- When reporting large numbers in general expressions (see above).

ORDINAL NUMBERS

AMA Manual of Style

Spell out ordinal numbers one through nine and use numerals for ordinals 10 and higher: first, not 1st; 15th, not fifteenth.

CBE Style Manual

All ordinal numbers should be expressed as numerals, even in headings: 2nd, not second; The 4th Annual Congress.

SPACING OF UNITS OF MEASUREMENT

- Use the percent sign, even in the text, without a space between the numeral and the sign: 34%.
- Space between the numeral and its unit of measurement: 136 mm Hg.

DECIMALS

AMA Manual of Style

Use a zero before the decimal (for example, 0.24 ng/mL) except:

- When reporting *P* values or correlation coefficients, where the maximum value of 1 is almost never obtained: $P = .04$; $r = .45$.

CBE Style Manual

Use a zero before all decimals, including *P* values and correlation coefficients: $P = 0.04$; $r = 0.45$.

REPORTING RANGES OF NUMBERS

Use the term *to* or *through*—and never a hyphen—to report a range of numbers: 2 to 5 mL, not 2-5 mL.

- However, a hyphen is used to indicate a range of pages in a reference citation: Ann Intern Med 1996;2:13-9.
- Units need be presented only at the end of the range: 200 to 240 mg/dL.
- Ranges involving percentages should include the percent sign with both numbers: 200% to 240%.
- Do not omit duplicate digits when reporting ranges: from 925 to 988 patients, not 925 to 88 patients.
- However, duplicate digits can be omitted in the ending page numbers of a reference citation: Ann Intern Med. 1996;2:13-9.

RATES, PROPORTIONS, AND FRACTIONS

Use the virgule (/) for proportions and rates and a colon (:) for ratios:

- About 1/3 of the samples.
- The infection rate averaged 50/100 000 people.
- The ratio of men to women was 3:4.5.

Spell out common fractions when they modify nouns: half the cases; a two-thirds majority.

Appendix 4

Spelling of Statistical Terms and Tests

The spelling of statistical tests does not appear to be standardized. Some spellings are more common than others, but many do not conform to the conventional rules of punctuation, particularly those that involve possessives and hyphens.

We have used the possessive form when only a single name is associated with a test (for example, Spearman's rank-order correlation coefficient) and the nominative form (preceded by an article) when two or more names are associated (for example, the Kruskal-Wallis test). Hyphens are used according to the usual rule: to connect double modifiers. Proper nouns are capitalized, the rest of the terms in the name generally are not.

Differences between our suggested spellings and the perhaps more common spellings found in the statistical literature are, in fact, trivial. Throughout this book, we have followed the rules outlined above and use the spellings given below.

analysis of variance
Bonferroni's correction
Breslow's generalized Wilcoxon test
the chi-square test
the Cochran-Mantel-Haenszel test
the Cox-Mantel test
Duncan's multiple-range procedure
Dunn's procedure
Dunnett's procedure
the *F* test
Fisher's exact test
Fisher's least-significant-difference method
Friedman's test
Hartley's test
the Kaplan-Meier method
Kendall's rank-correlation coefficient
the Kolmogorov-Smirnov test
the Kruskal-Wallis test
the log-rank test
the Mann-Whitney *U* test
the Mantel-Haenszel test
McNemar's test
Neuman-Keuls procedure
Pearson's product-moment correlation coefficient
the sign test
Scheffe's procedure
Spearman's rank-order correlation coefficient
Student-Neuman-Keuls procedure
Student's *t* test
Tukey's procedure
Wilcoxon's rank-sum test
Wilcoxon's signed-rank test
Yates' correction for continuity

Bibliography

(The letters a, b, c, d after the years are for reference to Part 3 only. References with these letters are in chronological rather than in alphabetical order.)

Abrams K, Ashby D, Errington D. Simple Bayesian analysis in clinical trials: a tutorial. Control Clin Trials. 1994;15(5):349-59.

Abramson NS, Kelsey SF, Safar P, Sutton-Tyrrell KS. Simpson's paradox and clinical trials: what you find is not necessarily what you prove. Ann Emerg Med. 1992;21(12): 1480-2.

Ad Hoc Working Group for Critical Appraisal of the Medical Literature. A proposal for more informative abstracts of clinical articles. Ann Intern Med. 1987;106(4):598-604.

Adams ME, McCall NT, Gray DT, Orza MJ, Chalmers TC. Economic analysis in randomized control trials. Med Care. 1992;30(3): 231-43.

Altman DG. Statistics and ethics in medical research. VI—Presentation of results. BMJ. 1980a;281(6254):1542-4.

Altman DG. Statistics and ethics in medical research. VII—Interpreting results. BMJ. 1980b;281(6255):1612-4.

Altman DG. Statistics and ethics in medical research. VIII—Improving the quality of statistics in medical journals. BMJ. 1981; 282 (6257):44-6.

Altman DG. Statistics in medical journals. Stat Med. 1982;(1):59-71.

Altman DG, Gore SM, Gardner MJ, Pocock SJ. Statistical guidelines for contributors to medical journals. BMJ. 1983a;286(6376):1489-93.

Altman DG, Bland JM. Measurement in medicine: the analysis of method comparison studies. Statistician. 1983b;32:307-17.

Altman DG, Dore CJ. Randomisation and baseline comparisons in clinical trials. Lancet.1990; 335(8682):149-53.

Altman DG. Statistics in medical journals: developments in the 1980s. Stat Med. 1991a;10(12): 1897-913.

Altman DG, Bland JM. Improving doctors' understanding of statistics. J R Statis Soc A. 1991b;154: 223-67.

Ambroz A, Chalmers TC, Smith H, Schroeder B, Frieman JA, Shareck EP. Deficiencies of randomized control trials [Abstract]. Clin Research. 1978; 26:280A.

American Medical Association. Attributes to Guide the Development of Practice Parameters. Chicago: American Medical Association; 1994: 1-11.

American Medical Association. Manual of Style. Chicago: American Medical Association; 1989.

Andersen JW, Harrington D. Meta-analyses need new publication standards [Editorial]. J Clin Oncol. 1992;10(6):878-80.

Anonymous. Significance of significant [Editorial]. N Engl J Med. 1968;278(22):1232-3.

Anonymous. Statistical errors [Editorial]. Br Med J. 1977;8(6053):66.

Anonymous. Methodologic guidelines for reports of clinical trials [Editorial]. Am J Clin Oncol. 1986;9:276.

Anonymous. Presenting statistics [Editorial]. Aust N Z J Surg. 1987;57:417-19.

Arroll B, Schecter MT, Sheps SB. The assessment of diagnostic tests: a comparison of medical literature in 1982 and 1985. J Gen Intern Med. 1988;3(5):443-7.

Ashby D, Machin D. Stopping rules, interim

analyses and data monitoring committees [Editorial]. Br J Cancer. 1993;68(6):1047-50.

The Asilomar Working Group on Recommendations for Reporting Clinical Trials in the Biomedical Literature. Checklist of information for inclusion in reports of clinical trials. Ann Intern Med. 1996;124(8):741-3.

Audet AM, Greenfield S, Field M. Medical practice guidelines: current activities and future directions. Ann Intern Med. 1990;113(9):709-14.

Avram MJ, Shanks CA, Dykes MH, Ronai AK, Stiers WM. Statistical methods in anesthesia articles: an evaluation of two American journals during two six-month periods. Anesth Analg. 1985;64(6):607-11.

Badgley RF. An assessment of research methods reported in 103 scientific articles from two Canadian medical journals. Can Med Assoc J. 1961;85:246-50.

Bailar JC III. Science, statistics, and deception. Ann Intern Med. 1986;104(2):259-60.

Bailar JC III, Mosteller F. Guidelines for statistical reporting in articles for medical journals. Amplifications and explanations. Ann Intern Med. 1988;108(2):266-73.

Basinski SH. Standards, guidelines and clinical policies. The Health Services Group. Can Med Assoc J. 1992;146(6):833-7.

Bates AS, Margolis PA, Evans AT. Verification bias in pediatric studies evaluating diagnostic tests. J Pediatr. 1993;122(4):585-90.

Begg CB. Biases in the assessment of diagnostic tests. Stat Med. 1987a;6(4):411-23.

Begg CB, Pocock SJ, Freedman L, Zelen M. State of the art in comparative cancer clinical trials. Cancer. 1987b;60(11):2811-5.

Begg CB. Selection of patients for clinical trials. Semin Oncol. 1988a;15(5):434-40.

Begg CB. Methodologic standards for diagnostic test assessment studies [Editorial]. J Gen Intern Med. 1988b;3:(5)518-20.

Begg CB. Suspended judgment. Significance tests of covariate imbalance in clinical trials. Control Clin Trials. 1990;11(4):223-5.

Begg CB. Advances in statistical methodology for diagnostic medicine in the 1980s. Stat Med. 1991;10(12):1887-95.

Begg C, Cho M, Eastwood S, Horton R, Moher D, Olkin I, et al. Improving the quality of reporting of randomized controlled trials: The CONSORT Statement. JAMA. 1996;276(8):637-9.

Bero L, Rennie D. The Cochrane Collaboration. Preparing, maintaining, and disseminating systematic reviews of the effects of health care. JAMA. 1995;274(24):1935-8.

Berry G. Statistical guide-lines and statistical guidance [Editorial]. Med J Aust. 1987;146(8):408-9.

Bland JM, Jones DR, Bennett S, Cook DG, Haines AP, MacFarlane AJ. Is the clinical trial evidence about new drugs statistically adequate? Br J Clin Pharmacol. 1985;19(2):155-60.

Borzak S, Ridker PM. Discordance between meta-analyses and large-scale randomized, controlled trials. Examples from the management of acute myocardial infarction. Ann Intern Med. 1995;123(11):873-7.

Bourne WM. "No statistically significant difference." So what? [Editorial]. Arch Ophthalmol. 1987;105(1):40-1.

Bracken MB. Reporting observational studies. Br J Obstet Gynaecol. 1989;96(4):383-8.

Braitman LE. Confidence intervals assess both clinical significance and statistical significance [Editorial]. Ann Intern Med. 1991;114(6):515-7.

Brett AS. Treating hypercholesterolemia: How should practicing physicians interpret the published data for patients? N Engl J Med. 1989;321(10):676-80.

Brown GW. Standard deviation, standard error. Which "standard" should we use? Am J Dis Child. 1982;136(10):937-41.

Brown GW. Statistics and the medical journal [Editorial]. Am J Dis Child. 1985;139(3):226-8.

Browner WS, Newman TB. Confidence intervals [Letter]. Ann Intern Med. 1986;105(6):973-4.

Bulpitt CJ. Confidence intervals. Lancet. 1987; 28(8531):494-7.

Bulpitt CJ, Fletcher AE. Economic assessments in randomized controlled trials. Med J Aust. 1990;153(Supp):S16-9.

Bulpitt CJ, Fletcher AE. Measuring costs and financial benefits in randomized controlled trials. Am Heart J. 1990;119(3 Part 2):766-71.

Bunce H III, Hokanson JA, Weiss GB. Avoiding ambiguity when reporting variability in biomedical data. Am J Med. 1980;69(1):8-9.

Center for Drug Evaluation and Research. Guideline for the format and content of the clinical and statistical section of new drug applications. Food and Drug Administration,

Washington, D.C.: US Department of Health, Education, and Welfare; July 1988.

Chalmers I, Adams M, Dickersin K, Hetherington J, Tarnow-Mordi W, Meinert C, et al. A cohort study of summary reports of controlled trials. JAMA. 1990;263(10):1401-5.

Chalmers TC, Smith H Jr, Blackburn B, Silverman B, Schroeder B, Reitman D, et al. A method for assessing the quality of a randomized control trial. Control Clin Trials. 1981;2: 31-49.

Cho MK, Bero LA. Instruments for assessing the quality of drug studies published in the medical literature. JAMA. 1994;272(2):101-4.

Christensen E, Juhl E, Tygstrup N. Treatment of duodenal ulcer. Randomized clinical trials of a decade (1964 to 1974). Gastroenterology. 1977;73(5):1170-8.

Cleveland WS. Graphs in scientific publications. Am Statistician. 1984;38(4):261-9.

Committee on Data for Science and Technology. Biologists' guide for the presentation of numerical data in the primary literature. Paris: International Council of Scientific Unions, Report No. 25; November 1977.

Concato J, Feinstein AR, Holford TR. The risk of determining risk with multivariable models. Ann Intern Med. 1993;118(3):201-10.

Connett JE. Biostatistical red flags [Editorial]. Transfusion. 1994;34(8):651-3.

Cooper GS, Zangwill L. An analysis of the quality of research reports in the Journal of General Internal Medicine. J Gen Intern Med. 1989;4(3): 232-6.

Cooper LS, Chalmers TC, McAlly M, Berrier J, Sacks HS. The poor quality of early evaluations of magnetic resonance imaging. JAMA. 1988;259:3277-80.

Council of Biology Editors Style Manual Committee. Scientific Style and Format. The CBE Manual for Authors, Editors, and Publishers, 6th ed. Cambridge, UK: Cambridge University Press, 1994.

Crane VS, Gilliland M, Tuthill EL, Bruno C. The use of a decision analysis model in multidisciplinary decision making. Hosp Pharm. 1991;26(4):309-25.

Cruess DF. Review of use of statistics in the American Journal of Tropical Medicine and Hygiene for January—December 1988. Am J Trop Med Hyg. 1989;41(6):619-26.

Cruess DF. Statistics in journals [Letter]. Lancet. 1991;337(8738):432.

Dar R, Serlin RC, Omer H. Misuse of statistical tests in three decades of psychotherapy research. J Consult Clin Psychol. 1994;62(1): 75-82.

Davis NM, Cohen MR. Medication Errors: Causes and Prevention. Philadelphia: George Stickley Company; 1981.

DerSimonian R, Charette LJ, McPeek B, Mosteller F. Reporting on methods in clinical trails. N Engl J Med. 1982;306(22):1332-7.

Detsky AS, Naglie IG. A clinician's guide to cost-effectiveness analysis. Ann Intern Med. 1990;113(2):147-54.

Diamond GA, Forrester JS. Clinical trials and statistical verdicts: probable grounds for appeal. Ann Intern Med. 1983;98(3):385-94.

Dickersin K. The existence of publication bias and risk factors for its occurrence. JAMA. 1990;263 (10):1385-9.

Dickersin K, Berlin JA. Meta-analysis: state-of-the-science. Epidemiol Rev. 1992;14:154-76.

Dunn HL. Application of statistical methods in physiology. Physiol Rev. 1929;9:275-398.

Eddy DM. Probabilistic reasoning in clinical medicine: problems and opportunities. In: Kahneman D, Slovic P, Tversky A, eds. Judgment Under Uncertainty: Heuristics and Biases. Cambridge, UK: Cambridge University Press; 1982: 249-67.

Eddy DM. Clinical decision making: from theory to practice. Designing a practice policy. Standards, guidelines, and options. JAMA. 1990; 263(22):3077-84.

Eddy DM. Clinical decision making: from theory to practice. Cost-effectiveness analysis: is it up to the task? JAMA. 1992;267(24):3342-8.

Ehrenberg AS. Rudiments of numercy. J R Statist Soc. 1977;140:277-97.

Ehrenberg AS. The problem of numeracy. Am Statistician. 1981;35(2):67-71.

Eisenberg MJ. Accuracy and predictive values in clinical decision-making. Cleve Clin J Med. 1995;62(5):311-6.

Eisenhart C. [Letter]. Science. 1968;162:1332-3.

Elenbaas RM, Elenbaas JK, Cuddy PG. Evaluating the medical literature. Part II: Statistical analysis. Ann Emerg Med. 1983a;12(10):610-20.

Elenbaas JK, Cuddy PG, Elenbaas RM. Evaluating the medical literature. Part III: Results and

discussion. Ann Emerg Med. 1983b;12(11): 679-86.
Emerson JD, Colditz GA. Use of statistical analysis in the New England Journal of Medicine. N Engl J Med. 1983;309(12):709-13.
Evans DB. What is cost-effectiveness analysis? Med J Aust. 1990a;153(Supp):S7-9.
Evans DB. Principles involved in costing. Med J Aust. 1990b;153(Supp):S10-2.
Evans M, Pollock AV. Trials on trial. A review of trials of antibiotic prophylaxis. Arch Surg. 1984;119(1):109-13.
Evans M. Presentation of manuscripts for publication in the British Journal of Surgery. Br J Surg. 1989;76(12):1311-14.
Feinstein AR, Spitz H. The epidemiology of cancer therapy. I. Clinical problems of statistical surveys. Arch Intern Med. 1969;123(2):171-86.
Feinstein AR. Clinical biostatistics XXV. A survey of the statistical procedures in general medical journals. Clin Pharmacol Ther. 1974; 15(1):97-107.
Feinstein AR. Clinical biostatistics XXXVII. Demeaned errors, confidence games, nonplussed minuses, inefficient coefficients, and other statistical disruptions of scientific communication. Clin Pharmacol Ther. 1976;20(5):617-31.
Feinstein AR. Clinical biostatistics XXXIX. The haze of Bayes, the aerial palaces of decision analysis, and the computerized Ouija board. Clin Pharmacol Ther. 1977;21(4):482-96.
Feinstein AR. X and ipr_p: an improved summary for scientific communication. J Chron Dis. 1987;40(4):283-8.
Felson DT, Cupples LA, Meenan RF. Misuse of statistical methods in arthritis and rheumatism. 1982 versus 1967-68. Arthritis Rheum. 1984;27(9):1018-22.
Felson DT, Anderson JJ, Meenan RF. Time for changes in the design, analysis, and reporting of rheumatoid arthritis clinical trials. Arthritis Rheum. 1990;33(1):140-9.
Felson DT. Bias in meta-analytic research. J Clin Epidemiol. 1992;45(8):885-92.
Fienberg SE. Damned lies and statistics: misrepresentations of honest data. In: Council of Biology Editors. Editorial Policy Committee. Ethics and Policy in Scientific Publication. Bethesda, MD: Council of Biology Editors; 1990:202-6.
Finney DJ, Clarke BC. Guest editorial: code for presentation of statistical analyses. Phil Trans R Soc Lond B. 1992;337:381-2.
Forrow L, Taylor WC, Arnold RM. Absolutely relative: how research results are summarized can affect treatment decisions. Am J Med. 1992;92(2):121-4.
Freiman JA, Chalmers TC, Smith H Jr, Kuebler RR. The importance of beta, the type II error and sample size in the design and interpretation of the randomized control trial. Survey of 71 negative trials. N Engl J Med. 1978;299(13): 690-4.
Ganiats TG, Wong AF. Evaluation of cost-effectiveness research: a survey of recent publications. Fam Med. 1991;23(6):457-62.
Ganiats TG. Practice guidelines movement. West J Med. 1993;158(5):518-9.
Garcia-Cases C, Duque A, Borja J, Izquierdo I, de la Fuente V, Torrent J, et al. Evaluation of the methodological quality of clinical trial protocols. A preliminary experience in Spain. Eur J Clin Pharmacol. 1993;44(4):401-2.
Gardner MJ. Understanding and presenting variation [Letter]. Lancet. 1975;25(7900):230-1.
Gardner MJ, Altman DG, Jones DR, Machin D. Is the statistical assessment of papers submitted to the British Medical Journal effective? BMJ. 1983;286(6376):1485-8.
Gardner MJ, Altman D. Confidence intervals rather than *P* values: estimation rather than hypothesis testing. BMJ. 1986a;292(6523): 746-50.
Gardner MJ, Machin D, Campbell MJ. Use of checklists in assessing the statistical content of medical studies. BMJ. 1986b;292(6523): 810-2.
Gardner MJ, Altman DG. Estimating with confidence. BMJ. 1988;296(6631):1210-1.
Gardner MJ, Bond J. An exploratory study of statistical assessment of papers published in the British Medical Journal. JAMA. 1990; 263(10):1355-7.
Gartland JJ. Orthopaedic clinical research. Deficiencies in experimental design and determination of outcome. J Bone Joint Surg [Am]. 1988; 70(9):1357-64.
Garvey WD, Griffith BC. Scientific communication: its role in the conduct of research and creation of knowledge. Am Psychol. 1971; 349-62.
Gehlbach SH. Interpreting the Medical Literature. 3rd ed. New York: McGraw-Hill; 1993.
Gelber RD, Goldhirsch A. Reporting and interpret-

ing adjuvant therapy clinical trials. Monogr Natl Cancer Inst. 1992;11:59-69.

Geller NL, Pocock SJ. Interim analyses in randomized clinical trials: ramifications and guidelines for practitioners. Biometrics. 1987; 43(1):213-23.

George SL. Statistics in medical journals: a survey of current policies and proposals for editors. Med Pediatr Oncol. 1985;13(2):109-12.

Gibbons JD, Pratt JW. *P* values: interpretation and methodology. Am Statistician. 1975;29(1): 20-5.

Gifford RH, Feinstein AR. A critique of methodology in studies of anticoagulant therapy for acute myocardial infarction. N Engl J Med. 1969;280 (7):351-7.

Gill TM, Feinstein AR. A critical appraisal of the quality of quality-of-life measurements. JAMA. 1994:272(8):619-26.

Glantz SA. Biostatistics: how to detect, correct and prevent errors in the medical literature. Circulation. 1980;61(1):1-7.

Glantz SA. It is all in the numbers [Editorial]. J Am Coll Cardiol. 1993;21(3):835-7.

Godfrey K. Comparing the means of several groups. N Engl J Med. 1985;313(23):1450-6.

Godfrey K. Simple linear regression in medical research. In: Bailar JC, Mosteller F, eds. Medical Uses of Statistics, 2nd ed. Boston: NEJM Books; 1992:201-32.

Goel V. Decision analysis: applications and limitations. The Health Services Research Group. Can Med Assoc J. 1992;147(4):413-7.

Goodman NW, Hughes AO. Statistical awareness of research workers in British anaesthesia. Br J Anaesth. 1992;68(3):321-4.

Goodman SN, Berlin J, Fletcher SW, Fletcher RH. Manuscript quality before and after peer review and editing at Annals of Internal Medicine. Ann Intern Med. 1994a;121(1):11-21.

Goodman SN, Berlin JA. The use of predicted confidence intervals when planning experiments and the misuse of power when interpreting results. Ann Intern Med. 1994b;121(3):200-6.

Gore SM, Jones IG, Rytter EC. Misuse of statistical methods: critical assessment of articles in BMJ from January to March 1976. BMJ. 1977; 1(6053):85-7.

Gore SM. Statistics in question. Assessing methods—confidence intervals. BMJ. 1981;283 (6292):660-2.

Gore SM, Jones G, Thompson SG. The Lancet's statistical review process: areas for improvement by authors. Lancet. 1992;340(8811):100-2.

Gotzsche PC. Methodology and overt and hidden bias in reports of 196 double-blind trials of nonsteroidal antiinflammatory drugs in rheumatoid arthritis. Control Clin Trials. 1989;10(1):31-56. [Erratum. Control Clin Trials. 1989;50(9): 356.]

Grant A. Reporting controlled trials. Br J Obstet Gynaecol. 1989;96(4):397-400.

Grimes DA. Randomized controlled trials: it ain't necessarily so [Editorial]. Obstet Gynecol. 1991;78(4):703-4.

Grimes DA, Schulz KF. Randomized controlled trials of home uterine activity monitoring: a review and critique. Obstet Gynecol. 1992; 79(1):137-42.

Griner PF, Mayewski RJ, Mushlin AI, Greenland P. Selection and interpretation of diagnostic tests and procedures. Principles and applications. Ann Intern Med. 1981;94(4 Part 2):557-92.

Gross M. A critique of the methodologies used in clinical studies of hip-joint arthroplasty published in the English-language orthopaedic literature. J Bone Joint Surg [Am]. 1988; 70(9):1364-71.

Guyatt GH, Tugwell PX, Feeny DH, Haynes RB, Drummond M. A framework for clinical evaluation of diagnostic technologies. Can Med. Assoc J. 1986;134(6):587-94.

Guyatt GH, Sackett DL, Cook DJ. Users' guides to the medical literature. II. How to use an article about therapy or prevention. A. Are the results of the study valid? The Evidence-Based Medicine Working Group. JAMA. 1993; 270(21):2598-601.

Guyatt GH, Sackett DL, Cook DJ. Users' guides to the medical literature. II. How to use an article about therapy or prevention. B. What were the results and will they help me in caring for my patients? The Evidence-Based Medicine Working Group. JAMA. 1994;271(1): 59-63.

Guyatt GH, Sackett DL, Sinclair JC, Hayward R, Cook DJ, Cook RJ. Users' guides to the medical literature. IX. A method for grading health care recommendations. The Evidence-Based Medicine Working Group. JAMA. 1995;274(22):1800-4.

Haines SJ. Six statistical suggestions for surgeons. Neurosurgery. 1981;9(4):414-8.

Hall JC, Hill D, Watts JM. Misuse of statistical

methods in the Australasian surgical literature. Aust N Z J Surg. 1982a;52(5):541-3.

Hall JC. The other side of statistical significance: a review of type II errors in the Australian medical literature. Aust N Z J Med. 1982b;12 (1):7-9.

Hall JC. Use of the *t* test in the British Journal of Surgery [Letter]. Br J Surg. 1982c;69(1):55-6.

Hall JC, Mooney G. What every doctor should know about economics. Part 2. The benefits of economic appraisal. Med J Aust. 1990;152(2): 80-2.

Hampton JR. Presentation and analysis of the results of clinical trials in cardiovascular disease. BMJ. 1981;282(6273):1371-3.

Hayden GF. Biostatistical trends in Pediatrics: implications for the future. Pediatrics. 1983;72(1): 84-7.

Haynes RB. How to read clinical journals: II. To learn about a diagnostic test. Can Med Assoc J. 1981;124(6):703-10.

Haynes RB, Mulrow CD, Huth EJ, Altman DG, Gardner MJ. More informative abstracts revisited. Ann Intern Med. 1990;113(1):69-76.

Hayward RS, Laupacis A. Initiating, conducting and maintaining guidelines development programs. Can Med Assoc J. 1993a;148(4):507-12.

Hayward RS, Wilson MC, Tunis SR, Bass EB, Rubin HR, Haynes RB. More informative abstracts of articles describing clinical practice guidelines. Ann Intern Med. 1993b;118(9): 731-7.

Hayward RS. Users' guides to the medical literature. VIII. How to use? clinical practice guidelines. A. Are the recommendations valid? The Evidence-Based Medicine Working Group. JAMA. 1995;274(7):570-4.

Healy MJ. Statistics from the inside. 5. Data structures. Arch Dis Child. 1992;67(4):533-5.

Hemminki E. Quality of reports of clinical trials submitted by the drug industry to the Finnish and Swedish control authorities. Eur J Clin Pharmacol. 1981;19(3):157-65.

Hemminki E. Quality of clinical trials—a concern of three decades. Methods Inf Med. 1982; 21(2):81-5.

Henry DA, Wilson A. Meta-analysis. Part 1: An assessment of its aims, validity and reliability. Med J Aust. 1992;156(1):31-8.

Hillman AL, Eisenberg JM, Pauly MV, Bloom BS, Glick H, Kinosian B, et al. Avoiding bias in the conduct and reporting of cost-effectiveness research sponsored by pharmaceutical companies. N Engl J Med. 1991;324(19):1362-5.

Hillman AL. Economic analysis of health care technology. A report on principles. The Task Force on Principles for Economic Analysis of Health Care and Technology. Ann Intern Med. 1995;123(1):61-70.

Hoffman JI. The incorrect use of chi-square analysis for paired data. Clin Exp Immunol. 1976; 24(1):227-9.

Horwitz RI, Feinstein AR. Methodologic standards and contradictory results in case-control research. Am J Med. 1979;66(4):556-64.

Hosmer DW, Taber S, Lemeshow S. The importance of assessing the fit of logistic regression models: a case study. Am J Public Health. 1991;81(12):1630-5.

Hughes, MD. Reporting Bayesian analyses of clinical trials. Stat Med. 1993;12(18):1651-63.

Hujoel PP, Baab DA, DeRouen TA. The power of tests to detect differences between periodontal treatments in published studies. J Clin Periodontal. 1992;19(10):779-84.

Huth EJ. How To Write and Publish Papers in the Medical Sciences. Philadelphia: ISI Press; 1982.

International Committee of Medical Journal Editors. Uniform requirements for manuscripts submitted to biomedical journals. N Engl J Med. 1991;324(6):424-8.

Irwig L, Tosteson ANA, Gastonis C, Lau J, Colditz G, Chalmers T, et al. Guidelines for meta-analyses evaluating diagnostic tests. Ann Intern Med. 1994;120(8):667-76.

Iverson C, Dan BB, Glitman P, King LS, Knoll E, Meyer HS, et al, editors. American Medical Association Manual of Style. 8th ed. Baltimore, MD: Williams & Wilkins; 1983:305-9.

Jaeschke R, Guyatt GH, Sackett DL. Users' guides to the medical literature. III. How to use an article about a diagnostic test. A. Are the results of the study valid? The Evidence-Based Medicine Working Group. JAMA. 1994a;271(5):389-91.

Jaeschke R, Guyatt GH, Sackett DL. Users' guides to the medical literature. III. How to use an article about a diagnostic test. B. What are the results and will they help me in caring for my patients? The Evidence-Based Medicine Working Group. JAMA. 1994b;271(9): 703-7.

Jamart J. Statistical tests in medical research. Acta Oncol. 1992;31(7):723-7.

Jekel JF. Statistical significance versus importance [Letter]. Pediatrics. 1977;60(1)125-6.

Jewett DL. Reporting negative results [Letter]. Audiology. 1991;30(3):183-4.

Jones DR. Meta-analysis of observational epidemiological studies: a review. J R Soc Med. 1992;85(3):165-8.

Jonson, ME. Everyday diagnostics—a critique of the Bayesian model. Med Hypotheses. 1991; 34(4):289-95.

Joseph M, editor. Man is the Only Animal that Blushes . . . Or Needs To. The Wisdom of Mark Twain. New York: Random House; 1970.

Journal of the American Medical Association. Instructions for preparing structured abstracts. JAMA. 1993;271(2):162-4.

Journal of Hypertension. Statistical guidelines for the Journal of Hypertension. J Hypertens. 1992;10(1):6-8.

Juhl E, Christensen E, Tygstrup N. The epidemiology of the gastrointestinal randomized clinical trial. N Engl J Med. 1977;296(1):20-2.

Kanter MH, Taylor JR. Accuracy of statistical methods in Transfusion: a review of articles from July/August 1992 through June 1993. Transfusion. 1994;34(8):697-701.

Kanter MH, Petz L. The validity of statistical analyses in the transfusion medicine literature with specific comments concerning studies of the comparative safety of units donated by autologous, designated and allogenic donors [Editorial]. Transfus Med. 1995;5(2):91-5.

Kaplan RM, Feeny D, Revicki DA. Methods for assessing relative importance in preference based outcome measures. Qual Life Res. 1993; 2(6):467-75.

Kassirer JP, Moskowitz AJ, Lau J, Pauker SG. Decision analysis: a progress report. Ann Intern Med. 1987;106(2):275-91.

Kassirer JP. Clinical trials and meta-analysis. What do they do for us? [Editorial]. N Engl J Med. 1992;327(4):273-4.

Kassirer JP, Angell M. The journal's policy on cost-effectiveness analyses. [Editorial]. N Engl J Med. 1994;331(10):669-70.

Kaufman NJ, Dudley-Marling C, Serlin, RL. An examination of statistical interactions in the special education literature. J Special Ed.1986; 20(1):31-42.

Kawachi I, Malcom LA. The cost-effectiveness of treating mild-to-moderate hypertension: a reappraisal. J Hypertens. 1991;9(3):199-208.

Koes BW, Bouter LM, van der Heijden GJ. Methodological quality of randomized clinical trials on treatment efficacy in low back pain. Spine. 1995;20(2):228-35.

Kupersmith J, Holmes-Rovner M, Hogan A, Rovner D, Gardiner J. Cost-effectiveness analysis in heart disease, part I: general principles. Prog Cardiovasc Dis. 1994;37(3):161-84.

Lagakos S. Statistical analysis of survival data. In: Bailar JC, Mosteller F, eds. Medical Uses of Statistics. 2nd ed. Boston: NEJM Books; 1992: 281-92.

Lau J, Antman EM, Jimenez-Silva J, Kupelnick B, Mosteller F, Chalmers TC. Cumulative meta-analysis of therapeutic trials for myocardial infarction. N Engl J Med. 1992;327(4):248-54.

Laupacis A, Sackett DL, Roberts RS. An assessment of clinically useful measures of the consequences of treatment. N Engl J Med. 1988; 318(26):1728-33.

Laupacis A, Naylor CD, Sackett DL. How should the results of clinical trials be presented to clinicians? [Editorial]. ACP Journal Club. 1992a; (May/June):A-12-4.

Laupacis A, Feeny D, Detsky AS, Tugwell PX. How attractive does a new technology have to be to warrant adoption and utilization? Tentative guidelines for using clinical and economic evaluations. Can Med Assoc J. 1992b;146(4):473-81.

Laupacis A, Wells G, Richardson WS, Tugwell P. Users' guides to the medical literature. V. How to use an article about prognosis. The Evidence-Based Medicine Working Group. JAMA. 1994;272(3):234-7.

Lavori PW, Louis TA, Bailar JC, Polanski M. Designs for experiments—parallel comparisons of treatment. In: Bailar JC, Mosteller F, eds. Medical Uses of Statistics, 2nd ed. Boston: NEJM Books; 1992:61-82.

Leape LL. Practice guidelines and standards: an overview. QRB Qual Rev Bull. 1990; 16(2):42-9.

LeBlond RF. Improving structured abstracts [Letter]. Ann Intern Med. 1989;111(9):764.

Lee JT, Sanchez LA. Interpretation of "cost-effective" and soundness of economic evaluations in the pharmacy literature. Am J Hosp Pharm. 1991;48(12):2622-7.

Lee KL, McNeer F, Starmer CF, Harris PJ, Rosati RA. Clinical judgment and statistics. Lessons from a simulated randomized trial in coronary artery disease. Circulation. 1980;61(3): 508-15.

Lee KL, Bicknell NA, Pieper KS. Response to Palmas et al. [Letter]. Ann Intern Med. 1993; 118(3):231-2.

Leis HP Jr, Robbins GF, Greene FL, Cammarata A, Hilfer SE. Breast cancer statistics: use and misuse. Int Surg. 1986;71(4):237-43.

Levine M, Walter S, Lee H, Haines T, Holbrook A, Moyer V. Users' guides to the medical literature. IV. How to use an article about harm. The Evidence-Based Medicine Working Group. JAMA. 1994;271(20):1615-9.

Lewis RJ, Wears RL. An introduction to the Bayesian analysis of clinical trials. Ann Emerg Med. 1993;22(8):1328-36.

Liberati A, Himel HN, Chalmers TC. A quality assessment of randomized control trials of primary treatment of breast cancer. J Clin Oncol. 1986;4(6):942-51.

Light RJ, Pellimer DB. Summing Up: The Science of Reviewing Research. Cambridge, MA: Harvard University Press; 1984.

Lionel ND, Herxheimer A. Assessing reports of therapeutic trials. BMJ. 1970;3(723):637-40.

Longnecker DE. Support versus illumination: trends in medical statistics [Editorial]. Anesthesiology. 1982;57(2):73-4.

MacArthur RD, Jackson GG. An evaluation of the use of statistical methodology in the Journal of Infectious Diseases. J Infect Dis. 1984; 149(3):349-54.

Mahon WA, Daniel EE. A method for the assessment of reports of drug trials. Can Med Assoc J. 1964;90:565-9.

Mainland D. Chance and the blood count. Can Med Assoc J. 1934;(June):656-8.

Mainland D. Problems of chance in clinical work. Br Med J. 1936;2:221-4.

Mainland D. Statistical ritual in clinical journals: is there a cure?—I. Br Med J. 1984;288(6420): 841-3.

Mantha S. Scientific approach to presenting and summarizing data [Letter]. Anesth Analg. 1992;75:469-70.

Marks RG. Proper statistical analysis and documentation considerations for published research articles. Occup Ther Ment Health. 1987; 7(4):51-68.

Marks RG, Dawson-Saunders EK, Bailar JC, Dan BB, Verran JA. Interactions between statisticians and biomedical journal editors. Stat Med. 1988;7(10):1003-11.

Mason J, Drummond M, Torrance G. Some guidelines on the use of cost effectiveness league tables. BMJ. 1993;306(6877):570-2.

Maynard A. The design of future cost-benefit studies. Am Heart J. 1990;119(3 Part 2):761-5.

McGill R, Tukey JW, Larsen WA. Variation of box plots. Am Statistician. 1978;32(1):12-6.

McPherson K. Statistics: the problem of examining accumulating data more than once. N Engl J Med. 1974;290(9):501-2.

Meinert CL, Tonascia S, Higgins K. Content of reports on clinical trials: a critical review. Control Clin Trials. 1984;5(4):328-47.

Metz CE. Basic principles of ROC analysis. Semin Nucl Med. 1978;8(4):283-98.

Mike V, Stanley KE, editors. Statistics in Medical Research. New York: John Wiley & Sons; 1982:532-9.

Mills JL. Data torturing [Letter]. N Engl J Med. 1993;329(16):1196-9.

Moher D, Dulberg CS, Wells GA. Statistical power, sample size, and their reporting in randomized controlled trials. JAMA. 1994; 272(2):122-4.

Moher D, Olkin I. Meta-analysis of randomized controlled trials. A concern for standards. JAMA. 1995;274(24):1962-4.

Montgomery DC. Design and Analysis of Experiments. 2nd Ed. New York: John Wiley and Sons, 1984.

Morgan PP. Confidence intervals: from statistical significance to clinical significance [Editorial]. Can Med Assoc J. 1989;141(9):881-3.

Morris RW. A statistical study of papers in the Journal of Bone and Joint Surgery [Br] 1984. J Bone Joint Surg [Br]. 1988;70(2):242-6.

Moses LE. Statistical concepts fundamental to investigations. In: Bailar JC, Mosteller F, eds. Medical Uses of Statistics, 2nd ed. Boston: NEJM Books; 1992:5-26.

Moskowitz G, Chalmers TC, Sacks HS, Fagerstrom RM, Smith H Jr. Deficiencies of clinical trials of alcohol withdrawal. Alcohol Clin Exp Res. 1983;7(1):42-6.

Mosteller F. Communications: Should mechanisms be established for sharing among clinical trial investigators experiences in handling problems in design, execution, and analysis? Problems of omission in communications. Clin Pharmacol Ther. 1979; 25(5 Part 2):761-4.

Mosteller F, Gilbert JP, McPeek B. Reporting

standards and research strategies for controlled trials. Control Clin Trials. 1980;1:37-58.
Murray GD. The task of a statistical referee. Br J Surg. 1988; 75(7):664-7.
Murray GD. Confidence intervals [Editorial]. Nucl Med Commun. 1989;10(6):387-8.
Murray GD. Statistical aspects of research methodology. Br J Surg. 1991a;78(7):777-81.
Murray GD. Statistical guidelines for the British Journal of Surgery. Br J Surg. 1991b;78(7):782-4.
Naylor CD, Chen E, Strauss B. Measured enthusiasm: does the method of reporting trial results alter perceptions of therapeutic effectiveness? Ann Intern Med. 1992;117(11):916-21.
Naylor CD, Guyatt GH. Users' guides to the medical literature. X. How to use an article reporting variations in the outcomes of health services. The Evidence-Based Medicine Working Group. JAMA. 1996;275(7):554-8.
Nierenberg AA, Feinstein AR. How to evaluate a diagnostic marker test. Lessons from the rise and fall of dexamethasone suppression test. JAMA. 1988;259(11):1699-1702.
Nord E. Methods for quality adjustment of life years. Soc Sci Med. 1992;34(5)559-69.
O'Brien PC, Shampo MA. Statistics for clinicians. 1. Descriptive statistics. Mayo Clin Proc. 1981a;56(1):47-9.
O'Brien PC, Shampo MA. Statistics for clinicians. 7. Regression. Mayo Clin Proc. 1981b; 56(7):452-4.
O'Brien PC, Shampo MA. Statistics for clinicians. 11. Survivorship studies. Mayo Clin Proc. 1981c; 56(11):709-11.
O'Brien PC, Shampo MA. Statistics for clinicians. 12. Sequential methods. Mayo Clin Proc. 1981d;56(12):753-4.
O'Fallon JR, Duby SD, Salsburg DS, Edmonson JH, Soffer A, Colton T. Should there be statistical guidelines for medical research papers? Biometrics. 1978;34(4):687-95.
Oliver D, Hall JC. Usage of statistics in the surgical literature and the "orphan P" phenomenon. Aust N Z J Surg. 1989;59(6):449-51.
Ottenbacher KJ. Statistical conclusion validity and type IV errors in rehabilitation research. Arch Phys Med Rehabil. 1992;73(2):121-5.
Oxman AD, Guyatt GH. A consumer's guide to subgroup analyses. Ann Intern Med. 1992; 116(1):78-84.
Oxman AD. Evidence-based care: 2. Setting guidelines: how should we manage this problem? The Evidence-Based Care Resource Group. Can Med Assoc J.1994;150(9):1417-23.
Palmas W, Denton TA, Diamond GA. Publication criteria for statistical prediction models [Letter]. Ann Intern Med. 1993;118(3):231-2.
Pauker SG, Kassirer JP. Decision analysis. N Engl J Med. 1987;316(5):250-8.
Peace KE. The alternative hypothesis: one-sided or two sided? J Clin Epidemiol. 1989;42(5): 473-6.
Peterson HB, Kleinbaum DG. Interpreting the literature in obstetrics and gynecology: II. Logistic regression and related issues. Obstet Gynecol. 1991;78(4):717-20.
Phelps CE, Mushlin AI. On the (near) equivalence of cost-effectiveness and cost-benefit analyses. Int J Technol Health Care. 1991;7(1): 12-21.
Pocock SJ, Hughes MD, Lee RJ. Statistical problems in the reporting of clinical trials. A survey of three medical journals. N Engl J Med. 1987;317(7):426-32.
Prihoda TJ, Schelb E, Jones JD. The reporting of statistical inferences in selected prosthodontic journals. J Prosthodont. 1992;1(1):51-6.
Raju TN, Langenberg P, Sen A, Aldana O. How much "better" is good enough? The magnitude of treatment effect in clinical trials. Am J Dis Child. 1992;146(4):407-11.
Ransohoff DF, Feinstein AR. Problems of spectrum and bias in evaluating the efficacy of diagnostic tests. N Engl J Med. 1978;299(17): 926-30.
Raskob GE, Lofthouse RN, Hull RD. Methodological guidelines for clinical trials evaluating new therapeutic approaches in bone and joint surgery. J Bone Joint Surg. 1985;67-A(8):1294-7.
Raykov T, Tomer A, Nesselroade JR. Reporting structural equation modeling results in Psychology and Aging: some proposed guidelines. Psychol Aging. 1991;6(4):499-503.
Redelmeier DA, Rozin P, Kahneman D. Understanding patients' decisions; Cognitive and emotional perspectives. JAMA. 1993; 270(91): 72-6.
Reed JF, Slaichert W. Statistical proof in inconclusive "negative" trials. Arch Intern Med. 1981;141(10):1307-10.
Reid MC, Lachs MS, Feinstein AR. Use of methodologic standards in diagnostic test research. JAMA. 1995;274(8):645-51.

Reiffenstein RJ, Schiltroth AJ, Todd DM. Current standards in reported drug trials. Can Med Assoc J. 1968;99(23):1134-5.

Reizenstein P, Delgado M, Gastiaburu J, Lomme L, Ogier C, Pals H, et al. Efficacy of and errors in randomized multicenter trials. A review of 230 clinical trials. Biomed Pharmacotherapy. 1983;37(1):14-24.

Rennie D. Vive la difference ($P < 0.05$) [Editorial]. N Engl J Med. 1978;299(15):828-9.

Reznick RK, Guest CB. Survival analysis: a practical approach. Dis Colon Rectum. 1989: 32(10):898-902.

Richardson WS, Detsky AS. Users' guides to the medical literature. VII. How to use a clinical decision analysis. A. Are the results of the study valid? The Evidence-Based Medicine Working Group. JAMA. 1995a;273(16):1292-5.

Richardson WS, Detsky AS. Users' guides to the medical literature. VII. How to use a clinical decision analysis. B. What are the results and will they help me in caring for my patients? The Evidence-Based Medicine Working Group. JAMA. 1995b;273(20):1610-3.

Riegelman RK, Hirsch RP. Studying a Study and Testing a Test: How to Read the Medical Literature, 2nd ed. Boston, MA: Little, Brown and Company; 1989.

Rochon PA, Gurwitz JH, Cheung MC, Hayes JA, Chalmers TC. Evaluating the quality of articles published in journal supplements compared with the quality of those published in the parent journal. JAMA. 1994;272(2):108-13.

Ross OB. Use of controls in medical research. JAMA. 1951;145:72-5.

Rothman KJ. Significance questing [Editorial]. Ann Intern Med. 1986;105(3):445-7.

Sackett DL. How to read clinical journals: V. To distinguish useful from useless or even harmful therapy. Can Med Assoc J. 1981;124(9): 1156-62.

Sackett DL. Interpretation of diagnostic data: 5. How to do it with simple maths. Can Med Assoc J. 1983;129(9):947-54.

Salsburg DS. The religion of statistics as practiced in medical journals. Am Statistician. 1985:39(3):220-3.

Savitz DA. Measurements, estimates, and inferences in reporting epidemiologic study results [Editorial]. Am J Epidemiol. 1992;135(3):223-4.

Savitz DA, Tolo KA, Poole C. Statistical significance testing in the American Journal of Epidemiology, 1970–1990. Am J Epidemiol. 1994; 139(10):1047-52.

Scherer RW, Dickersin K, Langenberg P. Full publication of results initially presented in abstracts. A meta-analysis. JAMA. 1994;27(2): 158-62. [Erratum. JAMA. 1994;272(18)1410].

Schoolman HM, Becktel JM, Best WR, Johnson AF. Statistics in medical research: principles versus practices. J Lab Clin Med. 1968;71(3): 357-67.

Schor S, Karten I. Statistical evaluation of medical journal manuscripts. JAMA. 1966;195(13): 1123-8.

Schor S. Statistical reviewing program for medical manuscripts. Am Statistician. 1967;(Feb): 28-31.

Schor S. Statistical proof in inconclusive "negative" trials [Editorial]. Arch Intern Med. 1981; 141(10):1263-4.

Schultz KF, Chalmers I, Grimes DA, Altman DG. Assessing the quality of randomization from reports of controlled trials published in journals of obstetrics and gynecology. JAMA. 1994;272(2):125-8.

Schultz KF, Chalmers I, Hayes RJ, Altman DG. Empirical evidence of bias. Dimensions of methodological quality associated with estimates of treatment effects in controlled trials. JAMA. 1995a;273(5):408-12.

Schultz KF. Subverting randomization in controlled trials. JAMA. 1995b;274(18): 1456-8.

Schwartz D, Lellouch J. Explanatory and pragmatic attitudes in therapeutical trials. J Chronic Dis. 1967;20(8):637-48.

Schwartz WB, Gorry GA, Kassirer JP, Essig A. Decision analysis and clinical judgment. Am J Med. 1973;55(3):459-72.

Sheehan TJ. The medical literature. Let the reader beware. Arch Intern Med. 1980;140(4):472-4.

Sheps SB, Schechter MT. The assessment of diagnostic tests. A survey of current medical research. JAMA. 1984;252(17):2418-22.

Shott S. Statistics in veterinary research. J Am Vet Med Assoc. 1985;187(2):138-41.

Shuster JJ, Binion J, Walrath N, Grassmuck D, Mahnks D, Schmidt J. Statistical review process. Recommended procedures in biomedical research articles [Editorial]. JAMA. 1976; 235(5):534-5.

Simel DL, Feussner JR, Delong ER, Matchar DB. Intermediate, indeterminate, and uninterpretable diagnostic test results. Med Decis Making. 1987;7(2):107-14.

Simes J. Meta-analysis: its importance in cost-effectiveness studies. Med J Aust. 1990;153 (Suppl):S13-16.

Simon G, Wagner E, Vonkorff M. Cost-effectiveness comparisons using real world randomized trials: the case of new antidepressant drugs. J Clin Epidemiol. 1995;48(3):363-73.

Simon R, Wittes RE. Methodologic guidelines for reports of clinical trials. Cancer Treat Rep. 1985;69(1):1-3.

Simon R. Confidence intervals for reporting results of clinical trials. Ann Intern Med. 1986; 105(3):429-35.

Simpson RJ Jr, Johnson TA, Amara IA. The boxplot: an exploratory analysis graph for biomedical publications. Am Heart J. 1988;116(6 Part 1):1663-5.

Smith DG, Clemens J, Crede W, Harvey M, Gracely EJ. Impact of multiple comparisons in randomized clinical trials. Am J Med. 1987; 83(3):545-50.

Sonis J, Joines J. The quality of clinical trials published in The Journal of Family Practice, 1974-1991. J Fam Pract. 1994;39(3):225-350.

Sonnenberg FA, Beck JR. Markov models in medical decision making: a practical guide. Med Decis Making. 1993;13(14):322-38.

Sox HC Jr. Probability theory in the use of diagnostic tests. An introduction to critical study of the literature. Ann Intern Med. 1986;104(1): 60-6.

Squires BP. Statistics in biomedical manuscripts? what editors want from authors and peer reviewers [Editorial]. Can Med Assoc J. 1990; 142(3):213-4.

The Standards of Reporting Trial Group. A proposal for structured reporting of randomized controlled trials. JAMA. 1994; 272:1926-31. Correction: JAMA. 1995;273:776.

Stefadouros MA. A new system of visual presentation of analysis of test performance: the double-ring diagram. J Clin Epidemiol. 1993; 46(10):1151-8.

Stoddart GL. How to read journals: VII. To understand an economic evaluation (Part A). Can Med Assoc J. 1984b;130(11):1428-34.

Stoddart GL. How to read journals: VII. To understand an economic evaluation (Part B). Can Med Assoc J. 1984a;130(12):1542-9.

Stoto MA. From data analysis to conclusions: a statistician's view. In: Council of Biology Editors Editorial Policy Committee. Ethics and Policy in Scientific Publication. Bethesda, MD: Council of Biology Editors; 1990:207-18.

Style Manual Committee, Council of Biology Editors. Scientific Style and Format. The CBE Manual for Authors, Editors, and Publishers. 6th ed. Cambridge, UK: Cambridge University Press, 1994.

Sumner D. Lies, damned lies—or statistics? J Hypertens. 1992;10(1):3-8.

Testa MA, Simonson DC. Assessment of quality-of-life outcomes. N Engl J Med. 1996;334(13): 835-40.

Trobe JD, Fendrick AM. The effectiveness initiative. I. Medical practice guidelines. Arch Ophthalmol. 1995;113(6):715-7.

Tugwell PX. How to read clinical journals: III. To learn the clinical course and prognosis of disease. Can Med Assoc J. 1981;124(7):869-72.

Tyson JE, Furzan JA, Reisch JS, Mize SG. An evaluation of the quality of therapeutic studies in perinatal medicine. J Pediatr. 1983;102(1): 10-3.

Udvarhelyi IS, Colditz GA, Rai A, Epstein AM. Cost-effectiveness and cost-benefit analyses in the medical literature. Are the methods being used correctly? Ann Intern Med. 1992;116(3): 238-44.

Vaisrub N. Manuscript review from a statistician's perspective [Editorial]. JAMA. 1985;253 (21):3145-7.

Vrbos LA, Lorenz MA, Peabody EH, McGregor M. Clinical methodologies and incidence of appropriate statistical testing in orthopaedic spine literature. Are statistics misleading? Spine. 1993;18(8):1021-9.

Wainapel SF, Kayne HL. Statistical methods in rehabilitation research. Arch Phys Med Rehabil. 1985;66(5):322-4.

Wainer H. How to display data badly. Am Statistician. 1984;38(2):137-47.

Wald N, Cuckle H. Reporting the assessment of screening and diagnostic tests. Br J Obstet Gynaecol. 1989;96(4):389-96.

Walker AM. Reporting the results of epidemiological studies. Am J Public Health. 1986;76 (5):556-8.

Walker RD, Howard MO, Lambert MD, Suchinsky R. Medical practice guidelines. West J Med. 1994;161(1):39-44.

Wallenstein S, Zucker CL, Fleiss JL. Some statistical methods useful in circulation research. Circ Res. 1980;47(1):1-9.

Walter SD. Methods of reporting statistical results from medical research studies. Am J Epidemiol. 1995;141(10):896-906.

Ware JH, Mosteller F, Delgado F, Donnelly C, Ingelfinger JA. *P* values. In: Bailar JC, Mosteller F, eds. Medical Uses of Statistics. 2nd ed. Boston: NEJM Books; 1992:181-200.

Warner KE. Issues in cost effectiveness in health care. J Public Health Dent. 1989;49(5 Spec No): 272-8.

Wasson JH, Sox HC, Neff RK, Goldman L. Clinical prediction rules. Applications and methodological standards. N Engl J Med. 1985;313 (13):793-9.

Wasson JH, Sox HC. Clinical prediction rules. Have they come of age? JAMA. 1996;275(8):641-2.

Watts GT. Statistics in journals [letter]. Lancet. 1991;337(8738):432.

Wears RL. What is necessary for proof? Is 95% sure unrealistic? [Letter]. JAMA. 1994;271(4):272.

Weech AA. Statistics: use and misuse. Aust Paediatr J. 1974;10(6):328-33.

Weinstein MC, Stason WB. Foundations of cost-effectiveness analysis for health and medical practices. N Engl J Med. 1977;296(13):716-21.

Weinstein MC. Principles of cost-effective resource allocation in health care organizations. Int J Technol Assess Health Care. 1990;6(1): 93-103.

Weiss GB, Bunce H. Are we ready for statistical guidelines for medical research papers? [Letter]. Biometrics. 1979;35:911.

Weiss W, Dambrosia JM. Common problems in designing therapeutic trials in multiple sclerosis. Arch Neurol. 1983;40(11):678-80.

Welch HG. Comparing apples and oranges: Does cost-effectiveness analysis deal fairly with the old and young? Gerontologist. 1991;31(3):332-6.

West RR. A look at the statistical overview (or meta-analysis). J R Coll Physicians Lond. 1993; 27(2):111-5.

White SJ. Statistical errors in papers in the British Journal of Psychiatry. Br J Psychiatry. 1979;135: 336-42.

Wilson A, Henry DA. Meta-analysis. Part 2: Assessing the quality of published meta-analyses. Med J Aust. 1992;156(3):173-87.

Wilson MC, Hayward RS, Tunis SR, Bass EB, Guyatt GH. Users' guides to the medical literature. VIII. How to use clinical practice guidelines. B. What are the recommendations and will they help you in caring for your patients? The Evidence-Based Medicine Working Group. JAMA. 1995;274(20):1630-2.

Working Group on Recommendations for Reporting Clinical Trials in the Biomedical Literature. Call for comments on a proposal to improve reporting clinical trials in the biomedical literature: a position paper. Ann Intern Med. 1994;121:894-5.

Wulff HR. Confidence limits in evaluating controlled therapeutic trials [Letter]. Lancet. 1973; 2(835):969-70.

Wulff HR, Andersen B, Brandenhoff P, Guttler F. What do doctors know about statistics? Stat Med. 1987;6(1):3-10.

Yancy JM. Ten rules for reading clinical research reports [Editorial]. Am J Surg. 1990;159(6): 553-9.

Young MJ, Bresnitz EA, Strom BL. Sample size nomograms for interpreting negative clinical studies. Ann Intern Med. 1983;99(2):248-51.

Yusuf S, Wittes J, Probstfield J, Tyroler HA. Analysis and interpretation of treatment effects in subgroups of patients in randomized clinical trials. JAMA. 1991;266(1):93-8.

Zelen M. Guidelines for publishing papers on cancer clinical trials: responsibilities of editors and authors. J Clin Oncol. 1983;1(2):164-9.

The Zitter Group. Outcomes Backgrounder: An Overview of Outcomes and Pharmacoeconomics. San Francisco, CA: The Zitter Group; 1994:1-56.

Zivin JA, Bartko JJ. Statistics for disinterested scientists. Life Sci. 1976;18(1):15-26.

INDEX

For more terms, or for more detailed information about terms listed here, see Part 2, Guide to Statistical Terms and Tests.

D

About the Authors

Thomas A. Lang, MA, is Manager of Medical Editing Services at The Cleveland Clinic Foundation, where he supervises the editing of scientific manuscripts for publication in peer-reviewed journals. He received his master's degree in Communications Management from the Annenberg School of Communications at the University of Southern California. A medical writer and editor since 1975, he has co-authored a college text on personal health, taught classes in communications and technical writing at several universities, and leads workshops on medical writing throughout the U.S. and Canada. He has been a member of the American Medical Writers Association since 1979 and a Fellow of the Association since 1993. In 1994 he received the group's Golden Apple Award for Outstanding Workshop Leader.

Michelle Secic, MS, is a Senior Biostatistician in the Department of Biostatistics and Epidemiology at The Cleveland Clinic Foundation, where she assists researchers in designing, analyzing, and interpreting medical research studies. She received her master's degree in Statistics from Bowling Green State University. From 1989 through 1992 she participated in the American Statistical Association's Quantitative Literacy Program, a project that assists high school teachers in learning statistics and incorporating statistical concepts into their classrooms. She has been an invited speaker for Career Days at many local high schools and colleges to promote the understanding of statistics.